ART, MIND, AND BRAIN

ART, MIND, AND BRAIN

A COGNITIVE APPROACH
TO CREATIVITY

HOWARD GARDNER

BasicBooks
A Division of HarperCollins*Publishers*

Library of Congress Cataloging in Publication Data

Gardner, Howard.
  Art, mind, and brain.

  Bibliography: p. 369
  Includes index.
  1. Creative ability. 2. Creative ability in children.
3. Creation (Literary, artistic, etc.) 4. Creative
thinking. 5. Brain—Localization of functions.
I. Title.
BF411.G37   1982   700'.1'9   82–70846
ISBN 0-465-00444-X (cloth)
ISBN 0-465-00445-8 (paper)

To my colleagues at

Harvard Project Zero

and

to the agencies which have generously

made possible our collaboration

CONTENTS

Contents

PART III

ON EDUCATION AND MEDIA: THE
TRANSMISSION OF KNOWLEDGE

PART IV

THE BREAKDOWN OF THE MIND

Contents

PART V

THE HEIGHTS OF CREATIVITY

PREFACE

FOR the last fifteen years I have been studying human creative processes, particularly as they are manifest in the arts. I have done so principally from the vantage point of cognitive psychology, that aspiring discipline which seeks to uncover the basic laws of human thought. My views have of course changed over the years (as have the audiences addressed), but my impulse has remained essentially the same—to gain insight into creative processes and products, be they from the hand of an autistic graphic artist (like the amazing young English girl, Nadia), a writer who sustained brain damage (like Baudelaire), or a composer at the height of his powers (like Mozart). My current thoughts on this topic, and many of the steps that led to them, are presented in this collection of essays.

One of my professors in graduate school, a brilliant but insidious fellow, once taunted me: "Why study creativity? The psychologists who have done so are a notably dull lot." He was right in a sense, because the list of individuals who have studied the creative process is distressingly long in comparison with the handful who have actually illuminated it. But my professor was just as certainly wrong. The greatest psychologists—from William James to Sigmund Freud, from B. F. Skinner to Jean Piaget—have all recognized the importance and the appeal of a study of the creative processes. They have all sought to explain how human beings can fashion comprehensive theories in science or powerful works of art. And if they have not fully succeeded in providing a coherent and cogent account of this most puzzling of areas, it is not for want of trying.

There are autobiographical keys to the course I have followed. As a bright but somewhat isolated child, I was singled out by others for two reasons: first, I did well in school; second, I played the piano with some skill and flair. My pleasures as a youth came from reading, writing, and thinking as well as from my involvement with music. I did some creative writing, nearly all of it trite, including numerous stories and poems in high school and an execrable novel of more than a thousand pages shortly after my graduation from college. I have also tried my hand at composing. On my bar mitzvah I received my first *ex libris*—a triptych consisting of a book, a musical score, and a hoe (for gardener!). At that pivotal time, more than one elder confidently predicted that my life would be forever enmeshed with scholarship and the arts.

No surprise, then, that when I first began to study developmental psychology, I was soon struck by certain limitations in the field. The child was seen by nearly all researchers as an exclusively rational creature, a problem-solver—in fact, a scientist in knickers. This bias could be traced principally to the tremendous (and mostly beneficent) influence of Jean Piaget and, to a somewhat lesser extent, the impact of other prominent developmental psychologists, such as Jerome Bruner in the United States and Lev Vygotsky and Alexander Luria in Russia. Little attention was paid to social, moral, personality, or emotional development, except among psychoanalytically oriented observers, among whose ranks was Erik Erikson, whom I was fortunate enough to have had as a tutor when I was in college.

A second and related limitation was the focus, within the cognitive arena, on certain forms of logical-rational thought. As a onetime dedicated pianist, and as one who has continued to gain major solace from the arts, I knew instinctively that there was something wrong with this perspective. While a first-year graduate student, I elected to direct my own research toward a developmental psychology of the arts and, if possible, to persuade my colleagues about the desirability—no, the necessity—for a concern with artistic forms of thinking. I had the good fortune to become a charter member of a research team that as its assignment sought to unravel the nature of artistic thinking. Noting that next to nothing was known about this topic, its founder Nelson Goodman pointedly dubbed our group "Project Zero." My work during the last fifteen years as a member (and, more recently, as co-director) of this project led to numerous experimental studies and to my first book, *The Arts and Human Development* (1973)*; many other writings since then, including the present collection, have espoused the cause of development and the arts. For the last decade I have also spent part of each working day conducting neuropsychological investigations

---

* Bibliographical information for all cited works is given in the Reference section at the back of this book.

of the effects of brain damage on mental activity, especially in the arts. If I have been guilty of the contemporary psychologists' sin of excessive focus on cognition, I hope to have at least contributed to broadening the notion of what "counts" as mind and perhaps, in the process, also to have touched upon personality, the emotions, and the cultural context in which all mental processes necessarily unfold.

A scholar *is* his teachers, his own masters, poorly or artfully reconstructed and recombined. It seems proper to introduce readers to my area of concern in the same way that I arrived there—through a consideration of certain key ideas that arose in the social sciences during the last few decades. Accordingly, this collection begins with tributes to three giants of the cognitive sciences—the psychologist Jean Piaget, the linguist Noam Chomsky, and the anthropologist Claude Lévi-Strauss. Each of these individuals has explored with exemplary seriousness the assumptions that the human mind is highly organized and that, through a study of human behaviors and products, one can decipher the principal structures of thought. Lévi-Strauss displays the additional virtue of an explicit concern with the arts, and so he doubles as a link to a second group of masters—Ernst Cassirer, Susanne Langer, Nelson Goodman, and Ernst Gombrich—who embraced a cognitive or, more precisely, a symbolic approach to the arts and who provided many clues about how to conduct a psychological study of the artistic process.

From Piaget (as well as other structuralists), I have evolved my views of human development and many of my methods of inquiry. From Goodman (as well as other students of symbolism), I have adopted the conviction that the arts entail the use of various symbol systems and that each artistic symbol system merits separate inquiry. As a result of studying these masters and reviewing other work in the social sciences, I have become convinced of the importance of exploring artistic mastery from as wide a set of perspectives as possible. Indeed, each "lens" on the mysteries of artistic creation holds promise of illuminating a slightly different portion of the puzzle. Accordingly, in the main sections of this collection I examine the components of artistic production and mastery from numerous vantage points—that of the normal child, the gifted child, the child who exhibits pathology, the normal adult, the brain-damaged adult, and the individual from a different cultural background, as well as several artists at the heights of their powers. These elements are the pieces of mastery—the constituent building blocks out of which someday, I hope, we will be able to construct a comprehensive psychology of creative processes.

My ultimate goal has always been to illuminate artistry at its greatest heights. For reasons that are spelled out in various essays, however, it has seemed best not to make a direct onslaught on the accomplished artist. My preferred approach has been through a study of the working activities of the young child who is in the process of developing artistic competences.

I have long enjoyed working with children and contemplating their artwork, and so it has been natural for me to favor this lens in investigating mastery. Yet, in addition to personal predilection, I have also been struck and animated by a central enigma: the many apparent links between the seemingly casual productions of young children and the masterworks of accomplished artists. If there is a single theme that haunts this book and, indeed, my scholarly life, it has been the similarities *and* the differences between "child art" and Art.

Having introduced this central enigma at the beginning of Part II, "Artistic Development in Children," I proceed to assemble the pieces of mastery from numerous perspectives. This survey includes a consideration of different art forms, different age groups, and different kinds of child populations. In Part III, "On Education and Media: The Transmission of Knowledge," I consider the role (both positive and negative) of various educational interventions upon the "natural" course of artistry and also the effects of the various media of communication (most notably, television) upon the creative processes in both children and adults. Part IV, "The Breakdown of the Mind," treats the disintegration of high-level cognitive skills under various conditions of brain damage; along the way, I attempt to place into proper perspective the bold claims about creativity, artistry, and "the two halves of the brain." Each of the parts begins with an introduction, which establishes the rationale for its particular "lens" and the way it has been adapted in this collection.

As I have already suggested, the task of describing artistry and creativity in their full-blown forms lies largely in the future. A clear asset of working with children, and also with brain-damaged adults, is that these populations hold hope of illuminating aspects of artistic mastery without at the same time proving of such overwhelming complexity and intricacy as to defy analysis. Still, given my central concern with the genuine masters and masterpieces of art, I have not been able to resist the temptation of describing the consummate creator. As a kind of dessert to the main course of scholarship in the earlier pages and as a sort of appetizer to future work, I conclude this collection with two short pieces on the heights of creative achievement.

In conducting the research described in the present collection, I have had the opportunity to experience at least one aspect of the creative process—the sense of working in a new area of study where virtually "zero" was known, and of having the opportunity to push forward, at least in the direction of +1. In this effort I have had the privilege of collaboration with exceptional colleagues. There is no way in which I can adequately thank, or even give the names of, all of the individuals who have made it possible for me to undertake productive research in this area. Still, I want to mention those individuals with whom I have worked most directly and ask them to stand for the much larger group. At the Boston Veterans Administration Medical Center and the Boston University School of Medicine, Harold Goodglass and Edgar Zurif; at Harvard Project Zero, Nelson Goodman and David Perkins (who were there at its creation), Vernon Howard, Laurene Meringoff, and Tom Carothers. Two long-time and treasured colleagues, Ellen Winner and Dennie Wolf, were kind enough to permit me to reprint essays which we co-authored.

I have been equally fortunate in receiving generous support from a large group of funding agencies. These essays were not, for the most part, supported directly by these institutions but, clearly, they could not have been written without their help and flexibility. It is with a deep and abiding sense of gratitude that I thank the Spencer Foundation and its President, H. Thomas James; the Markle Foundation and its President, Lloyd Morrisett; the Carnegie Corporation and its Vice-President, Barbara Finberg; the Sloan Foundation and its Program Officer, Kenneth Klivington; the National Institute of Education and its long-term Program Officer, Martin Engel; the National Science Foundation and the director of its Linguistics Program, Paul Chapin; and the National Institute of Neurological Diseases, Communication Disorders, and Stroke and its Program Officer, Christy Ludlow. I am indebted in different but important ways to the Veterans Administration, where much of my research has been conducted, to the Harvard Graduate School of Education, the Boston University School of Medicine, the Bernard van Leer Foundation, the MacArthur Foundation, and to Howard Muson and Jack Nessel of *Psychology Today*. Finally, for their help in preparing this collection for publication, I wish to thank Jane Isay, my admirable editor, Maureen Bischoff, Linda Carbone, Vincent

Torre, and Annabel Tyrrell of Basic Books; and Jasmine Hall and Eve Mendelsohn of Harvard Project Zero.

Thanks to the generosity of these individuals and these institutions, it has been possible for me to participate in what I consider to be a remarkable and highly privileged calling—the opportunity to conduct research, without artificial barriers or stimulants, in order to try to understand better the workings of the human mind and eventually to found improved practice upon this knowledge. I have the good fortune of being able to present the initial fruits of these studies in this collection. Alas, at a time when support for this kind of effort has virtually disappeared in this country, I hope this book will not have to serve as an epitaph for research on artistry. Rather, it is my fervent hope that the research community will somehow find a way to survive so that the various pieces that are scattered here might some day be brought together into a more coherent account of artistic mastery.

HOWARD GARDNER
Cambridge, Massachusetts
June 1982

ACKNOWLEDGMENTS

The author gratefully acknowledges permission to reprint the following drawings and photographs.

Page 28. Drawing by David Levine. Reprinted with permission from *The New York Review of Books.* Copyright © 1967 N.Y. Rev. Inc.

Page 62. Permission granted by Nelson Goodman and Hackett Publishing Company, Inc., Indianapolis, Indiana.

Page 66, Figure 7.1. Wall Painting: Figures in a Funeral Procession. Copy in tempera. From the tomb of Ramose, Dynasty XII-Prov.: Thebes. Expedition, The Metropolitan Museum of Art, 1930. All rights reserved, The Metropolitan Museum of Art.

Page 67, Figure 7.2. Cimabue. *Madonna and Child Enthroned with Angel and Prophets.* c. 1275–1280. Uffizi, Florence. Photo: Alinari/EPA.

Page 68, Figure 7.3. Giotto. *Madonna and Child Enthroned with Saints and Angels.* c. 1310. Uffizi, Florence. Photo: Alinari/EPA.

Page 69, Figure 7.4. John Constable, *Wivenhoe Park, Essex.* National Gallery of Art, Washington, Widener Collection.

Page 70, Figure 7.5. Dürer. *Draftsman Drawing a Reclining Nude.* c. 1525. Besitzvermerk: Staatliche Museen Preussischer Kulturbesitz Kupferstichkabinett, Berlin.

Page 72, Figure 7.6. E. H. Gombrich, *Art and Illusion: A Study in the Psychology of Pictorial Representation,* Princeton, N.J.: Princeton University Press, 1960.

Page 76, Figure 7.7. Dürer. *Group of Six Nude Figures.* c. 1515. Städelsches Kunstinstitut Frankfurt a. Main.

Acknowledgments

Page 77, Figure 7.8. Kulmbach. *Studies of Men in Bondage*. Nationale Forschungs und Gedenkstätten, Weimar. Figure appears in J. Rosenberg, *On Quality in Art*, Bollingen Series 35:13, copyright © 1967 by the Trustees of the National Gallery of Art, Washington, D.C.

Page 143. Picasso. *Study for the Horse*, study for *Guernica*. 1937. © Museo del Prado, Madrid. © SPADEM, Paris/ VAGA, New York, 1982.

Pages 186–89. With permission from *Nadia: A Case of Extraordinary Drawing Ability in an Autistic Child*. 1977. L. Selfe. Copyright 1977 Academic Press Inc. (London) Ltd.

Page 322. R. Jung, *Psychiatrie Der Gegenwart* (2nd ed., vol. I/2, p. 899; first published in 1974) Berlin-Heidelberg-New York: Spring 1980.

For permission to reproduce his own previously published articles, he gratefully acknowledges the following publishers.

Essay 1. "Jean Piaget: The psychologist as Renaissance man" © 1980 by The New York Times Company. Reprinted by permission.
"Jean Piaget—Review of the Grasp of Consciousness" © 1976 by The New York Times Company. Reprinted by permission.

Essay 2. "Cognition comes of age." Introduction to M. Piatelli-Palmarini, ed., *On Language and Learning*. Cambridge, Mass.: Harvard University Press, 1980, and reprinted from *Psychology Today* Magazine. Copyright © 1979 Ziff-Davis Publishing Company.

Essay 5. *"Philosophy in a New Key* Reconsidered" by Howard Gardner. From *Human Nature*, November 1978. Copyright © 1978 by Human Nature, Inc. Reprinted by permission of the publisher.

Essay 6. "Gifted worldmakers." Reprinted from *Psychology Today* Magazine. Copyright © 1980 Ziff-Davis Publishing Company.

Essay 8. © 1979 by The New York Times Company. Reprinted by permission.

Essay 9. *Journal of Communication*, Vol. 29, No. 4 (1979): 146–56.

Essay 10. "How children learn: Three stages of understanding art." Reprinted from *Psychology Today* Magazine. Copyright © 1976 Ziff-Davis Publishing Company.

Acknowledgments

Essay 11. "Artistic Symbols in Early Childhood" by Howard Gardner, Dennie Wolf, and Ann Smith in *New York University Education Quarterly* 6 (1975): 13–21.

Essay 12. "Children's art: The age of creativity." Reprinted from *Psychology Today* Magazine. Copyright © 1980 Ziff-Davis Publishing Company.

Essay 13. "Do babies sing a universal song?" Reprinted from *Psychology Today* Magazine. Copyright © 1981 Ziff-Davis Publishing Company.

Essay 14. Reprinted from *Psychology Today* Magazine. Copyright © 1979 Ziff-Davis Publishing Company.

Essay 15. "The making of a storyteller." Reprinted from *Psychology Today* Magazine. Copyright © 1982 Ziff-Davis Publishing Company.

Essay 16. "Children's art: Nadia's challenge." Reprinted from *Psychology Today* Magazine. Copyright © 1979 Ziff-Davis Publishing Company.

Essay 17. Reprinted from *Psychology Today* Magazine. Copyright © 1981 Ziff-Davis Publishing Company.

Essay 18. "Unfolding or training: Of the optimal approach to art education." From *The Arts, Human Development, and Education* by Elliot W. Eisner et al., eds. (Berkeley, Calif.: McCutchan Publishing Corporation, 1976), pp. 100–10. © 1976 McCutchan Publishing Corp. Permission granted by the publisher.

Essay 19. Howard Gardner, "Illuminating Comparisons in the Arts." In Mary Henle, ed., *Vision and Artifact.* Copyright © 1976 by Springer Publishing Company, Inc., New York. Used by permission.

Essay 20. Reprinted from *Psychology Today* Magazine. Copyright © 1979 Ziff-Davis Publishing Company.

Essay 21. "Reprogramming the media researchers." Reprinted from *Psychology Today* Magazine. Copyright © 1980 Ziff-Davis Publishing Company.

Essay 22. Gardner, H. and Jaglom, L. "How Kids Learn TV." Reprinted from *The Dial*, August 1981.

Essay 23. "Does television stimulate or stultify?" Copyright © 1982 *TV Guide* (Canada) Inc. Used by permission.

Essay 24. "On becoming a dictator." Reprinted from *Psychology Today* Magazine. Copyright © 1980 Ziff-Davis Publishing Company.

Acknowledgments

Essay 25. "Brain damage: A gateway to the mind." Copyright © 1975 by *Saturday Review*. All rights reserved. Reprinted by permission.

Essay 26. © 1978 by Harvard Magazine. Reprinted by permission.

Essay 27. "The loss of language" by Howard Gardner. From *Human Nature*, March 1978. Copyright © 1978 by Human Nature, Inc. Reprinted by permission of the publisher.

Essay 28. "Developmental dyslexia and the forgotten case of Monsieur C." Reprinted from *Psychology Today* Magazine. Copyright © 1973 Ziff-Davis Publishing Company.

Essay 29. "How the split brain gets jokes." Reprinted from *Psychology Today* Magazine. Copyright © 1981 Ziff-Davis Publishing Company.

Essay 31. "The lives of Alexander Luria." Reprinted from *Psychology Today* Magazine. Copyright © 1980 Ziff-Davis Publishing Company.

Essay 33. "Composing symphonies and dinner parties." Reprinted from *Psychology Today* Magazine. Copyright © 1980 Ziff-Davis Publishing Company.

PART I

MASTERS

INTRODUCTION

STRUCTURES AND SYMBOLS

TWENTY YEARS AGO psychology seemed a rather remote and sterile area to individuals interested in the full and creative use of the mind. The field harbored a trio of uninviting specializations. There was academic psychology, featuring the use of contrived laboratory apparatus to study the perception of visual illusions or the memorization of long lists of nonsense syllables. Such lines of study bore little evident relationship to human beings engaged in thought. There was behaviorism, the approach that emerged from work with rats and pigeons. Behaviorists claimed that we act in the way we do because we are reinforced for doing so and, given their focus on overt activity, these scholars denied inner life—no thoughts, no fantasies, no aspirations. Finally, there was psychoanalysis, which offered not only a controversial method of treatment but also an overarching theory of human nature. While psychoanalysis had a grandeur and depth that eluded both academic psychology and behaviorism, it strongly accentuated human personality and unconscious motivation while saying little about rational thought processes or conscious problem-solving.

The cognitive revolution came in two parts. First, there was the frank recognition that one could—one must—take seriously human mental processes, including thinking, problem-solving, and creating. Study of the mind once again became a proper scientific undertaking. Second, there was the demonstration by several researchers that human thought processes were characterized by considerable regularity and structure. Not all of this cogitation took place in full view, nor could such cognitive processes always be either related to external stimuli or confirmed by introspection. But there was structure to thought processes, a structure the careful analyst could help lay bare.

Many of us who were studying the behavioral sciences in the 1960s were swept up—and have remained inspired—by this revolution. For some, the appeal lay in computer programming and artificial intelligence—the design of machines that display intelligence. For others, the thrill came in conducting careful laboratory experiments in which one could trace, on a millisecond-by-millisecond basis, an individual's mental processes as he carried out a multiplication problem, reasoned through a logical syllogism, or rotated an image of a geometrical form in his head. Still others took roads that went through pedagogy, through anthropology, or through the neurosciences. In my own case, I found especially appealing the approach to the mind put forth by structuralists working in the cognitive regions of several social sciences.

In the opening set of essays I lay out the principal assumption of this structuralist approach as it was exemplified by the developmental psychologist Jean Piaget, the linguist Noam Chomsky, and the anthropologist Claude Lévi-Strauss. These thinkers share a belief that the mind operates according to specifiable rules—often unconscious ones—and that these can be ferreted out and made explicit by the systematic examination of human language, action, and problem-solving. There are many intriguing differences among their approaches as well, and I review several of these: still, one finds throughout a surprisingly (and reassuringly) common vision of what the human mind is like and how it can best be described for scientific purposes.

The structuralist approach to the mind has limitations. Those that are most germane, given my own concern with artistic knowledge, derive from the essentially closed nature of structuralist systems. Though creative thought has not escaped their attention, each of the major cognitive structuralists views the options of human thought as in some way preordained, limited in advance. This makes their work especially problematic for a study of mind where the major focus falls on innovation and creation, as in the fashioning of original works of art.

To my mind the limitation implicit in the standard structuralist stance can be circumscribed by a recognition of one special feature of human thought—its ability to create and sponsor commerce through the use of various kinds of symbol systems. These symbol systems—these codes of meaning—are the vehicles through which thought takes

4

place: by their very nature they are creative, open systems. Through the use of symbols the human mind, operating according to structuralist principles, can create, revise, transform, and re-create wholly fresh products, systems, and even worlds of meaning.

These ideas were persuasively laid forth in modern times by the German philosopher Ernst Cassirer. He was perhaps the first to articulate the vision that I have just introduced—the belief that the key to various forms of creation lies in an understanding of how humans use symbol systems. Further articulation of this pregnant vision was performed in the philosophical area by one of his students, Susanne Langer, and more recently by the philosopher Nelson Goodman. In explicating the work of these two individuals, we come to see how the structuralist methods and approach toward the mind might be oriented toward lines of thought other than those of a purely logical-rational variety. At the same time we make a transition from a philosophical treatment of symbolization to a set of approaches that lend themselves to empirical investigation—for example, through studies in developmental psychology and neuropsychology. Important additional inputs to this process can come from scholars in the arts who have taken seriously the wedding of the philosophical and psychological traditions. An exemplary instance of this approach comes from the art historian Ernst Gombrich, whose investigation of creative work in the visual arts provides a connecting link to the studies of specific art forms introduced in later parts of this book.

1

JEAN PIAGET: PSYCHOLOGIST, EDUCATOR, AND GENETIC EPISTEMOLOGIST

JEAN PIAGET, the renowned student of human growth, himself experienced a most unusual personal and scientific development. A child prodigy who published his first research paper at age eleven, Piaget realized a scientific career of unsurpassed fecundity. He risked a number of sharp career shifts, turning to psychology only after having received his doctorate in biology, and later, in middle age, training himself in logic and physics. Internationally honored as a young man for his pathbreaking studies of children (he received an honorary doctorate during Harvard's tercentenary while still in his thirties), he was nevertheless for many years regarded as an anachronism and only recently regained a dominant position in the social sciences. Indeed, unlike most scientists whose seminal contributions occur early, Piaget made some of his most important discoveries in the later decades of his life and continued his feverish pace until his death in 1980 at the age of eighty-four. By his own example, this proud Swiss confirmed his country's capacity to spawn creative scientists as well as competent clockmakers.

Even within the field of psychology, Piaget was a maverick. Where most researchers favor large populations of subjects and powerful statistics, Piaget habitually used small samples (often his own three children) and rarely computed even the simplest statistic. Where most psychologists defend their field and its claims to scientific respectability, Piaget preferred to term himself a genetic epistemologist—one who studies the origins of human knowledge. Where his principal equals in influence and notoriety—Sigmund Freud and B. F. Skinner—wrote with great skill and passion, often reaching over the heads of skeptical colleagues to more receptive lay audiences, Piaget's writings were workaday at best and often posed difficulties for colleagues and translators. And where those psychologists with the greatest followings have focused either (like Skinner) on overt, often striking behaviors or (like Freud) on bizarre personality configurations and emotional reactions, Piaget selected as his topic an intangible, passionless, and at one time highly obscure domain—the operations of a child's mind. Indeed, Piaget's claim to greatness lay chiefly in his detailed description of the clockwork regularity with which the mind of every normal child develops.

Any effort to assess Piaget's contribution and to evaluate his later writings must build upon some familiarity with the problems he originally confronted, the procedures he evolved, and the program he attempted to realize. As a brilliant young biologist in the early 1920s, Piaget sought a biological account of the nature and development of knowledge, or intelligence. His own research had been with mollusks, but before writing a synthesis, Piaget felt it might be useful to "take off a few years" to study young children. The detour lasted for the rest of his scholarly life, and his magnum opus *Biology and Knowledge*, which finally appeared in 1967, was admittedly only an interim effort.

In accounting for the unexpected immensity of Piaget's task, we confront directly the nature of his enterprise. First of all, in the early 1920s very little was known about children's intellective processes. In fact, to the extent that this topic was even considered, most researchers regarded the child as a "little adult" who perhaps knew less than an adult but reasoned in essentially the same way. Piaget began to question children in depth, listened carefully to their responses, focused especially on the strategies they used and the errors they made, and came up with a (then) startling conclusion—children at different ages construe the world in ways that are fundamentally different from those of adults. Piaget's early fame derived from his arresting demonstration of these characteristic mental operations and qualitatively different "cognitive stages" of childhood.

Following these initial demonstrations, Piaget's work in the 1930s took two related yet unanticipated turns. In order to test his hypothesis that all knowledge derives from human actions upon the world, Piaget began to investigate the earliest signs of human intelligence during the opening weeks and months of life. And indeed, in studying such humble activities as sucking and looking, he confirmed to his satisfaction that the infant's first motor acts and sensory discriminations constitute the earliest manifestations of intellect. At the same time, however, Piaget was not content merely to sketch out a general set of developmental stages. Rather, he wanted to probe the development of knowledge in each of the major domains defined by Western thought—number, causality, time, geometry, and the like. And so, not unlike the watchmaker who patiently assembles each wheel of the instrument, Piaget launched a large set of "domain-specific" studies, in which the stages of knowledge could be mapped and their place located within the human mind. These studies documented that actions could eventually occur "within the head"—in fact, such "mental operations" form the "mainsprings" of what is usually called *thought*.

One large dividend of these studies was the identification of four major stages of mental development. The first—that of *sensorimotor intelligence*—covers roughly the first two years of life. At this time the child "knows" the world exclusively through his own perceptions and actions upon it. The second stage—that of *intuitive* or *symbolic* thought—spans the preschool years. Now the child is able to use language, mental images, and other kinds of symbols to refer to the world which he* had previously known only directly through acting upon it. Yet the knowledge through symbols is still static: for example, the child cannot manipulate the "images" that he carries about in his head.

The capacity to manipulate such mental images and other forms of symbolic knowledge arises at the beginning of the school years, when the child becomes capable of *concrete operational* thought. The child of seven or eight can appreciate a certain state of affairs—for example, how a set of objects looks to him—not only from his present perspective, but, through the use of "internal actions" or "mental operations," from the vantage point of another person situated elsewhere. And he can in his mind proceed back and forth between two perspectives on the same scene through the use of the central operation of reversibility.

* For expositional purposes, the word *he* will be used in its generic sense throughout this book.

Finally, during the period of *formal operations,* which begins in early adolescence, the child becomes able to perform mental actions upon symbols as well as upon physical entities. He can write equations, utter propositions, and perform logical manipulations upon strings of symbols, for example, combining them, contrasting them, negating them. More generally, he becomes able to pose and solve scientific problems that require the manipulation of relevant variables. Piaget viewed this sequence of four stages as both invariant and universal. Given sufficient interaction with a normal environment and sufficient time, every normal child should realize this sequence. It is part of the human blueprint.

Like nearly all of Piaget's writings, this overall description of the theory is somewhat abstract. It is possible to secure a more textured portrait of the child's mind by following a single example of knowledge—an example that particularly fascinated Piaget—through the first decade and a half of the child's life.

As our glimpse into the ways of knowing first discerned by Piaget, let us consider how the child knows, or "cognizes," a ball of clay. Harking back to the beginning of life, we find that the infant's sensorimotor knowledge is restricted to the physical actions he can perform on a ball of clay. He can suck the clay, bite it, grasp it, knead it into various shapes. But he lacks any understanding apart from his actions, and once the ball is out of sight, he is unable to think about it at all.

A decisive event occurs in the second year of life. At about eighteen months the child comes to realize that the ball exists even when he is not looking at it. The child will search persistently for the ball when it has disappeared and will be able to imagine where it has gone if it is thrown in a certain direction: his knowledge now includes an awareness of the object's permanence.

Soon afterward, in the preschool years, the child becomes able to use various kinds of symbols with reference to the ball. He learns the word *ball* and uses it more or less appropriately to refer to round objects. He engages in play with dolls and may toss them a pretend ball. He may dream via mental imagery of round objects, and he can imitate the various motions of a ball, even hurtling his own body across the room.

Yet he fails to understand certain principles about how a ball behaves: for example, he does not realize that a ball of clay can change its shape and still remain the same in amount; he does not appreciate that a set of five balls arranged in a circle is equivalent to a set of five balls laid out in a straight line; restricted to static imagery and to his own perspective, he cannot anticipate how the ball appears to someone sitting elsewhere in a room. As Piaget put it, the child is still mired in an intuitive or preoperational stage.

During the early years of school, the child becomes able to appreciate these and other principles governing the behavior of objects. He can "conserve" numbers because he can "reverse" the operation of "bringing the balls in a circle" and appreciate that the original array can be readily reconstituted. In addition to acquiring a sense of quantity, of number, and of the perspectives of other people, he can now give a simple definition of the word *ball*, and he appreciates that an object can be at once a ball, a toy, and a round thing. Shown five red balls and two white balls, he is able to affirm that there are more balls than there are red balls. Now at the concrete-operational stage, he is beginning to be able to reason with words and to conduct simple experiments.

But only at the time of adolescence does the child become capable of abstract thought with reference to the world of the ball. Now, in addition to anticipating what will happen to a ball under various conditions, he can discuss it in terms of scientific laws, make predictions, and test hypotheses. Capable of formal operational thought, the youth can explain the reason a billiard ball shot against a surface at one angle will rebound at a complementary angle. He can solve reasoning problems of the sort: ball A is fatter than ball B; ball B is thinner than ball C; which ball is the thinnest? He has the capacity to write an essay about spheres and to appreciate Newtonian (and even Einsteinian) principles about the behavior of spherical objects.

Beyond question, Piaget provided the most crucial information that we have about what children know, how they come to their knowledge, what they are likely to be able to learn, and what is completely beyond their grasp at various stages of development. Yet it may seem that these kinds of insights are remote from the kinds of practical problems that generally attract the public to the work of child psychologists.

In my view Piaget's findings can contribute significantly to the understanding of numerous matters involving children. To be sure, Piaget himself modestly disclaimed any ambition to be an educational policymaker, and it is true that he is far from having devised curricula or platforms. Yet I think that once one has understood Piaget well—to use his term, once one has assimilated his theory—one should be able to approach children in a much better informed and more appropriate manner.

Let me mention a few insights about children that derive from Piaget's writings. Most parents—not to mention most children—remember the terrible fuss made when youngsters are presented with a cookie and the cookie accidentally breaks in half. In the eyes of an adult, the amount of cookie is the same and so the fuss is pointless. However, for the "preoperational child," quantity inheres in a specific item— that particular chocolate-chip cookie. There is no appreciation that two cookies of different appearance could contain the same amount of dough and chocolate bits—in fact, the whole notion of "same amount" has little meaning for the four- or five-year-old.

We all know some teachers, and some parents, who are extremely successful at conveying new kinds of information, even as other adults of equal intelligence and skill are woefully unsuccessful. While many factors contribute to such differences, one lesson from Piaget's work is particularly germane. Piaget argued that development must take place at its own pace and cannot be rushed. All the same, there occur certain points of "disequilibrium" in development—times when the child is becoming aware of contradictory ideas and is therefore especially sensitive to examples that suggest a resolution.

Suppose, therefore, that the mother of our fussy child feels he has recently become uncertain about what happens when the cookie splits. Blindfolding her youngster, she demonstrates to him that he cannot taste the difference between the broken and the intact cookie. After trying this exercise a few times, she may find that he has acquired a new appreciation of conservation of matter.

Consider one further illustration, this time involving children of a much older age. Many adolescents become intensely involved in ideological movements—they respond to the appeal of a religious sect, a school of philosophy, or the sway of a spellbinding orator. They master the ideas being touted, they engage in endless argumentation, they are prepared to devote all their energies—perhaps even their lives— to The Cause.

The capacity to become enwrapped in such movements seems a direct product of two cognitive revolutions at adolescence. First, a youngster at this time becomes able to reason in purely verbal terms: no longer in need of concrete demonstrations or vivid images, he can be convinced for the first time simply by the power of the word. Second, and relatedly, the youth can now conceive of all possible ramifications of a position. He is able to view all the world through one set of lenses, to think of the utopias that might come to pass if a certain set of ideas becomes dominant. He can also don another set of lenses and imagine a contrasting view of the world. No wonder some youngsters are eager to substitute absolutist visions for the murky compromises that mark the mundane existence of those about them. Adults who wish to deal with such youths might help them realize that any road taken involves certain benefits and certain costs.

This example illustrates the virtue of Piagetian analysis in the practical arena. It is an analysis that does not dictate what parents should do, but it may help them understand better what their offspring are up to—and why.

But Piaget did not consider himself a psychologist or an educator. A biologist by training and a synthetic thinker by inclination, Piaget viewed himself as founder of a new field of knowledge—that of genetic epistemology. The goal of this discipline was to illuminate the nature of the basic categories of scientific thought through investigation of the origins (or genesis) of this knowledge. This task was inherently interdisciplinary, and Piaget labored for decades, first alone and later with like-minded colleagues, in an effort to lay out the core aspects of our conceptions of number, logic, space, time, causality, and other Kantian building blocks of knowledge. Key in this effort were experts from each field of science as well as genetic psychologists—experimental researchers trained by Piaget to uncover the origins and development of basic scientific concepts in the young child. Also included in a research team were philosophers, who defined the concepts, and historians of science, who chronicled the growth of knowledge over the centuries within each scientific field. When the insights from this team of scholars were put together, they would yield the fullest possible account of the particular scientific concept in question.

No one can question the grandeur—or the hubris—of this undertaking. Piaget sought no less than to forge a great chain of mental being, which proceeded from the elementary functioning of genes and nerve cells, through the actions of young children upon the physical objects of the world, to the internal operations of thought in the minds of normal adults and innovative scientists—a chain that culminated in fundamental changes in the structure of a science. How matter could give rise to new—and valid—ideas: this was Piaget's guiding passion, one as synoptic as those of Freud and Skinner and, indeed, reminiscent of the vision of the greatest thinkers of the past.

While many others might have doubted the feasibility of this enterprise, both from a scientific and a philosophical point of view, Piaget kept any misgivings under firm control, set up his experiments, and ploughed ahead. Displaying the discipline, energy, and organizational capacity associated with genius, he produced dozens of books and countless papers, each time revisiting the same core concerns in the light of his most recent findings. In the middle fifties he founded the International Center of Genetic Epistemology, and, aided by an energetic group of students and collaborators, raced against time until the end to sketch out the principal lines of his vision. And it seems to me that it is in the light of this vision—first fathomed as a teenager and rarely deviated from thereafter—that Jean Piaget must be evaluated.

In an age of fragmented specialization, Piaget was indubitably a Renaissance man. Nowhere is this more poignantly evident than in *Logic and Scientific Knowledge* (1967), an encyclopedia he planned, edited, and largely wrote, which surveyed all of the sciences from the perspective of genetic epistemology. To prepare for this massive work, Piaget held seminars with experts from every field of knowledge, often collaborating with them for upwards of a year. He rose early each morning and worked through the evening, tutoring himself in the discipline of that year and ultimately mastering at least the basic conceptual issues. The undertaking of such encyclopedic assignments was Piaget's method of bridging his own science with every other one. Indeed, it was his way of pursuing his own religion—the passion for truth, the search for the totality of knowledge.

But this herculean effort has as yet had little impact. An encyclopedia largely from the hand of one man, no matter how brilliant, seems a throwback to a Johnsonian age. The flaws are too evident. Piaget did not have the necessary firsthand familiarity with the phenomena of other sciences, or the sympathy with the history and cultural background of other disciplines, or the sophistication in the philosophical analysis of concepts. He lacked the intuitions on which he so readily drew in his investigation of the mollusks in the lakes of Switzerland and the children in the classrooms of Geneva. Yet what slips through in the 1,250-odd pages is the sense of wonder and exploration that gives rise to knowledge. Till the end, the child—and the adolescent—in Piaget were never stilled. Like Sigmund Freud, he was by temperament a passionate speculator and integrator, who sought ruthlessly to suppress his speculative nature, but, fortunately, never wholly succeeded in doing so.

Still, it is as a scientist that Piaget himself would most wish to be assessed, and any ultimate assessment must examine the core of his research program. In my view, there is little doubt that Piaget defined the major psychological issues concerning the child and cognition, even as he created a viable new area of study—genetic epistemology. To be sure, young (and not-so-young) Turks are already finding fault with experiment X or with operation Y; in all likelihood significant portions of the Piagetian enterprise will have to be revised. But the overall edifice seems reasonably secure. Revisions will likely be made within the framework laid out and the questions first posed by Piaget.

Yet in adopting a certain conception of thought—that form of logical rationality valued by Descartes and glorified in recent centuries by Western science—Piaget may have neglected central aspects of human cognition. To be sure, science and mathematics involve sophisticated forms of thinking. But so do literature, art, and music, and Piaget had little to say about them. Indeed, these areas of thought prove difficult even to envision in his array of "cognitive domains." Relatedly, in his zeal for capturing the operations of the mind, Piaget consistently neglected the realm of feeling. We learn much from his writings about children's conceptions of water, but little about their fear of floods, their love of splashing, their desire to be minnows, mermaids, or mariners. So, too, some aspects of consciousness may be captured in a child's verbal reflections upon his physical actions. But the subtle and perennial tensions among conscious, preconscious, and unconscious processes are missed. Vast realms of awareness—occasions of existential anxiety, peak experiences, the often overpowering imagery of daydreams and nightmares—are bypassed in this "civilized," streamlined, and even somewhat mechanistic view of human consciousness.

Piaget's contributions need no defense. Like nearly all social scientists, I have learned much from him—indeed, his work has guided my choice of research topics and the ways in which I investigate them. Nor have his contributions been merely academic. For instance, much of the recent interest in child-centered learning and in "open instruction" has been directly inspired by Piaget's views of mental development and the nature of thought. Finally, it would be misleading to suggest that Piaget was oblivious to the limitations mentioned here. It was with explicit intent—and perhaps a twinge of regret—that he elected to fix his powerful intellect upon scientific thought and thus to neglect realms of imagination, emotion, and "lived" experience.

Still the image of the Swiss watchmaker poring over an unassembled instrument remains haunting and disturbingly apt. Piaget's own orderly habits of mind and thought allowed him, like the watchmaker, to prepare an astonishing number of the component parts and to make significant progress in constructing a well-balanced, working instrument. It may turn out that other forms of thought, in their dialectical, turbulent, or aesthetic facets, eluded even a master craftsman. The human mind, which for more than sixty years fascinated Piaget, and which in his own case gave rise to an inspiring and strikingly original body of thought, may not be like a watch at all.

2

ENCOUNTER AT ROYAUMONT:

THE DEBATE BETWEEN

JEAN PIAGET AND

NOAM CHOMSKY

IN OCTOBER 1975 a confrontation of considerable importance to the temper of future intellectual discourse took place at a chateau in the Parisian suburb of Royaumont. The principal participants in this debate were Jean Piaget, the renowned Swiss psychologist and epistemologist, and Noam Chomsky, the noted American linguist and political activist. Their subject was no less than the nature of the human mind itself.

For a number of years, Piaget had hoped that such a meeting could be arranged. Sensitive to currents in contemporary social science, he had known about the threat to his position represented by the work of Chomsky and his collaborators. Chomsky had also been reading Piaget's works and had commented upon them critically. While less eager than Piaget for a personal encounter, he accepted the invitation proffered by the late Nobel laureate Jacques Monod, president of the Center for the Study of Man, to join together in a symposium dubbed (and later published as) "On Language and Learning."

The Piaget-Chomsky Debate

The encounter at the Abbaye de Royaumont was historically important for several reasons. To begin with, Chomsky and Piaget were recognized leaders of two of the most influential (possibly *the* most influential) schools of contemporary cognitive studies. Taken seriously by all scientists in their respective fields of linguistics and developmental psychology, they had achieved international reputations that far transcended their areas of specialization. Accompanied by colleagues who were associated in varying degrees with their own programs of research, Piaget and Chomsky presented their ideas to an illustrious gathering of scholars: Nobel laureates in biology, leading figures in philosophy and mathematics, and several of the most prominent behavioral scientists in the world today. Those in attendance listened critically to the arguments and joined vigorously in the ensuing discussion, seldom hesitating to make pronouncements and take sides. It was almost as if two of the great figures of the seventeenth century—Descartes and Locke, say—could have defied time and space to engage in discussion at a joint meeting of the Royal Society and the Académie Française.

The Royaumont meeting may well have had additional significance. Possibly for the first time figures at the forefront of such relatively "tender-minded" disciplines as psychology and linguistics succeeded in involving a broad and distinguished collection of "tough-minded" scholars in debates formulated by the behavioral scientists themselves—with scarcely a hint of condescension by the representatives of such firmly entrenched disciplines as biology and mathematics. Equally noteworthy, the protagonists represented the cognitive sciences—a field hardly known (and not even christened) two decades ago, and one far less familiar to both the general public and the scholarly community than many other pockets of the behavioral sciences.

The stakes in the exchange were also considerable, for the outcome of the Royaumont meeting might very well influence the future awarding of research funds; the interests of the brightest young scholars; and, indeed, the course of subsequent investigations of human cognition—arguably the most important line of inquiry in the social sciences today. Would the next generation of scholars be more attracted to pursuing the method of Piaget, observing children as they slowly construct knowledge of the physical world, or, inspired by Chomsky, would they find more challenge in formulating abstract characterizations of the presumably innate knowledge that a child has in such rule-governed domains as language, music, or mathematics?

The Royaumont meeting brought together two men who not only

represent different approaches but who were also dissimilar in background and style. On the one hand there was Noam Chomsky, the intense, urban intellectual, forty-six years old, employed for many years in the highly technical study of linguistics, and long engaged in political commentary and disputation about United States foreign policy. Chomsky had, with his devastating critiques, almost singlehandedly discredited two dominant schools of social science—behavioral psychology and traditional structural linguistics. And on the other hand there was Jean Piaget, thirty-two years Chomsky's senior, a European savant in the grand tradition, involved for half a century in widely known studies of the growth of children's thought. While equally proud, Piaget, a relatively nonpolitical citizen of that most neutral of all countries, had always avoided drawing hard battle lines between himself and other investigators. Indeed, to use one of his own terms, he had filled the role of "perpetual assimilator," eager to make contact with those of apparently opposing points of view and to assimilate their ideas to his own or, if necessary, accommodate his to theirs.

If the two men's styles and backgrounds were different, their ideas seemed, at least from a distance, remarkably akin. Both had vigorously opposed those who believed in a science built up of elements, those who mistrusted theoretical constructs, and those who felt that overt behavior was all that should be studied. Both were firmly in the rationalist tradition, worthy successors to René Descartes and Immanuel Kant. Believers in the organized human mind as an appropriate subject for study, Chomsky and Piaget were eager to discover universal principles of thought, convinced of the severe constraints built into human cognition, and relatively uninterested in social and cultural influences and in differences among individuals. Both believed in the importance of a biological perspective, but both were equally attracted to the formulation of logical models of the human mind.

Indeed, their deepest similarity lay in a belief (shared with Freud) that the important aspects of the mind lie beneath the surface. One could never solve the mysteries of thought by simply describing overt words or behaviors. One must, instead, search for the underlying structures of the mind: in Chomsky's view, the laws of universal grammar; in Piaget's, the mental operations of which the human intellect is capable.

Why, then, given this common enterprise (at least Piaget saw it that way), was there need for a debate? And why was there such a heated dispute at Royaumont about the proper future course for the sciences of the intellect? The answer is that there were important differences in the basic assumptions and methods by which the two men arrived at their respective models of human thought.

It is instructive that neither Piaget nor Chomsky was a psychologist by training, nor would either have answered readily to the label of cognitive scientist. Originally trained as a biologist, Piaget long stressed the continuity of the evolution of the species and the development of human intellect. As an adolescent he was intrigued by alterations in the shape of mollusks placed into lakes of differing climates and turbulences; he observed the same adaptiveness at work in the young infant gradually exploring the physical objects of the world. Moreover, Piaget realized that adaptation is never a simple reaction to the environment; rather, it is an active constructive process, in which problem-solving proceeds at first through the exercise of one's sensory systems and motor capacities, but eventually evolves to the height of cognition through logical operations "in the head."

All individuals pass through the same stages of intellectual development, Piaget proposed, not because we are "programmed" to do so but rather because, given the interaction of our inborn predispositions with the structure of the world in which we live, we are inevitably going to form certain hypotheses about the world, try them out, and then modify them in light of the feedback we receive. The image of thought that motivated Piaget was that of an active, exploring child systematically seeking solutions to a puzzle until he ultimately hits upon the right one, and then moves on to a yet more challenging puzzle. The "nativist" notion that all intellect is present at birth, waiting only to unfold, was anathema to Piaget, as was the rival empiricist view that all knowledge already exists in the world, just waiting to be etched into the blank infant mind.

And that was where the issue was joined with Noam Chomsky. A linguist from his earliest student days, ever committed to rigorous philosophical analysis and formal logical-mathematical methods, Chomsky's lifelong pursuit has been to understand the core of human language—the syntax that undergirds our verbal output. Chomsky views human language as marvelous and self-contained; he sees it, in fact, as a separate region of the mind. The phenomena that have intrigued Chomsky are the deep differences between superficially similar sentences: how we know instantly that "John is easy to please" functions differently from "John is eager to please"; how we recognize at once the underlying affinities between superficially different sentences, such as "The girl hit the boy," and "The boy was hit by the girl"; how we turn a statement effortlessly into a question or a question into a command.

But how did Chomsky move from these highly particularistic observations to a theory of mind? His route involved a demonstration that linguistic understanding requires mental work of a highly abstract sort. One must somehow be able to represent in one's mind the content of sentences at a level far removed from the surface properties of an utterance. Indeed, convinced early on of the inadequacy of previous attempts to explain language, Chomsky introduced into linguistics a set of wholly novel concerns. In fact he reformulated an agenda for scientific linguistics: to find a (and preferably *the*) set of grammatical rules that would generate syntactic descriptions of all of the permissible and none of the impermissible sentences in any given language. Such a grammar would constitute a valid description of the knowledge that a language user must employ when producing and understanding the sentences of his language.

Chomsky put forth a set of specific proposals concerning the formal nature of a grammatical system that could fulfill these goals. Because it is so difficult to determine how a child, exposed only to the surface structure of language, could ever "construct" these abstract representations, Chomsky arrived at a strong but highly controversial conclusion: knowledge of certain facets of language (and, by extension, of other intellectual "faculties") must be an inborn property of mind. Such knowledge requires, to be sure, a triggering environment (exposure to speech). But there is no need for active construction by the child or for more specific social or cultural input—the plan is all there. Nor are there separate stages of development based on changes in the child's mental capacities and on interaction with the environment: language unfolds in us in as natural a manner as the visual system or the circulatory system. The model lurking behind Chomsky's position, then, is that of a totally preprogrammed computer, one that needs merely to be plugged into the appropriate outlet.

And so we encounter the heart of the dispute between the two redoubtable thinkers. Whereas Piaget saw the child's efforts as engaging the full range of inventive powers as he stalks ahead from one stage to the next, Chomsky viewed the child as equipped with requisite knowledge from the beginning, only needing time to let that knowledge unfold.

At the conference both men made statements that were true to form in their examples, style of argument, and vision of science. Piaget characteristically focused on the arresting behavioral phenomena of children that he and his collaborators had discovered—the understanding of the permanence of objects, which does not occur until the end of infancy; the general capacity to symbolize, which is said to underlie both linguistic and pretend-play activities; the ability to appreciate the conservation of matter, which arises only during the early school years. Although Piaget criticized his old nemeses, the behaviorists and the nativists, for the most part he remained eager to convert others to his general picture of universal human development—a portrait attractive and convincing in its overall outlines but difficult to formulate in terms sufficiently precise for ready confirmation or disconfirmation.

Chomsky also offered a number of intriguing specific examples to support his point of view, but his overall approach was markedly different. Unlike Piaget's, his examples were not of dramatic behavioral phenomena; rather he pointed to abstract internal rules that seem necessary to account for certain regularities of linguistic output. For instance, he returned a number of times to the following illustration. When we transform the sentence "The man who is here is tall" into a question, we unfailingly produce the query "Is the man who is here tall?" rather than: "Is the man who here is tall?" Somehow we know that the relative phrase "the man who is here" must be treated as a single unit rather than broken up in the course of changing the order of the words.

Such rules are discovered by examining the features of correct linguistic utterances and of certain incorrect but "possible" syntactic constructions that seem never to appear. Once pointed out, such regularities are evident, and further experimentation to demonstrate their validity seems superfluous. Accordingly, Chomsky relied heavily on such examples to discount alternative rules and rival points of view. Disenchanted with accounts that had even a tinge of empiricism, he displayed little patience with the version of genetic-environmental contact that stands at the core of Piaget's interactionism. What impelled Chomsky's stance was a vivid image of what scientific practice should be like: metaphoric or impressionistic accounts must be avoided in favor of more precise statements phrased in a sufficiently formal manner to allow clear testing and decisive disconfirmation.

A number of other crucial differences emerged in the course of the debate. Perhaps the most dominant issue at Royaumont was one that took its original formulation from the pages of Shakespeare and has constituted a continuing source of contention between philosophers on opposite sides of the English Channel: whether (as Chomsky held) knowledge is largely inborn, part of the individual's birthright, a form of innate ideas existing in the realm of "nature"; whether (as traditional empiricists like Skinner have contended) knowledge is better conceived of as a product of living in an environment, a series of messages of "nurture" transmitted by other individuals and one's surrounding culture, which become etched onto a *tabula rasa;* or whether (as Piaget insisted) knowledge can be constructed only through interaction between certain inborn modes of processing available to the young child and the actual characteristics of physical objects and events. This issue of genetic versus cultural contributions to the mind was pointedly phrased by the convener of the conference, Jacques Monod: "In asking myself the vast question, 'What makes man man?' it is clear that it is partially his genome and partially his culture. But what are the genetic limits of culture? What is its genetic component?"

Whether by design or happenstance, considerable time was spent discussing Chomskian nativism versus Piagetian "interactionism," a conflict that at Royaumont centered particularly on questions pertaining to the origins of language. At issue was whether human linguistic capacities can in any interesting sense be considered a product of general "constructed" intellectual development (as Piaget contended), or whether they are a highly specialized part of human genetic inheritance, largely separate from other human faculties and more plausibly viewed as a kind of innate knowledge that has only to unfold (as Chomsky insisted).

To be sure, whether language is interestingly dependent on certain nonlinguistic capacities is crucial, and this question was discussed at a sophisticated level during the conference. Yet the specific debate between nativism and interactionism strikes many observers, including me, as unnecessary and sterile. Within the biological sciences many feel it is no longer fruitful to attempt to sort out hereditary from environmental influences, and within the behavioral sciences even those seduced by this question often have difficulty agreeing on just what counts as evidence in favor of one side or the other. That Chomsky and Piaget could draw such different conclusions from equally pertinent bodies of data about early cognitive and linguistic milestones and that they occasionally shifted positions on what might count as evidence for their positions indicates to me that the reason this issue was so extensively reworked was that the two spokesmen had strong views on it, rather than that either of them was likely to convince the other or skeptical "others."

Topics more susceptible to solution were also addressed at Royaumont. In particular, three related and recurring issues are worth citing, for they underline pivotal differences between the two protagonists and, unlike the nature/nurture miasma, may well be resolved in the coming years. A first argument centers on the Rousseauan dilemma of the relationships between child and adult thought: whereas Piaget and his followers believed in the utility of stages, with children as they become older attaining qualitatively different (and increasingly more powerful) modes of reasoning, Chomsky and his colleague Jerry Fodor argued strongly that such an account of stages of thought is logically indefensible. In fact, according to Fodor, it is in principle impossible to generate more powerful forms of thought from less powerful ones; essentially, all forms of reasoning that an individual will eventually be capable of are specified at birth and emerge via a maturational process during development.

A second discussion concerned the nature of the mental representations by which we conceive of our experiences, including the objects and persons of the world. In the Piagetian view, the ability to represent knowledge to oneself and to others is a constructive process that presupposes a lengthy series of actions upon the environment. Mental representation awaits the completion of sensorimotor development at age two; its emergence makes possible symbolic play, dreams, mental images, language—in fact the whole gamut of symbolic capacities. Chomsky and his colleagues, on the other hand, expressed doubts about the legitimacy of grouping together a family of representations, and of referring to a symbolic function that is supposed to emerge at a certain point in development. In their view, language as a symbol system should be radically dissociated from other symbolic forms.

The final issue, intimately related to the first two, involved the generality of thought and of thought processes. According to Piaget, thought is an extremely broad set of capacities: identical mental operations underlie one's encounters with a wide range of cognitive materials and topics (space, time, morality, causality), and the roots of later forms of thought (for example, reasoning in language) can be located in earlier forms (such as sensorimotor problem-solving by the one-year-old). From Chomsky's radically different point of view, language is divorced from other (and earlier) forms of thinking. Moreover, each intellectual faculty is *sui generis*—a separate domain of mentation, possibly located in a discrete region of the brain, exhibiting many of its own processes and maturing at its own rate. Indeed, Chomsky repeatedly invoked the striking, if somewhat bizarre, metaphor of the mind as a collection of organs, rather like the liver or the heart. We do not speak of the heart as learning to beat but rather as maturing according to its genetic timetable. So, too, we should conceive of language (and other "organs of the mind" such as those that account for the structure of mathematics or music) as mental entities that are programmed to unfold over time. Just as the physiologist dissects the heart in order to unravel its anatomy and its mechanisms, the linguist must perform analogous surgery on the human faculty of language.

The positions taken by the protagonists on these issues conveyed their general intellectual styles and substance, facets of their intellectual bequest that came across with increasing clarity and finality as the discussions progressed. Although both Piaget and Chomsky paid homage to models provided by biology and logic, they were fundamentally interested in quite different kinds of examples and explanations. Piaget was fascinated by the behaviors children emitted—and, more specifically, the errors they made—when solving the challenging puzzles he posed. He had developed an elaborate technical vocabulary, rooted in biology, to describe these phenomena—a rich description of the stages through which children pass in each of these realms of achievement. He also developed his own logical formalism to describe the affinities underlying structurally related behaviors and the differences that obtain across discrete mental stages. The phenomena he discerned offer a convincing series of snapshots of how development proceeds, but the specific terms he devised and the models he formulated have fared less well in the face of rigorous criticism. At most, Piaget's adventures into technical vocabulary and formal models offer a convenient way of synthesizing the enormous amount of data he accumulated. In the end, it is his overall *vision* of how capacities relate and of how knowledge in its varied forms develops that inspires workers in the field.

Though similar in certain respects, Chomsky's achievement is of a fundamentally different order. Rather than being struck by behavioral phenomena that he feels compelled to describe, Chomsky is driven by a powerful vision of how linguistic science should be pursued and by a belief in the way this analytic approach should be extended across the human sciences. In his view, the student of linguistics should construct models of human linguistic competence and thereby specify the "universals" of language. Stating the rules, steps, and principles with utmost (mathematical) precision becomes a prerequisite for work in this area. And so, even as Chomsky has high regard for models stated in such a way that they can be definitively tested, he dismisses more general and more allusive "positions," "schemas," and "strategies." Those domains of thought that are susceptible to study must be investigated in the way that a linguist studies language: the analyst must propose a formal system of rules that will either generate just the acceptable behaviors in that domain or will be shown in principle to fail (because, for example, they generate too many, too few, or the wrong behaviors), and he must strive to discover just those rules that the human mind actually follows.

Given those different approaches and philosophies of science, it is not surprising that, when the two scholars faced each other, there was serious and continuing disagreement. At the beginning of the discussion, each man paid homage to the other: Piaget noted "all the essential points in this about which I think I agree with Chomsky." And Chomsky acknowledged "Piaget's interesting remarks." As the discussion proceeded and became increasingly heated, the tone became distinctly less friendly. Piaget criticized the nativist position as "weak" and "useless," even as Chomsky described certain Piagetian assertions as "false," "inconceivable," and (in a mathematical sense) "trivial." Not surprisingly, neither of the scholars conceded that he might be wrong, even as each of their "seconds" rallied strongly to their positions. My reading of the interchanges suggests that most of the disinterested natural scientists were more swayed by Chomsky's presentation, but it is difficult to determine whether they were persuaded by Chomsky's rigor or were simply "turned off" by Piaget's old-fashioned, Lamarckian views on biological evolution. The social scientists in attendance at Royaumont seem to have been divided equally between the two camps.

It is too early to say which of these competing perspectives will carry the day in the burgeoning discipline of human cognition. While the issues at Royaumont are being widely discussed, the energies of future scholars have yet to be fully marshaled in either man's behalf. My own guess is that the kind of rigorous formal treatment espoused by the Chomsky circle will be increasingly embraced, but that it will be applied to the kinds of data, and addressed to the sorts of problems, that concerned Piaget and his colleagues. The academic journals of 1990 may well be filled with Chomsky-style grammars representing the child's knowledge at different stages of development. In other words, some kind of illuminating synthesis of the two men's theories may well be possible in the future.

In reading the transcript, I was struck by the grandeur of each perspective. No finer minds in our time have confronted the problem of the nature of thought: each exemplifies the power of his views both in formal presentations and informal exchanges.

At the same time, however, I was disturbed by a paradox. Piaget insisted throughout on the active exploratory nature of human intelligence; yet he offered a description of intellect that applies equivalently to all individuals and takes no account whatsoever of the heights of creative thought—the kind of inventiveness epitomized by his own work. For his part, Chomsky gave ample illustration of the creative genius of human language—the ways in which all of us are able to produce and understand sentences that have never before been uttered. Yet, at the same time, his assertion that we "know it all" in the beginning seems to leave remarkably little room for the flowering of genuinely new ideas—like those of Chomsky himself. As with many theorists, the works—and the lives—of the two men belie their own efforts to produce an overarching account of their field of inquiry.

In fact, to my mind the keynote for the conference at Royaumont was set by the biologist Guy Céllerier. After hearing the two presentations, Céllerier proposed a metaphor that he felt described the growth of intellect: he compared the development of the mind to climbing a hill. Extending that metaphor, we can assume that the broad steps of the journey are preordained but that the steps that one will actually take—the footholds gained, the heights one will ultimately reach, one's perspective at the end of the journey—cannot be anticipated.

Yet in their heroic effort to explain all of human thought, Piaget and Chomsky seem to have underestimated the extent to which such an exploration is open, impossible to predict, reducible neither to one's birthright nor to an inevitable sequence of stages. Perhaps the most apt metaphor for the colloquy on the regal mountain is the Sisyphean task—which each human is destined to repeat in his own turn and his own way—of striving to attain the summits of knowledge.

3

CLAUDE LÉVI-STRAUSS:

TOWARD THE STRUCTURES

OF ART

THE CONTRAST, an irresistible one, has been cleverly caricatured by David Levine. On the one side is the highly educated French savant Claude Lévi-Strauss, knowledgeable about classical philosophical traditions and deeply steeped in anthropological lore about numerous cultures in the world; on the other, a rendering of Rousseau's noble savage, plucked directly from the state of nature—humanity in untrammeled form. The two are sipping from their respective martini glasses while perhaps engaged in deep discussion in an elegant French salon. The caricature suggests Claude Lévi-Strauss's principal contribution to the social-science conversation of our time: his assertion that the human mind, be it in civilized or savage garb, is everywhere the same, reflecting the same principles, operating on the same kinds of content.

Indeed, Lévi-Strauss has devoted the better part of a long and distinguished scholarly career to defending the proposition that all members of our species think in the same way and fashion comparable products. Whether it be myth or science, kinship exchange or input-output models, paleolithic cave art or realistic academic masterpieces, each involves similar degrees of subtlety and comparable forms of complexity. The savage mind is the mind of us all.

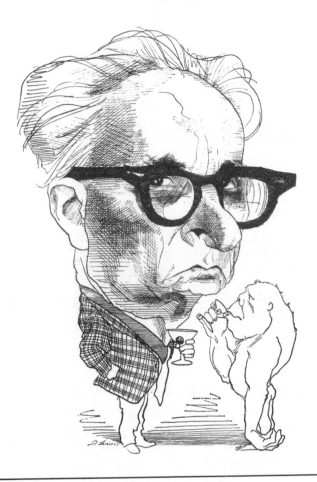

Figure 3.1. Drawing by David Levine. Reprinted with permission from *The New York Review of Books*. Copyright © 1967 N.Y. Rev. Inc.

Though his interest in the exotic dates back to his childhood, Lévi-Strauss was not a prodigy. Unlike Jean Piaget and Noam Chomsky, who arrived at their principal insights during their twenties and were already quite famous before reaching Biblical middle life, Lévi-Strauss did not select his calling (or was not "selected," as he would put it) until he was almost thirty. It was in 1934, when an acquaintance telephoned him and asked him whether he would be interested in accepting the post of Professor of Sociology at São Paulo University in Brazil, that Lévi-Strauss first thought of doing anthropological field

28

work. Thereupon he began the four years of travels among the Indian tribes of central Brazil which constitute his major field work.

Lévi-Strauss was forever changed by these travels. He had started upon his journeys with the usual European inclination to view primitives as wild, different, romantic. He thought he had found Rousseau's pristine state when he reached the long-isolated Nambikwara of the Amazon. But he was gradually disabused of this stereotype. As he spent more time with these folk, he became impressed by their sense of humor, their petty rivalries, the political acumen of their chief; and he came to the realization that the similarities between the Nambikwara and himself made any differences trivial, that, like himself, they were "nothing but human beings." Having searched for infinite variety, for a natural society reduced to its simplest form, whether of blood-thirsty cannibals or noble savages, Lévi-Strauss instead discovered the common humanity of savages and savants and, coincidently, the central themes of his scholarly work.

Until he had gone to the bush, Lévi-Strauss had been a French intellectual of the purest sort. He had attended school with Simone de Beauvoir and Maurice Merleau-Ponty and was just a few years junior to the most famous French intellectual of the era, Jean-Paul Sartre, whom Lévi-Strauss came to dislike and eventually to supplant some decades later as the most prominent (or notorious) French intellectual. Like others in his cohort, Lévi-Strauss was critical of French society, but rather than opposing it from within, he took his stand by embracing peoples who were superficially very different from himself, and by arguing their case and their importance in the Collège de France. This was done most effectively and persuasively in his autobiographical travelogue *Tristes Tropiques*, a classic of the genre and the book that propelled Lévi-Strauss to enormous acclaim in France in the mid-1950s. (Paradoxically, while other intellectuals became increasingly estranged from the political drift in their country, Lévi-Strauss has in later years become a relatively conservative member of the French establishment.)

Lévi-Strauss concedes in *Tristes Tropiques* that, while he was tremendously affected by his experiences in the Brazilian hinterlands, he did not know what scientific sense to make of what he had discovered. Insight on how to organize his many thoughts and findings came to him in the early 1940s when, as a refugee scholar, he found himself at the New School for Social Research in New York City. There he chanced upon the lectures of another *émigré* scholar, the Slavic linguist

Roman Jakobson. In another of the epiphanous experiences to which Lévi-Strauss refers in his autobiography, he saw in the "revelation of structural linguistics" the way to a scientific or "structural" study of anthropology.

Working with colleagues in the "Prague school" of linguistics, Jakobson had devised a method of linguistic analysis which held promise of placing linguistics on a firm scientific footing. Jakobson put forward two key notions. First of all, he claimed that one could discover, underneath the apparently infinite surface variations of different languages, a number of key elements, or building blocks. For example, to make any sound, an individual must choose between having the vocal tract open or closed, the lips together or apart, the nasal passage blocked or free. The choices made on each of these small number of "distinctive features" would determine which sound of which language was enunciated. The structure or organization in language resulted from an identification of these "distinctive features," followed by a study of how they were combined in various ways to constitute the sounds of language.

But how to go from sound to meaning? That is where Jakobson's second notion came in. The basic elements of language acquired significance only in the light of their relationship to one another. Thus the phoneme *p*, as in *pa* or *pin*, is meaningless in itself, but it acquires significance when compared to a contrasting phoneme *b*, as in *bin*. Similarly the word *pa* is just a sound until it acquires meaning, first by being related to an entity in the world, but more importantly, by its relation to other words of the same class that can occupy the same place in a sentence (e.g., *mother, uncle*) and by its susceptibility to combination with other kinds of words (e.g., *wants, cries, likes, is, dies*). Through focusing on the relations among the linguistic elements, and the relations that obtain *among the relations*, Jakobson ultimately provided a way to think about language at all levels, from phonology and syntax through semantics and poetics. It was a scholarly tour de force and it had a profound and lifelong effect upon the still unformed young anthropologist.

Lévi-Strauss declared that anthropologists must follow the lead of their linguistic brethren. They must undertake a structural analysis of cultural phenomena analogous to the structural decoding of linguistic phenomena undertaken by the Prague school. Stated in programmatic terms, this involved the realization that one must study the

unconscious infrastructure (the distinctive features) of cultural phenomena rather than their surface manifestations: one must focus not
on the terms, or the units, of the realm but rather on the relationships
between those units. Only then could their meaning, or significance,
be discovered. Finally, one must regard the entire domain (like language
or kinship) as an organized system governed by general laws. Whether
confronting a kinship pattern, a social organization, a program of classification, or a myth, the anthropologist must look for the units of meaning and discover how they relate to one another within a coherent
and organized system.

That, then, was Lévi-Strauss's program, conceived of in the early
1940s in New York and carried out over the next four decades in a
far-reaching set of studies which cover the range of cultural phenomena
that have occupied anthropologists.

Lévi-Strauss turned his energies first to the most classic areas of anthropological analysis—kinship studies and social structure. Invading
the enclaves that had been most thoroughly studied by representatives
of earlier anthropological schools—functionalists like Malinowski and
structural functionalists like Radcliffe-Brown—Lévi-Strauss put forward
a number of iconoclastic assertions and embraced a novel analytic
approach.

First of all, he introduced rigor through the use of algebraic methods,
mathematical formulas, and other paraphernalia of the more objective
sciences. Substantively, he argued that anthropologists had selected
the wrong units or building blocks for analysis. For example, instead
of focusing on individual kinship terms or the relationship between
members of the nuclear family (as a surface analysis of the kinship
realm might dictate), he proposed a study of the "avunculate," the
set of relationships that obtain among eight relatives, including the
maternal uncle. The elementary structure that he uncovered was a
global system in which the relationship (or attitude) between maternal
uncle and nephew was to that between brother and sister as the relationship between father and son was to that between husband and wife.
By discovering the attitudes held by certain relatives in the avunculate,
it would be possible to infer the remaining ones. And so Lévi-Strauss
claimed that, through a discovery of the "real" underlying structural
units, he could account for a much wider variety of phenomena and
surface manifestations than had proved feasible through the traditional
analyses of terms and relations in the nuclear family.

Again, in the area of social organization, another classic preserve of cultural anthropology, Lévi-Strauss introduced distinctions and methods of the sort devised initially by Jakobsonian linguists. For example, he challenged the views of both anthropologists and natives that a large number of societies consisted of dual organizations—two parallel kinds of clans, often exogamous, existing within the same village. Lévi-Strauss provided evidence that these "dual organizations" were actually a rationalization which reflected neither the actual kinship and social relations nor the terminology of the social system. Instead, certain underlying structural relations having to do with the exchange of women and other commodities transcended both dual and non-dual organizations. These structural relations accounted more parsimoniously and more completely for the social functioning of these groups.

In the early 1950s Lévi-Strauss attended a conference of linguists and anthropologists at which he delivered a paper on "Linguistics and Anthropology." In this paper, which had an electrifying effect on the audience, he pointedly remarked that there was present an "uninvited guest which has been seated during this Conference beside us and which is the *human mind*" (p. 71). Lévi-Strauss felt that, in their focus on the material aspects of culture, anthropologists had been neglecting the most important feature of understanding any culture—namely, the ways in which the human mind takes in, classifies, and interprets information. Lévi-Strauss elected henceforth to devote his anthropological career to a study of the human mind in its raw form. In pursuing this study, he necessarily came to rely upon his own ingenious mind and his ability to read the minds of savages. As if to justify his hubris in pretending to speak for all men and women, he has referred to his own "neolithic intelligence" and in a well-known and oft-quoted passage in *The Raw and the Cooked* (p. 13) declared: "It is in the last resort immaterial whether in this book the thought processes of the South American Indians take shape through the medium of my thought, or whether mine take place through the medium of theirs."

Lévi-Strauss has approached the savage mind from three distinct vantage points. Initially he examined the ways in which individuals from primitive cultures classified the materials of their world. Challenging the accepted wisdom that the primitive mind operates differently from the civilized mind, Lévi-Strauss accrued a mass of beguiling evidence to indicate that the principal feature of all minds is to classify and that primitives classify along much the same lines as do members of more advanced cultures. He described the classifying practices of primitive groups as a "science of the concrete." In a famous analogy, he compared the mind of the savage with the practices of a handyman, or *bricoleur:* in both cases, instead of starting with a preordained theory from which one makes deductions (in the manner of a trained engineer), the individuals work inventively with what is at hand (or in the ready accesses of their minds) in order to solve problems that happen to arise. Individuals devise concepts and comparisons not because they satisfy basic biological urges (not because they are good to "eat with," as a functionalist might argue) but rather because they satisfy cognitive constraints (they are good to "think with").

By no means is there an unlimited number of ways in which the human mind can work. Rather, we human beings are strictly limited in the kinds of combinations we can make, the kinds of distinctive features or oppositions we can play with. As Lévi-Strauss declared in *Tristes Tropiques* (p. 60):

The ensemble of a people's customs has always its particular style: they form into a system. I am convinced that the number of these systems is not unlimited, and that human societies, like individual human beings (at play, in their dreams, or in moments of delirium), never create absolutely; all they can do is to choose certain combinations from a repertoire of ideas which it should be possible to reconstitute.

Shades of Jakobson on the distinctive features of language!

The most extensive search for the rules of human cognition undertaken by Lévi-Strauss is described in his massive study of mythmaking, called *Mythologiques.* In it he analyzed no fewer than 800 American Indian myths drawn from different eras and from diverse cultures dispersed over two continents. All this was in the service of the claim that there is, in fact, one seamless chain of mythological being, a single logic of myth, which can be observed in all of its manifestations by studying a large corpus of myths.

Lévi-Strauss believes that the simple empirical categories that populate myths—percepts of smell, sound, silence, light, darkness, hunger, or thirst—are best conceived of as conceptual tools for approaching the more abstract ideas with which individuals everywhere must grapple: dilemmas like the relationship between nature and culture, the status of the incest taboo, the importance of certain kinship and social arrangements. These ideas may be expressed in terms of logical propositions; and, indeed, if myths are to be properly understood, these logical terms and relationships must be specified. Moreover, the relationships among the myths are seen as quasi-biological in character, analogous to the physical transformations of anatomy and physiology which relate animal species to one another. To use another analogy (and Lévi-Strauss never hesitates to multiply metaphors), mythmaking can be compared with the way in which a composer manipulates themes of a fugue so that they are all variations of the same underlying "subject."

Mythologiques represents Lévi-Strauss's most sustained effort to demonstrate that all human patterns and behaviors are codes. The mind's inherent structuring tendency determines the form taken by key social phenomena, such as differences in status, networks of friend-ships, feelings of hostility, and so on. Such relations are confronted and treated in myths by means of codes relating to such empirical categories as food, landscapes, seasonal changes, climates, celestial bod-ies, shelter, and animal and plant life. The specific terms or objects that appear may differ across myths and cultures, but the underlying laws of discourse and the operating constraints of combination and transformation do not vary. Myths deal with problems of human exist-ence that must be confronted even though (or perhaps because) they seem insoluble. They embody such dilemmas in structured narrative form and thereby make these puzzles intelligible ("good to think").

Lévi-Strauss had another agenda. In addition to making sense of myths in their own terms, he was intent on demonstrating that one could analyze the experiences of the senses in a logical way. Noting that the standard scientific approach has been to ignore qualitative aspects of experience as much as possible and to focus upon measurable quantities, Lévi-Strauss sought to create a logic that will capture and retain the particular qualities of experiences. For the experiencing per-son, and perhaps particularly for primitive individuals, objects are "charged" with affect and with penumbras of connotation: the opera-tion of myths and of mind will be comprehensible only if these qualita-tive aspects are somehow retained in one's analysis. *Mythologiques* may be thought of as a massive experiment to determine whether the sciences can elucidate qualitative and aesthetic phenomena.

During the 1970s Lévi-Strauss devoted his attention to ritual masks gathered from a circumscribed set of Northwest Indian tribes. Charac-teristically, Lévi-Strauss claimed that no individual mask had any deci-pherable meaning in itself, and that the meaning the masks bore as an ensemble could be discerned only by taking into account the masks produced by other groups—groups from the same region which, how-ever, differed from a given tribe in terms of era, geographical location, and/or social situation. Borrowing a tool from structural linguistics,

Lévi-Strauss broke down masks into distinctive features—for example, facial features that were "protruding" or "involuted"—and scored each mask in terms of its value for that feature. He concluded that if the form of the mask remained the same across groups, its semantic function would alter; whereas if the mask changed with respect to certain features, its semantic function would remain the same.

In focusing on masks, Lévi-Strauss came closer than ever before in his professional work to an explicit statement of his attitudes toward the arts. In his view, the individuating features of a work of art or craft arose because of the deep need of each clan or lineage to define itself in relationship to other ones. That is, style *is* a statement by a culture that it differs from other cultures, which in turn have made their own choices in the way in which their masks are constituted: choices which are taken from the same set of options but which reflect the differences as perceived (at least at an unconscious level) by the members of the cultures themselves. Lévi-Strauss ended his discussion of masks by asserting that the entire Western belief in individual creativity is an illusion. However liberating and stimulating this illusion may be to the practicing artist, one cannot follow the path of creation by oneself. One inevitably declares oneself in relationship to all other users of the language of an art form.

On the one hand, Lévi-Strauss is the compleat Cartesian, the prototypical French intellectual. He is a believer in logic, in the rational possibilities of language and thought. He seeks to identify basic elements within a domain, to trace the proper relations among those elements, and to express them in logical formulae. Again faithful to the French tradition, he is ever the systematizer, organizing networks of kinship and of social organization, grouping masks, myths, and even entire classification systems. In these ways Lévi-Strauss can be readily absorbed into the Piaget-Chomsky camp. Indeed, the three men share a belief in the importance of postulating mental representations, a faith that similarities between individuals are far deeper than differences, a conviction that much of the explanation of cognition will ultimately derive from human genetics and biology, a sympathy with formal mathematical or logical representations of behavior, impatience with notions of "learning" and "environmental causes," and an antipathy to various "isms," including behaviorism, empiricism, and functionalism (though not, of course, to structuralism).

Yet while Piaget and Chomsky are centrally and virtually exclusively oriented toward rational and scientific accounts of experience, Lévi-

Strauss is equally involved in and sympathetic to the arts. His own background is richly embedded in artistry. His father was a painter, and he himself paints and has considerable literary gifts as well. He is certainly the only one of our structuralists who can be called a stylist, and his writing is much admired throughout the French literary world. Lévi-Strauss is also fascinated, indeed obsessed, by music and has written far more about music and how it functions than he has about the other art forms. His most riveting aesthetic experiences have come from music, from listening to Wagner, Debussy, Stravinsky. He goes so far as to claim that it is because of his congenital inability to compose a musical work that he has been driven to study myths, which he sees as in many ways exploiting the same principles of human cognition as does music. Perhaps because of this deep-seated belief in the similarities between myth and music, Lévi-Strauss planned the entire *Mythologiques* according to an elaborate musical framework; this is reflected in such whimsical section titles as "Recitative Theme and Variations," "A Short Sonata in Well-Tempered Anatomy," "Rustic Symphony in Three Movements," and "A Fugue of the Five Senses."

In addition to an explicit concern with music and art in his anthropological writings, Lévi-Strauss has also shared with a wider audience some of his opinions about the contemporary art scene. As he perceives it, the arts have traditionally played an important role in cultures. They have allowed groups to define themselves and to assert their relationships to other groups, and they have provided a means whereby individuals within a group can affirm their own solidarity. These fruits can be recognized not only in preliterate societies but also in Greek art before the fifth century and in Italian art before the Sienese period, but art in the modern era has disrupted this traditional mission through its increasing focus on the individual artist and its insistent preoccupation with representational fidelity. Rather than being avowedly symbolic and communal, as most traditional art has been, modern art has become prone to the sins of imitating reality and glorifying single creators.

In Lévi-Strauss's view, contemporary art has reached an impasse. Having shown that they can achieve complete realism, modern artists have now redoubled their sins by producing completely abstract forms in both music and the visual arts: it is very difficult for individuals within the culture to relate in any way to such artworks. Also, instead of having a particular artistic language yoked to the culture, we now have spawned protean creators like Picasso and Stravinsky, who could assume any number of styles at will; but, while they appeared thereby to be citizens of the world, they had in fact cut themselves off from any identifiable group.

Lévi-Strauss does not deny that he finds a certain interest in contemporary musical, artistic, and literary experiments, but basically (or at least ideologically) he has an extreme aversion to them. He regards them as divorced from human experience and particularly from the crucial experiences that individuals in a group should share. Such experiments have thus lost any kind of symbolic importance: they are indistinguishable from pure mental games, on the one hand, or from "found" physical objects on the other. All humans require moorings in order to make sense of things; the contemporary arts undercut our moorings. As Lévi-Strauss once quipped, the abstract artist shows us the kind of painting he would make if, by chance, he were to make any. And contemporary serial music "is like a sailless ship, driven out to sea by its captain, who is privately convinced that by subjecting life aboard to the rules of an elaborate protocol, he will prevent the crew from thinking nostalgically either of their home port or of their ultimate destination" (*The Raw and the Cooked*, p. 25).

Lévi-Strauss has shared his own artistic values with readers. On the one hand, he admires simple groups where the arts exhibit a kind of integrity and wholeness which is lacking in our contemporary scene. He has also indicated his admiration for contemporary Japanese society, where harmony between man and nature seems to have been preserved, where family arrangements for fashioning products have been retained, and where the arts and crafts continue to function organically within the culture in a way in which they have long since ceased to do in the Western context. Lévi-Strauss confirmed his belief in the importance of traditional institutions within a culture by accepting membership in the French Academy, to which he was the first anthropologist ever elected.

But Lévi-Strauss did not participate in the debate at Royaumont (though he sat in during one of these sessions). Perhaps characteristically, he felt that such public confrontations were more likely to degenerate into dramatic showpieces than to yield useful insights. Nevertheless, we can indicate certain areas in which we might expect agreement or disagreement between Lévi-Strauss and the two structuralists who did attend. In my view, Lévi-Strauss and Piaget would have argued most vociferously about the issue of developmental stages, with Lévi-Strauss claiming that the child's mind operates in ways fundamentally similar to those of an adult, and Piaget stressing the qualitative differences in thought between individuals at different developmental levels. There would also have been conflict on the role of language in relation to thought. Lévi-Strauss sees language as the pre-eminent verbal system and as a model for all forms of thinking, whereas Piaget derives thought from action and attributes to language a secondary, if not a peripheral, role.

As to the hypothetical conversation between Lévi-Strauss and Chomsky, Lévi-Strauss would have no difficulty with Chomsky's belief in highly structured innate knowledge or with his skepticism concerning qualitatively discrete developmental stages in the course of childhood. Their views would diverge, however, on the relationship between language and other cognitive systems. Lévi-Strauss considers language as a model for all manner of sign systems, ranging from kin relations to ritual masks. Chomsky, on the other hand, is extremely skeptical of such semiotic analyses: he would acknowledge only "trivial parallels" between language and other sign systems.

But whatever differences might have emerged among these pioneers of structuralism, they shared one thing of import: an intensive interest in the operational principles of the mind, which makes them very special, if not unique, in the social sciences of our time. I see Piaget as preoccupied with one type of mind, that of the scientist; Lévi-Strauss as occupied with an opposing kind, the mind of the artist in the broadest sense, to include not only the painter, the poet, the musician, but also the mythmaker—the individual exploiting his sensory qualities and experiences in an effort to understand the central puzzles of his society. In this vein, Piaget and Lévi-Strauss serve as complements to one another, focusing on the two most important and pervasive aspects of human cognition. Chomsky's focus on language reveals yet a third perspective; however, he seems more open than Piaget or Lévi-Strauss to the possibility that the human mind consists of different faculties, which can be harnessed to divergent ends.

Every program of research has its limitations, and that includes structuralism as practiced by these three seminal thinkers. Most debilitating in my view is the limited potential of their respective systems to handle creative thought—innovations of the sort associated with major artists, scientists, political leaders, or inventors. To be sure, each of our structuralists has touched on this issue: Chomsky by calling attention to the creativity entailed in ordinary language; Piaget by searching for the roots of invention in elementary psychological and biological processes; Lévi-Strauss by challenging the whole concept of original invention. Nonetheless, there is something about their closed systems of exploration—their faith in the limited number of routes the mind can in fact follow—which makes it difficult to envision how one could ever account in a structuralist social science for the innovative work of an Einstein, a Shakespeare, or a Freud—or, for that matter, for the fecund imaginations of the three structuralists themselves.

Even if Lévi-Strauss is right in principle—that there is only a limited number of cultural forms—it may be that the amount of invention and creation that human beings can generate is, as a practical matter, unlimited. For some reason the research programs of the major structuralists, which grew out of the battles they were fighting with their predecessors, have not permitted them to recognize and embrace the open-endedness of human creation. Despite his protestations to the contrary, Lévi-Strauss has probably come the closest, for he acknowledges the importance of symbolic activity in human experience and he reveals a special attraction to issues of artistic invention. He falls short because he fails to appreciate the "generative" or "creative" aspects immanent in the use of various symbol systems.

To my mind, there is a crucial leap that a structuralist study of the mind must take. The leap involves a recognition that the basic unit of human thought is the symbol, and that the basic entities with which humans operate in a meaningful context are symbol systems. Attention to symbol systems is possible (indeed natural) within a structuralist framework, but such a focus opens up the possibility of the endless devising of meaningful worlds—in the arts, in the sciences, indeed in every realm of human activity. Insights into such worlds have been given most eloquent form by a series of philosophers to whose work I pay homage in the next set of essays—my mentors Ernst Cassirer, Susanne Langer, and Nelson Goodman. The key to an understanding of artistic creation lies, I believe, in a judicious wedding of structuralist approaches to philosophical and psychological investigations of human symbolic activity.

4

ERNST CASSIRER

AND THE SYMBOLIC APPROACH

TO COGNITION

ONE DAY in 1917 as he was mounting a streetcar to ride home, the German philosopher Ernst Cassirer had a grand vision: a comprehensive philosophical treatise on symbolic forms. By the time he had arrived home a few minutes later, the plan for a new multivolume work had already crystallized in his own mind, in approximately the form that it would assume a decade later.

Three years later Cassirer paid a casual visit to the Warburg Library in Hamburg. There he encountered an unsurpassed collection of materials drawn from art, philosophy, astrology, magic, folklore, myth, and literature, which chronicled the thought processes of individuals drawn from diverse cultures. In a "creative flash" reminiscent of his earlier revelation on the streetcar ride, Cassirer realized that this composite of materials could provide indispensable raw materials for his work on the philosophy of symbolic forms. As he commented at the time, "This library is dangerous. I shall either have to avoid it altogether, or imprison myself here for years. The philosophical problems involved are close to my own, but the concrete historical material which Warburg has collected is overwhelming" (Schilpp, p. 48).

Ernst Cassirer

Cassirer's original inspiration in 1917 and his later visit to the Warburg Library are moments of first importance in the history of modern philosophy. As a result of these experiences, Cassirer composed in the 1920s three epoch-making volumes, translated some years later as *The Philosophy of Symbolic Forms*. These works helped to bring about a major reorientation in philosophical work both in the United States and abroad. And inspiration from this work has spread in more recent years throughout the social sciences, including that investigation of artistic symbols which is our special concern here.

Few signs in Cassirer's early personal and scholarly life foreshadowed a magnum opus of this sort. Born in 1874 in Breslau to a wealthy Jewish family, Cassirer was a happy-go-lucky child beloved by all, but only an average performer in school. At his family's insistence he studied law but soon discovered that it did not satisfy a growing ardor to understand fundamental epistemological problems.

Like many another young student with a passing interest in philosophy, Cassirer was converted to serious scholarship by the experience of reading the works of Immanuel Kant, then the major figure in German philosophical circles. The budding scholar encountered in the works of Kant an inspiring concern with basic categories of knowledge—space, time, number, causality; a persuasive affirmation that our daily experience results from the organization that the active mind *imposes* upon reality; and the related realization that knowledge must be based upon objects and sensory data, but that these can never be known directly.

As an assiduous scholar, blessed with the gift of near total recall, Cassirer read widely in philosophy, ultimately presenting a thesis on Leibniz. His early heroes in philosophy were those figures concerned with logical-rational and mathematical thought, such as Leibniz, Kant, and Descartes. Moreover, his scholarship did not cease at the philosophical boundary of the humanities. In fact, one of Cassirer's early books was an exposition of Einstein's theory of relativity, written but a few years after that breakthrough had been initially propounded. Immersion in Einstein's work convinced Cassirer that changes in scientific understanding could bring about major revisions in our notions of such fundamental categories of thought as space and time.

While his interest in science and rationality was clearly dominant at this time, a close look at Cassirer's early life does yield scattered clues anticipating his later preoccupation with symbolic forms. Cassirer had a tremendous love for music from his earliest days. Once he became oriented toward scholarly work in his teenage years, the young Cassirer read widely not only in philosophy and science but also in literature and the arts. He loved poetry and drama and, because of his remarkable memory, could recite long sections from the German classics.

In retrospect, one can also discern hints of his later orientation in certain facets of his early scholarly career. Cassirer was very sensitive to contemporary strains in European intellectual life, such as the then recently invented distinction between the natural sciences and the sciences of the mind (or spirit). His immersion in problems of knowledge convinced him that one would have to include a wide range of forms of knowing—not only those valued in the sciences—in any comprehensive treatment of the subject. He also acquired a lifelong skepticism about substantive definitions (the essence of man is . . .) as opposed to functional descriptions (what human beings do is to . . .). In light of such insights, Cassirer was placed in an excellent, perhaps unique, position to attend to the wide range of human symbolic activities, including the forms of knowledge important in the arts. One has the impression that, like Sigmund Freud, Cassirer first voluntarily suppressed this "tender-hearted" interest in order to deal with the seemingly "more serious" concerns of logic, rationality, and science. Fortunately, however, as in the case of his Viennese counterpart, this decision in favor of "tough-minded" study was not irrevocable.

Thus in the course of his early training Cassirer was influenced profoundly by the Kantian revolution but was also prepared to question certain aspects of classical German dogma. Kant had assumed that categories of pure understanding were simply given to human beings as part of their birthright. He had taken it for granted that such concepts as the relationship between part and whole, the nature of identity, and the awareness of contradictions between A and not A, would be clear to every human being from the first. According to this dogma, man should inherently be capable of rational scientific thought. For his part, however, Cassirer became convinced that these rational constructions arose only late in the course of human history and always commingled with other less rationally oriented forms of thought. An examination of the human mind must take into account a much wider range of forms of thinking.

And what of the vision that first came to Cassirer on that fateful streetcar ride in 1917 and which later formed the core of the three volumes on the philosophy of symbolic forms? It involved the daring assertion that philosophical thought could describe and illuminate the most diverse products of human cognition. As Cassirer was later to express it in *An Essay on Man* (p. 71):

In the boundless multiplicity and variety of mythical images, of religious dogmas, of linguistic forms, of works of art, philosophical thought reveals the unity of the general function by which all these creations are held together. Myth, religion, art, language, even science, are now looked upon as so many variations on a common theme—and it is the task of philosophy to make this theme audible and understandable.

Thus, in Cassirer's view, our construction of reality was based upon the availability of a vast collection of mental conceptions or symbolic forms. The efforts of human beings to capture their experiences, and to express them in forms which can effectively communicate, depended upon an amalgam of these symbolic conceptions or forms.

This embracing of symbols ran counter to many philosophical ideas prevalent during the early part of the century. To begin with, the notion that myth, imagination, and other forms of "imprecision" or "ignorance" ought to be treated with the same seriousness as mathematics or science was abhorrent to many philosophers reared in the Descartes-Leibniz-Kant tradition. But Cassirer's thought appeared even more revolutionary to those committed to empiricism. Rather than presupposing a reality independent of symbolic forms, Cassirer claimed that our reality was *created* by symbolic forms, that language in fact *constitutes* rather than reflects reality. Contrary to a Lockean and Humean view, perception and meaning are not causally determined by or obtained from the objects in the external world; rather, meanings arise from within and are brought to bear upon the flux of objects and experiences.

Cassirer's conception challenged the establishment's philosophical view in yet another respect. Rather than there being a basic set of categories such as space, time, and number, which were apprehended by all human beings in the same way, one now encountered a far more complex state of affairs. Within each symbolic form there would be particular embodiments of space, time, and number, as well as particular forms of expression of these conceptions. In place of the absoluteness of space, time, and number, Cassirer substituted a far more pluralistic and relativistic picture reflecting different types and levels of symbolization.

And so, for Cassirer, symbols were not simply tools or mechanisms of thought. They *were* the functioning of thought itself, vital creative forms of activity, our sole ways of "making" reality and synthesizing the world. It proves impossible to think of symbolizing activity apart from human imagination and creativity: man lives in a symbolic universe. And in the process of symbolic activity, human beings inevitably engage in meaning-making, in imaginative problem-solving, and in equally creative problem production.

From such a philosophical-anthropological perspective, which takes human consciousness as a point of departure, man might well be thought of as *animal symbolicum.* Cassirer described the peculiar world of this symbolic animal:

Physical reality seems to recede in proportion as man's symbolic activity advances. Instead of dealing with the things themselves, man is, in a sense, constantly conversing with himself. He has so enveloped himself in linguistic forms, in artistic images, and mythical symbols or religious rights, that he cannot see or know anything except by the interposition of this artificial medium. He lives in the midst of imaginary emotions, in hopes and fears, in illusions and disillusions, in his fantasies and dreams. (*An Essay on Man,* p. 25)

The human mind, fortified with symbols, comes to re-create the physical world in its own symbolic image.

One can identify a revealing evolution in Cassirer's thinking over the decades. At the beginning of his scholarly career, he unquestionably endorsed the prevailing wisdom that scientific thought was the highest form of human cognition. True, one of his pivotal insights, already apparent in his earliest writings but crystallized in *The Philosophy of Symbolic Forms,* was that scientific thought must be considered in relationship to the other forms of thought, such as language and myth. Nonetheless, throughout *The Philosophy of Symbolic Forms* there remains the conviction that scientific thought is inherently superior to the other forms of symbolic expression.

That bias on behalf of science was evident in several respects. To begin with, Cassirer stressed that the requirements of science necessitate the introduction of symbols that in precision and fruitfulness surpass those of ordinary language. He also indicated that only in scientific work do individuals become aware of the symbols and notations they use. He discoursed at great length on the misconceptions of various "simpler" populations—such as brain-damaged individuals, children, and individuals who subscribe to myth; even though he exhibited much sympathy with these populations and sought to take seriously their own particular world views, he still displayed the scholar's relative disdain for "fuzzier" forms of thinking. He recognized these world views as qualitatively distinct ways of seeing, feeling, and conceiving.

In his last years, having wryly observed that "a big book is a big evil," Cassirer penned a far shorter work, *An Essay on Man* (1944), which summarized and reformulated the most important themes introduced in *The Philosophy of Symbolic Forms*. In this book Cassirer had clearly moved beyond a hierarchical notion of forms of thinking. He conceded that there were limitations in the sciences: the move toward mathematical and scientific thinking entailed an impoverishment of reality, with objects being reduced to mere formulae. In place of rank ordering Cassirer now embraced the view of a set of ways of knowing, each having its own strength: "All these functions complete and complement one another. Each one opens a new horizon and shows us a new aspect of humanity" (p. 228).

Indeed, if Cassirer secured one special niche within his circle of forms of knowing, it was now given to the arts. He recognized that art provided a richer, more vivid and colorful image of reality and offered as well more profound insight into its formal structure. He placed the highest value on spontaneous original work in which man fully explored his own universe. As he put it, "This form of originality is the prerogative and distinction of art: it cannot be extended to other fields of human activity" (p. 227). And he revealed the special power of artistic production by closing his *Essay* with a telling quotation from Immanuel Kant's *Critique of Judgment* (pp. 188–190):

Thus we can readily learn all that Newton has set forth in his immortal work in the *Principle of Natural Philosophy,* however great a head was required to discover it; but we cannot learn to write spirited poetry, however express may be the precepts of art and however excellent its model.

The philosophy of symbolic forms was no longer rank-ordered: it was now a conversation among equal symbolic forms.

The way first forged by Cassirer was soon followed by other imaginative scholars. The philosopher who did the most to bring Cassirer's work to the attention of a wider public, particularly in this country, was his colleague and translator Susanne Langer, most especially in her *Philosophy in a New Key* (1942). In that inspired treatise Langer sketched out the new directions in philosophical thinking which had been inspired by Cassirer's pioneering work and at the same time provided a foretaste of her own views on the philosophical basis of artistic thinking. She declared "a revolution in philosophy—the tendency of great minds to see philosophical implications in facts and problems belonging to other fields of learning—mathematics, anthropology, psychology, physics, history, and the arts" (Schilpp, p. 382). In Langer's view, Cassirer was instrumental in launching this revolution; in my view, Langer deserves major credit for helping to sustain it and give it direction. I have reflected on the tremendous impact that Langer's book had on my own thinking in my appreciation of *Philosophy in a New Key*, which comprises the next essay.

Langer developed Cassirer's intuitions on the differences between scientific and artistic thinking in her pregnant distinction between discursive and presentational symbols. The contemporary American philosopher Nelson Goodman has continued this effort at characterizing artistic symbolization and has introduced a much fuller and more precise delineation of various kinds of symbols in his *Languages of Art* (1968) and *Ways of Worldmaking* (1978). Goodman carried the Cassirer-Langer program forward by relating symbolic function to characteristics of particular notational systems. At the same time, he provided a rich set of concepts with which one is able to analyze the ways in which works of art function.

Goodman has himself sought to relate his work to the relevant scholarly traditions, and it is germane to quote his assessment as expressed in the preface to *Ways of Worldmaking* (p. *x*):

I think of this book as belonging to that mainstream of philosophy that began when Kant exchanged the structure of the world for the structure of the mind, continued when C. I. Lewis exchanged the structure of the mind for the structure of concepts, and now proceeds to exchange the structure of concepts for the structure of the several symbol systems of the sciences, philosophy, the arts, perception, and every-day discourse. The movement is from unique truth and the word fixed and found towards a diversity of right and even conflicting versions or worlds in the making.

I delineate further lines of Goodman's own thinking and suggest some ways in which these notions have guided my own program of research in the sixth essay of this collection.

In founding Project Zero at Harvard some fifteen years ago, Goodman embodied his belief (perhaps reflecting the *Zeitgeist*) that philosophical and psychological perspectives on the arts ought to be brought together in a coordinated program of research. Nearly all the studies described in subsequent sections of this book represent an effort to carry out this research program. As I see it, my colleagues and I have taken as our point of departure the philosophical distinctions introduced in the Cassirer-Langer-Goodman traditions. Then, guided by the cognitive agenda of the structuralists and employing the clinical methods fashioned by Piaget, we have sought to understand the nature, development, and breakdown of artistic processes in various human populations. Put differently, this work can be thought of as a coming together of three previously disparate strands: the principles embraced by a structuralist approach to the mind; the agenda of a philosophical school that is especially oriented to symbolic thoughts in the arts; and a set of experimental procedures that have proved appropriate for work with normal children and with brain-damaged adults.

I have already noted the individuals who have most directly influenced my own thinking in this effort. I have also profited immensely from reading works by those individuals of a philosophical bent who have focused in their writings on specific art forms and who have so posed issues that they prove susceptible to psychological analysis and experimentation. In the area of music, I am indebted to Leonard Meyer, who opened up psychological explorations of music in his book *Emotion and Meaning in Music,* and to Jeanne Bamberger, who has initiated path-breaking studies of children's representations of musical knowledge. In the literary arts I single out for attention the writings of I. A. Richards, Stanley Fish, and Norman Holland, each of whom in separate ways has made possible a psychologically informed approach to the analysis of literary experience. Finally, in the area of the visual arts, the writings of Rudolf Arnheim and Ernst Gombrich have assumed special importance for the works of my colleagues and me. I welcome the opportunity to indicate my indebtedness to both of these scholars: to Arnheim in essay 19, and to Gombrich in essay 7, the last in this section.

5

PHILOSOPHY IN A NEW KEY REVISITED: AN APPRECIATION OF SUSANNE LANGER

MUCH of what we learn, even within academic disciplines, is picked up as general wisdom, as ideas that are "in the air"; such knowledge can be absorbed simply as a part of breathing in an intellectual atmosphere. Certain ideas and concepts are acquired in more specific situations, in textbooks, discussion groups, or formal courses, only to have their sources forgotten once the "point" has been absorbed. Just a small part of our knowledge retains traces from the moment of original encounter—we remember certain "crystallizing" experiences, for instance, an occasional lecture, a powerful poem, painting, or piece of music, a passage from the Bible or the *Iliad*, and, infrequently, some pages from a path-breaking work of scholarship, perhaps Sigmund Freud's *On the Psychopathology of Everyday Life.*

In the early 1960s, I, like many other students of that time, encountered a book that had just such an enduring influence on me. The book itself was physically unimposing: a thin Mentor paperback, its cover bordered with bands of gold and decorated with an odd montage consisting of a lyre, a dragon, and a Socratic figure. But the book's content was riveting, its messages memorable. As I turned its pages with mounting excitement, I felt myself confronting a set of issues that I had but dimly sensed before, posed in a way that made sense to me. The work, *Philosophy in a New Key,* by philosopher Susanne Langer, led me to other books, including those by Langer's mentor, Ernst Cassirer, and to other courses, including one given by Nelson Goodman, and eventually helped determine my major scholarly interest—the study of human symbolic activity.

I think Langer's slender volume had an equally potent influence on dozens, perhaps hundreds, of other students. And yet the author is not widely cited; she is ignored or disparaged by a significant number of philosophers, and, despite an imposing shelf of books, she never gained a permanent position at a major university. These thoughts pervaded my consciousness as I returned to the book, several years after the initial encounter, to discover whether separation had diluted or reinforced the power it once held over me, and in the process to ponder the justice of the fate met by its author.

Writing in 1941, Susanne Langer surveyed the entire philosophical tradition, from the days of the pre-Socratic philosophers to the rise of science in the nineteenth century. As she saw it, a whole set of issues—the central philosophical agenda of days past—had been invalidated by the emphasis on science. The nature of truth, of value, of beauty, had been ruled "out of court," the bifurcation of mind and body was no longer taken seriously; with positivism at the helm, there was tolerance only for hard, material facts and no niche for ideas, emotions, values. Amid this impatience with anything immaterial, Langer spotted a paradox. The very empiricists who scorned all matters of mind held in special regard a group of individuals (mathematicians) who worked with the most abstract, least tangible of all elements—numerical symbols.

Mathematicians were "special" because they made no claim to be illuminating the issues of real life or the structure of the physical world. They dealt exclusively with another level of discourse—that of symbolic meaning. It was this symbolic domain that began, at the end of the nineteenth century, to take hold of the philosophical community. In fact, a dominant trend in philosophy at the time Langer was writing entailed an obsession with symbols, one as pervasive as earlier philosophers' preoccupation with the senses of man and the raw matter of the physical world.

The new agenda, the recently cut key of philosophy, consisted of a concern with all manner of symbols—words, numbers, and other abstract forms—and with the various meanings that underlie our dreams, fill our imaginations, and draw us to treasure works of civilization, ranging from the Parthenon to the string quartets of Beethoven. As Langer put it in *Philosophy in a New Key*, in an effort to contrast her vision of meaning with that of earlier times:

> But between the facts run the threads of unrecorded reality, momentarily recognized, wherever they come to the surface . . . the bright, twisted threads of symbolic envisagement, imagination, thought—memory and reconstructed memory, belief beyond experience, dream, make-believe, hypothesis, philosophy—the whole creative process of ideation, metaphor, and abstraction that makes human life an adventure in understanding. (pp. 236–237)

Now these ideas, this new key, were already in the air at the time Langer wrote. Few of the ideas she put forth in her work were wholly new. Indeed, Langer takes great care to cite and pay tribute to a raft of predecessors: semiotician Charles Peirce; neurologist Kurt Goldstein; the students of language, I. A. Richards and Wilbur Urban; philosophers Rudolf Carnap and Ludwig Wittgenstein; her own professor, the great logician and metaphysician, Alfred North Whitehead; and, above all, the man who had some dozen years before completed a three-volume study of symbolic forms, the redoubtable epistemologist Ernst Cassirer.

In fact, a trove of articles and books had been a prelude to this new key, but it would be a gross injustice to relegate Langer's work to the level of "mere" popularization. It was popularization, but it was much more. In the tradition of the finest educational syntheses, Langer drew illuminating connections among works whose relationships had not yet been seen, avoided the perils of arid formulas and moist metaphysics, and placed the entire movement in a historical and philosophical perspective that had not yet been articulated. Moreover—and here lies her claim to originality—Langer articulated concepts that clarified issues in a still uncharted philosophical region and raised questions that are still being pondered.

The basic argument of *Philosophy in a New Key* is disarmingly simple, and given the hindsight of today, it seems much less arresting than it was on publication or even at the time I first encountered it. Langer posited a basic and pervasive human need to symbolize, to invent meanings, and to invest meanings in one's world. It was a property of the human mind to search for and to find significances everywhere, to transform experience constantly to uncover new meanings.

But the symbols wrought by the human mind were not all of the same sort and Langer found it necessary to distinguish two kinds.

Consider, as an example, the proposition "George Washington chopped down a cherry tree." Its meaning can be conveyed in two contrasting ways. The first, called *discursive symbolism,* involves the expression of this idea in words or other kinds of "languages." One notes the meaning of each term, combines them according to accepted rules of syntax, and arrives at a commonly shared meaning. Most familiar ideas and notions could be expressed in such coin.

Opposed to discursive symbolism is another, less understood variety, which Langer labeled *presentational symbolism.* Here, an equivalent idea could be gleaned from a picture. Such pictorial symbols do not yield meaning through a sum of their parts, for there *are* no reliably discriminable parts. They present themselves and must be apprehended as a whole; moreover, they operate primarily through shades of meaning, nuances, connotations, and feelings (the appearance of the lad, the force of the blow, the ambience that day), rather than through a discrete, translatable message. Any consideration of the meanings with which our lives are wrapped must take into account at least these two kinds of symbol, the meanings they bear, how they work, their special geniuses.

For most readers the distinction between these two forms of symbol was the key concept of philosophy's new key. In introducing this contrast, Langer identified an important set of similarities (both express meanings) and differences (they operate in fundamentally contrasting ways) between words or mathematics on one hand, and pictures, sculpture, and dance on the other. She broached the possibility of analyzing feelings, emotions, and other intangible elements of human experience through the relatively public arena of symbol analysis. Clearly, she had helped to solidify an appealing intuition, and by categorizing and analyzing it, offered others the chance to dissect it.

This aspect of Langer's work has undergone considerable criticism at the hands of her colleagues in philosophy. Because she offered no strict definition, it is difficult to identify examples of the two forms of symbolism with reliability or to be certain that there are only two such forms. And, even more damagingly, Langer's own examples were wanting. Language itself can operate in a discursive or presentational way (compare a textbook with a poem), even as pictures may wear a different symbolic garb (compare a portrait with a map or diagram). Critics with a more finicky, less intuitive approach than Langer's have had a field day challenging this distinction. Even those with a much more sympathetic eye have gone on to adopt more carefully worked out distinctions among symbol systems, such as those introduced by the philosopher Nelson Goodman.

Langer's purpose, however, was less to glorify this distinction than to see where she could apply it. So she sought to identify the origins of the various symbols that pervade the life of our culture. In separate far-ranging chapters she examined the evolutionary beginnings of symbolic activity in the thought patterns of animals and young children; the cultural beginnings of symbolism in the realms of myth and ritual; and the heights achieved by presentational symbolism in such art forms as music. These chapters are at best uneven. Many analysts have despaired of accounting for the origin of myth or rituals because the possibility of verification is so slim. Investigation of the symbol systems used by children and animals, barely broached in 1940, is now sufficiently advanced to render her empirical statements dubious. An air of the treatises of the late nineteenth century, when authors felt compelled (and entitled) to comment on every aspect of the rise of civilization, is not entirely absent from Langer's synoptic work.

But amid these somewhat disappointing chapters stands one that has exerted a tremendous influence on many individuals: Langer's account of the significance of music. Langer rightly sensed that music was a symbolic system but that it did not directly communicate either reference (for example, the sound of waves) or feelings (for example, the composer's own sense of happiness or anger). She proposed that what music presented was the "forms of feelings"—the tensions, ambiguities, contrasts, and conflicts that permeate our feeling life but do not lend themselves to description in words or logical formulas. The composer presents in spaced tones his knowledge of the whole of human feeling life, and such nonarticulate symbols constitute the appeal and mystery of music. In a passage that conveys the seductive appeal as well as the maddening ambiguity of her prose, the philosopher suggests:

The real power of music lies in the fact that it can be "true" to the life of feeling in a way that language cannot; for its significant forms have that *ambivalence* of content which words cannot have. . . . Music is revealing, where words are obscuring, because it can have not only a content, but a transient play of contents. It can articulate feelings without becoming wedded to them. . . . The assignment of meanings is a shifting, kaleidoscopic play, probably below the threshold of consciousness, certainly outside the pale of discursive thinking. The imagination that responds to music is personal and associative and logical, tinged with affect, tinged with bodily rhythm, tinged with dream, but *concerned* with a wealth of formulations for its wealth of wordless knowledge, its whole knowledge of emotional and organic experience, of vital impulse, balance, conflict, the *ways* of living and dying and feeling. Because no assignment of meaning is conventional, none is permanent beyond the sound that passes; yet the brief association was a flash of understanding. The lasting effect is, like the first effect of speech on the development of the mind, to *make things conceivable* rather than to store up propositions. (pp. 206–207)

Taking music as the prototype of the arts, Langer suggested that this knowledge of feeling life constitutes the perennial attraction of artistic symbols; herein lie the reasons we treasure those statements and works that to the logical empiricist have no meaning at all.

Langer's concluding pages assessed trends in the world at the time of her writing. At the start of the most awful war in human history, it is scarcely surprising that Langer painted a gloomy portrait of "the fabric of meaning" in her society. She saw a world in which language was lauded above everything; where the inner life was disparaged, ignored, even destroyed. Drawing on her own analysis, she emphasized the importance, the necessity of an existence in which various levels of meanings and ranges of significance were tolerated. In place of "a philosophy that knows only deductive or inductive logic as reason, and classes all other human functions as 'emotive,' irrational or animal-ian," she proposed "a theory of mind whose keynote is the symbolic function . . . the continual pursuit of meanings—wider, clearer, more negotiable, more articulate meanings . . . the new world that humanity is dreaming of" (p. 246). Were I her editor, I might have been inclined to tone down these passages, but as a reader, particularly one thinking back to his college days, I resonate to these sentiments.

In large part Susanne Langer's work has accomplished its mission. Her ideas about symbolism, about meaning in art as well as in science, about the nature of different symbolic forms, are common coin; one need no longer read the little Mentor paperback (now reissued at several times the original price by Harvard University Press) to find out about them. Thus the book, reconsidered, has a historical importance—as one of that small set of pedagogical classics that has affected a multitude of students.

And yet the work retains a timeliness. Langer's graceful enthusiasm is engaging; the historical context in which the "revolution" is set helps place in perspective contemporary movements in the social sciences and the humanities; various distinctions introduced and various analyses offered constitute a genuine contribution to current discussions about human knowing. Because Langer intelligibly linked the old and new traditions in philosophy, because she legitimated a scholarly interest in symbolism and the arts, and because she foreshadowed research in psychology and philosophy that continues today, her work still carries a message.

And what of Susanne Langer herself? In succeeding years she went on to write an impressive set of books, volumes that plumbed with increasing depth the pivotal themes introduced in *Philosophy in a New Key*. This effort culminated in *Mind: An Essay on Human Feeling*, without doubt the most comprehensive attempt yet undertaken to establish a philosophical and *scientific* underpinning for aesthetic experience. Langer has gone her own way in these works; no longer in any sense popularizing, she has carefully studied relevant humanistic and scientific texts and has not hesitated to tackle the grand topics—mind, feeling, art—that frighten so many of her colleagues in philosophy. It is not surprising that she is more popular at small liberal arts colleges than at technologically oriented universities; more appreciated by old-fashioned humanists than by newfangled scientists. And it is not difficult to understand why, anticipated by earlier philosophers and succeeded by more disciplined minds, Susanne Langer has never broken into the charmed circle of mainstream philosophers. Yet this gifted philosopher, now nearing ninety, remains an inquiring mind in the best sense of the word—a scholar blessed with a powerful intuition, who knows no disciplinary bounds, who follows a problem wherever it will take her, and who has the gift of articulating the concerns of a generation of scholars and many generations of students. That she cannot be catalogued may explain why she has escaped certain honors— even as it suggests why she may transcend her time.

6

NELSON GOODMAN:

THE SYMBOLS OF ART

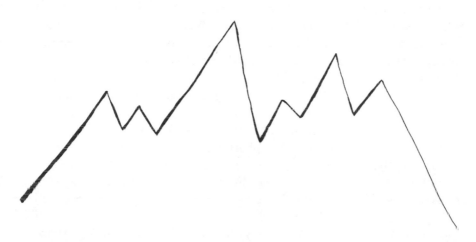

WE BEGIN with a squiggle, a simple zigzag line on a piece of paper. But is this line more than a squiggle? Is it a symbol? An artistic symbol? And if it attains the status of an artistic symbol, what is its worth?

According to the philosopher Nelson Goodman, the status of this squiggle depends entirely on how one chooses to construe it. If the squiggle stands for something—say a month-long record of the Dow Jones stock average—then it is functioning as a symbol. If it is part of a painting—say, the outline of a mountain range in a drawing by Hokusai—then it is functioning as an artistic symbol. The way in which one "reads" the squiggle depends upon the setting in which it is encountered, the graphic context which surrounds it, and the particular "mind set" of the viewer. And the determination of whether the symbol—be it taken from the artist's atelier or from the marketplace—is an effective one turns out to be the most challenging question of all.

Tackling difficult questions is nothing new for Nelson Goodman. The distinguished American scholar has for the last fifty years worked on some of the most intractable questions in the areas of logic, philosophy of science, and epistemology. Trained in the logical-analytic procedures of contemporary Anglo-American philosophy, he has bravely invaded far more subtle and elusive areas, such as psychology and the arts, and has brought his penetrating insights to the vexed issues there.

Goodman has the arts in his blood. Already a student of the fine arts during his undergraduate years at Harvard, Goodman ran an art gallery for fifteen years in the Boston area; he is married to the well-known painter Katherine Sturgis; and he has in recent years conceived and produced a number of multimedia productions. He also founded Project Zero, the group at Harvard that has conducted basic research in the arts and education since the mid-sixties. And in his book *Languages of Art*, Goodman almost singlehandedly converted the dreary field of the philosophy of art (or aesthetics) into a major and vigorous area of study.

Until the time of Goodman's writing, it is scarcely an exaggeration to say that the philosophy of art was mired in insoluble questions about value, beauty, and emotions. It is not that these issues are unimportant, but rather that philosophers were so overwhelmed by them that they had difficulty in making analytic progress: they fell into the trap of trying to clarify one obscure term (art) by other equally vexed ones (such as beauty, aesthetic, emotion). Goodman believed that it was more profitable to begin to analyze the arts in terms of elements that were relatively accessible and analyzable: that is, in terms of the artistic symbols that individuals create and perceive. His philosophy of art builds upon a recognition of types of symbols and how they function.

Goodman has acknowledged his considerable indebtedness to the Cassirer tradition. Cassirer's beliefs in the multiplicity of worlds, the creative power of understanding, the formative functions of symbols, are integral to Goodman's own thinking. But whereas Cassirer's account could be described as "countless worlds made from nothing, by use of symbols," Goodman declared in *Ways of Worldmaking:* "My approach is rather through an analytic study of types and functions of symbols and symbol systems" (pp. 1 and 5).

The analysis begins with the recognition that there are different kinds of symbols and symbol systems. Goodman then introduces his concept of a notational system—a symbol system that satisfies various syntactic and semantic criteria. Notationality is an ideal, and nearly all symbol systems in actual use violate at least one of the precise criteria of notationality. Still, it is possible to classify symbol systems according to the degree to which they approximate or deviate from notationality.

Such a classification reveals, for example, that Western musical notation basically fulfills the semantic and syntactic requirements of a notational system. Consistent with the rigorous demands of a notational system, it proves possible to go from the notation to the performed work and back again to the notation. Ordinary language fulfills the syntactic requirements in that one can recognize each of the constituent elements (words) and how they can be combined (syntax); but language does not fulfill the semantic requirements of notationality because the meaning universe of language is chock-full of ambiguity, redundancy, and other necessarily blurring features. Finally, such art forms as painting and sculpture violate all criteria of notationality. One cannot ascertain what the constituent elements are (there are no equivalents to words or notes in paintings), or how they might conceivably be combined, or what the elements of the work (or the work as a whole) stand for or represent. Painting is filled with multiple meanings at every possible level.

This delineation of the criteria of notationality accomplishes two important purposes. First of all, one can now examine and compare the whole range of symbol systems that human beings have devised in terms of a single and readily applicable set of criteria. That is a decided improvement over Cassirer's lack of criteria for distinguishing among symbol systems and Langer's overly simple dichotomy between presentational and discursive symbols. Second, and of greater importance for our concerns here, it is now possible to ask whether different psychological processes are involved in dealing with symbol systems of varying degrees of notationality. One may even investigate whether the processing of notational symbol systems might be undertaken by one region of the brain, while the processing of non-notational or partially notational systems might be undertaken by a different cerebral region.

Goodman turns his focus next to the question of how symbols function, how they in fact symbolize. Here again he acknowledges that symbols can stand for or denote objects, but he goes on beyond common consensus to recognize other equally important but relatively neglected modes of symbolization.

Goodman devotes special attention to the fact that symbols can exemplify various properties. We can gain a feeling for these functions by considering a work of music. Strictly speaking, a work of music does not represent or denote anything in the world. As Stravinsky (among others) insisted, music is, by its very essence, powerless to convey specific meanings. On the other hand, it is clear that music has available to it considerable communicative powers. A work of music may literally exemplify certain properties, such as speed or loudness, and may in the process illuminate those same aspects in our own daily experience. Far more tellingly, music can metaphorically exemplify or "express" numerous other properties, such as gaiety, anger, conflict, passion, pride, and pomp and circumstance. Of course those properties cannot be literally exhibited by music: pride is a property of persons, pomp of events. But music functions symbolically by metaphorically recreating those properties through the use of such resources as mode, rhythm, and timbre.

Similar analytic tools can be brought to bear on works in the visual arts. To return for a moment to our opening squiggle, this meagre line can denote elements ranging from an electrocardiogram to a road on a map, but if, for example, it is part of a painting, it can also express or exemplify certain properties. Our line can literally exemplify angularity or unevenness but it can also metaphorically express conflict, ambivalence, and other properties ordinarily associated with selves or situations.

In indicating some of the ways in which symbols *can* function, we approach the core of Goodman's assertions about art. Whether symbols function as artistic symbols depends upon *which* of the properties of the symbol one attends to. If, for example, one construes our squiggle simply as the Dow Jones average and pays attention only to the relative height on the ordinate of each of the points, then the symbol is only functioning in the denotational manner. Literal or metaphorical exemplificatory powers are irrelevant. If, on the other hand, the same squiggle is apprehended as a mountain range in a Hokusai drawing, one then focuses on an entirely different set of symbolic properties. Over and beyond the strictly denotational aspects of the mountain range (whether it is high or low, jagged or smooth, has two or three peaks), one notes literal exemplificatory properties (for example, its blackness) and its expressive properties (its gracefulness or grandeur). One attends as well to other properties of aesthetic symbols, such as the repleteness of the rendering—the fact that every detail, every nuance of the line contributes to the overall impact of the work. To the extent that these properties are noted and function in a significant manner in the work, that work is being construed as an artistic symbol.

Using Goodman's analytic scheme as a point of departure, we have been able to secure considerable evidence that these distinctions between various symbolic functions are not merely logical ones. One can show that children are much more sensitive to representational and denotational features than they are to aspects of repleteness and expressivity; at the same time, one can also demonstrate that, under certain conditions, children may also become sensitive to those aspects that prove of particular import in the arts. Similarly, studies with brain-damaged patients reveal that, in certain pathological conditions, the expressive and stylistic aspects of works of art become relatively more salient, whereas in other conditions it is the representational or object-related features which stand out.

Furthermore, a case can be made that the left hemisphere of the human brain is relatively more effective than the right at dealing with notational symbol systems (ones with distinct elements which can be combined according to syntactic principles), while the right hemisphere is more at ease in dealing with dense and replete non-notational systems (ones where fine gradations are important, and where an attempt to decompose the work into its components is likely to be misleading). Thus, out of an analysis that was devised primarily for philosophical purposes, consequences of genuine psychological import have emerged. To use the current psychological jargon, concepts like "notationality" and "expressivity" turn out to be "psychologically real."

Goodman rejects the classical question, "What is art?" in favor of the alluring formulation, "When is art?" This is not surprising, for, as we have seen in the foregoing discussion, the question of whether something functions as an art object is a question of how it is construed under certain circumstances, rather than a question of properties that inhere in the object or symbol itself. As Goodman declared in *Languages of Art:*

Just as an object may be a symbol—for instance, a sample—at certain times and under certain circumstances and not in others, so an object may be a work of art at some times and not in others. Indeed, just by virtue of functioning as a symbol in a certain way does an object become, while so functioning, a work of art. (p. 67)

Having made this point, Goodman does propose several "symptoms" of the aesthetic, criterial attributes that are likely to be in the foreground in cases where a symbol is functioning aesthetically, and likely to be minimized or absent in cases where it is not. The use of the word *symptom* is by no means casual. Goodman wishes to invoke the medical model here. While no single cue suffices to make the diagnosis accurately, the greater the number of cues pointing in the same direction, the more likely that the condition can be correctly identified.

Goodman nominates five symptoms of the aesthetic:

Syntactic density, where the finest differences may constitute a difference between symbols. An example would be a drawing in which the finest, most subtle differences between two lines may convey important distinctions.

Semantic density, where the referents of symbols are distinguished by fine differences in certain respects. For example, in ordinary English the meanings of words overlap one another in many subtle ways: it is impossible to say where "intentionally" or "deliberately" ends and "on purpose" begins.

Relative repleteness, where comparatively many aspects of a symbol are significant. Here the difference between the stock-market graph and the Hokusai drawing becomes germane. If the symbol functions repletely, one needs to attend to an indefinitely large number of aspects. If it is functioning in a non-replete manner, only the numerical values count.

Exemplification, where a symbol, whether or not it denotes, symbolizes by serving as a sample of properties that it literally possesses. In the musical example mentioned earlier, the tune literally exemplifies speed and metaphorically exemplifies gracefulness.

Multiple and complex reference: Here the symbol performs several integrated and interacting referential functions, some direct and some mediated through other symbols. Rather than having a simple unambiguous meaning which is readily accessible and which lends itself to paraphrase or translation, the symbol carries a penumbra of overlapping and difficult-to-separate meanings, each of which contributes to the work's effects. Goodman has described the set of circumstances which obtains when these properties are operating:

These properties tend to focus attention on the symbol rather than, or at least along with, what it refers to. Where we can never determine precisely just which symbol of a system we have or whether we have the same one on a second occasion, where the referent is so elusive that properly fitting a symbol to it requires endless care, where more rather than fewer features of the symbol count, where the symbol is an instance of properties it symbolizes and may perform many inter-related simple and complex referential functions, we cannot merely look through the symbol to what it refers to as we do in obeying traffic lights or reading scientific texts, but must attend constantly to the symbol itself as in seeing paintings or reading poetry. (*Ways of World-making*, p. 69)

Just what does this complex conceptual apparatus furnish to the student of the arts? To begin with, Goodman's scheme enables us to avoid many thorny issues upon which previous aestheticians have been impaled. For example, one can proceed deeply into analysis without confronting such issues as which work of art is better and has greater value, which is beautiful and which is not. One concentrates instead on identifying those aspects of a symbol that contribute to its functioning as an artistic work. One addresses a host of questions on how different artistic symbols function in specific art forms and works of art. Thus the study of the arts becomes far more manageable and far less elusive than in previous times.

There is also a more positive virtue in Goodman's scheme. In particular, Goodman's contributions are of great significance to those interested in psychological aspects of artistry. More so than any other commentator on the arts, he has provided a workable notion of the kinds of skills and capacities that are central for anyone who works in the arts—for anyone who traffics in artistic symbols. Goodman's artistic creator is the individual with sufficient understanding of the properties and functions of certain symbol systems to allow him to create works that function in an aesthetically effective manner—works that are replete, expressive, susceptible to multiple readings, and the like. By the same token, the artistic perceiver, whether audience member, critic, or connoisseur, must be sensitive to the properties of symbols that convey artistic meaning—to repleteness, expressivity, density, and plurisignificance. By following Goodman's analysis, one may secure a model of what the competent artistic practitioner can accomplish: in the light of this "artistic end state" one can examine the skills required to become sensitive to artistic works or to create artistic works in a competent fashion. Such an agenda has proved invaluable in planning my own research program, and its merits have been increasingly appreciated by other empirical workers as well.

Even if Goodman had merely stipulated the criteria of artistic symbols and functions and had altogether bypassed the question of aesthetic merit or value, his contribution would have been of signal importance for anyone who studies the arts. But in recent writings Goodman has not shirked from attacking the even more difficult question of what makes one artistic work more effective or more "right" than another. Goodman's solution to this issue grows directly out of his involvement in the Cassirer tradition, out of his recognition that there is no one real world against which to compare our various versions. He affirms, rather, the existence of an innumerable collection of worlds, each of which we construct and none of which can claim epistemological priority over another.

At first blush, Goodman seems to defend a total relativism. He refuses to give any priority to a material world or to a description in terms of physics. In his view, physics—be it the variety put forth by Aristotle, Newton, or Einstein—is but one version of the world. And this version is not inherently superior to versions of the world fashioned by Homer, Shakespeare, or James Joyce. As scientific or artistic creators, we do not solve the jigsaw puzzle of reality. Rather, we build endless realities out of Lego.

But while Goodman refuses to consider one domain of knowledge inherently superior to another, or to compare a given physicist with a given poet, he does not embrace total relativism. Instead, using a homey but revealing analogy, he provides a suggestive way to think about how one version of the world might be better than another. Suppose a tailor is asked to produce a sample from a given bolt of cloth. Almost any piece cut from the bolt can be called a sample. But, Goodman points out, only a select number of those pieces would count as a *fair sample.* For example, in the illustration reproduced here, five segments of equivalent size have been cut from the same bolt. But only the one in the lower right panel can serve as a fair sample, accurately reflecting the principal features of the entire bolt. Samples that omit the basic pattern altogether or present it at a misleading angle obviously cannot qualify as fair samples.

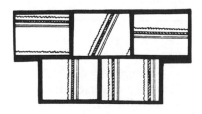

In Goodman's view, works of art can also be profitably viewed as samples. Just as certain fabric swatches accurately reflect the whole bolt, so may certain works of art accurately reflect, literally or metaphorically, important forms, feelings, affinities, and contrasts from the fabric of life. To put the matter perhaps too simply, versions of the world that strike us as being "fair" or "right" are those that seem to capture significant aspects of our own experiences, perceptions, attitudes, and intuitions.

Goodman himself is reluctant to designate certain artists or works as inherently "fairer" than others. Yet his writings indicate the kinds of criteria he would employ. For example, we might apply his reasoning to explain why, of the many versions of "The Last Supper" painted in the Renaissance, Leonardo's famous work on the wall of a church in Milan was "the fairest of them all." Assuming that all of the artists were striving to capture the drama of the pivotal moment when Christ revealed that one of his disciples would betray him, we might examine their works in terms of the range of emotions explored, the extent to which the tensions have been captured, and the care with which interpersonal dynamics are portrayed. In earlier versions, the disciples were typically aligned from left to right in a wooden manner, with practically no variation in expression. Leonardo, however, painted each with clear personality traits and definite facial expressions, talking, gesticulating, and eyeing one another—reflecting the drama of the moment.

To take a somewhat different example, consider the effect sometimes achieved by an artist whose vision is radically new. If, after looking at a variety of postimpressionist paintings, we see a Cézanne for the first time, we may begin to view the everyday world through fresh eyes. The artist may then be said to have fairly sampled the visual world—that is, to have created an experience that others ultimately recognize as an authentic version of reality. That the artist, in so doing, also *creates* reality is illustrated by a Picasso anecdote. When the artist unveiled his portrait of Gertrude Stein, an observer remarked that it did not look much like Stein. "No matter," Picasso said. "It will."

Goodman would be the last to insist that standards of rightness are unchanging. Indeed, a continuing function of works of art is to alter the way we conceive of experience and hence to change our attitudes about what is important and what feels right. But that is only to say that our versions of the world also continue to change. Just as the never-innocent eye comes to see the world in ever-changing ways, so, too, do the versions that we construct further influence and change our conceptions, at least as long as we allow them to do so. While refusing to attribute a unique status to the physicist's (or the artist's) version of reality, Goodman does furnish us with ways of judging among the versions fashioned *within* each creative domain. And so, beginning with apparently insubstantial differences between simple squiggles, Goodman provides us with entry points to hitherto mysterious questions about the essence of the arts and the relative merits of artistic works.

7

ERNST GOMBRICH:

WHY ART HAS A HISTORY

A TOUR through any major museum or any text on the history of art reveals an extraordinary progression in graphic art over the past three millennia. When we observe flattened "paper cutout" Egyptian wall painting (see figure 7.1) or the stilted, wooden madonna and child of the medieval master Cimabue (figure 7.2), we confront artwork that strikes us as being schematic and unrealistic. Then, with the arrival of the Renaissance, we encounter a clear contrast, one exemplified by Giotto's madonna (figure 7.3). A march had begun toward increasing realism, a march that continued from the fifteenth to the nineteenth century. By the time the English artist John Constable painted "Wivenhoe Park" in the early nineteenth century (figure 7.4), audiences had begun to encounter landscapes and scenes that rivaled photographs in their degree of depicted realism.

This trend reached its apogee with the arrival of impressionism, that still-treasured style of painting which attempts to capture light, color, texture, and other surface appearances at a specific moment in time. But impressionism also signaled the denouement of the march toward realism, for in the subsequent postimpressionist, cubist, and expressionist periods there was the rapid and near total collapse of any effort at depicting the world as it appears to the naked eye. And with the abstract expressionism of the forties and fifties, the breakdown was

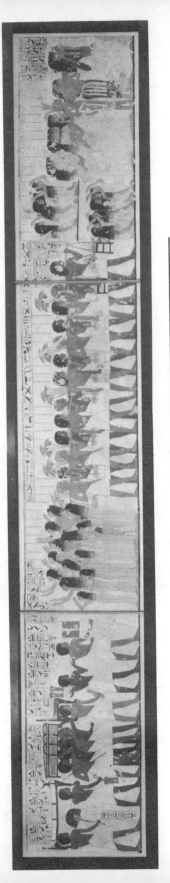

Figure 7.1. Expedition, The Metropolitan Museum of Art, 1930. All rights reserved, The Metropolitan Museum of Art.

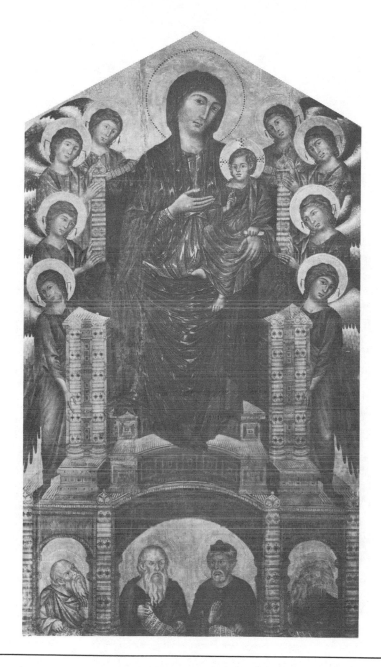

Figure 7.2. Cimabue. *Madonna and Child Enthroned with Angel and Prophets*

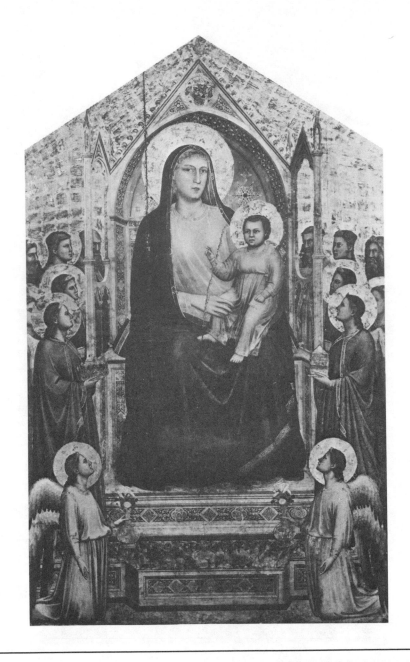

Figure 7.3. Giotto. *Madonna and Child Enthroned with Saints and Angels*

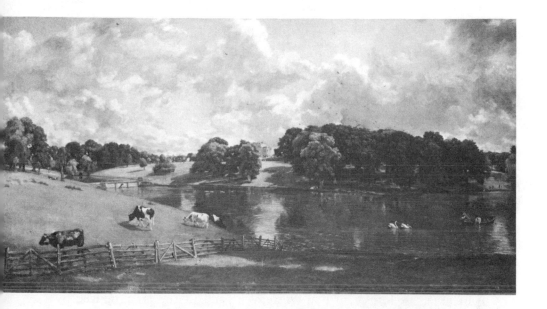

Figure 7.4. John Constable. *Wivenhoe Park, Essex.* National Gallery of Art, Washington, Widener Collection.

total. Artists produced jangled tangles of line, patches of color, and series of geometric forms remote from any scene in the everyday world. As a contemporary coda, we have the baffling potpourri of artistic styles of the past few decades—pop art, minimal art, conceptual art, and once again several varieties of preternaturally realistic art.

Examining these trends with the benefit of hindsight, nearly all observers would agree that this progression was not random. It could not simply have occurred in any order. With the exception of a brief flirtation with realistic effects during classical times, there seems to be a slow but measurable progression over the centuries toward retinal fidelity—pictures that look like the three-dimensional scenes they purport to portray. It is as if Albrecht Dürer's vision of painting an exact likeness of the nude behind the window of his study had come true (figure 7.5), and had then been shattered by a remarkable series of jolts.

But why *this* particular history of art? Can one offer a coherent account which at once explains the progress toward realism over the centuries *and* the chaos of the last century? What of analogous trends

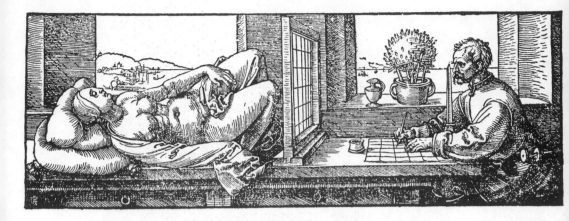

Figure 7.5. Dürer. *Draftsman Drawing a Reclining Nude*

in other art forms—in non-Western art and in the art produced by children? Finally, to take a slightly different tack, can we account for the selection, out of the countless works produced in each epoch's style, of the particular works that are considered worthy of inclusion in our chronicle of art?

The best guide to these issues is the Austrian-born art historian Sir Ernst Gombrich. Gombrich taught at Oxford, Cambridge, and Harvard and was until recently a professor at the Warburg Institute in London, the same research center that had served in the pre-Nazi era as the setting for Ernst Cassirer's study of symbolic forms. According to this versatile scholar, the quest for realism is a relatively recent phenomenon, one reflecting the secular trends of the Renaissance and post-Renaissance periods. Until that time most artists and observers did not demand retinal fidelity but simply schematic equivalence—the production of forms that can, in codelike fashion, be "read" as persons, objects, or scenes.

The first criterion for the production of realistic paintings is the motivation to do so, and perhaps the painters of the Middle Ages were not interested in recreating retinal appearances. But even with strong motivation to create a realistic painting, one may well fail. There is an enormous chasm between the ability to see accurately (as every normal person does) and the ability to draw realistically. And there is a fundamental reason for this: we unconsciously and automatically correct the images imprinted on our retinas—we read into them and regularize them. For example, a near and a distant person take up vastly different spaces on our retinas, yet we regard the two figures as roughly identical in size. Similarly, unless seen from a bird's-eye view, a table top forms an irregular parallelogram on the retina, yet we automatically correct it so that it appears rectilinear. Clearly it is difficult to become aware of our actual retinal images. But only if we do so can we hope to create a picture that achieves the illusion of realism.

Because it is so hard to experience our retinal images, even a gifted artist must begin with a simplified schema—a form or set of marks that "stand for" an object in the real world. Such schemas—two-dimensional equivalents of objects and their relations in a three-dimensional world—arise from a pair of sources: the movements and motions that we come naturally to make upon a piece of paper and the forms and formulas that other individuals have in the past devised for rendering certain aspects of the world. One reason for the late development of realism is that for a long time artists were simply content with such schemas. Only in the past few centuries did they begin to revise their schemas systematically so that they more closely resembled the images upon their retina.

Gombrich stands out as an art historian of the first rank who feels that answers to many historical puzzles about art lie in a study of human psychology. It is therefore not surprising that in his path-breaking study, *Art and Illusion,* Gombrich discerned the schematic origins of art in the graphic activities of young children. Young children produce circles, lines, and eventually a combination of them to yield the tadpole—the most elementary version of a human being. While serviceable and recognizable, this schema bears little resemblance to a real human being. It certainly does not arise from the child's looking at a human being and trying to draw that human as it is; rather, it is a formula, a symbolic equivalent that "stands for" objects in the world. Children's tadpole drawings eventually give way to somewhat more realistic renderings. Yet, according to Gombrich, these renderings owe much more to children's imitations of the drawings of older individuals than to any observation of the physical world. Children replace simpler symbols with more articulated graphic symbols; they rarely proceed by matching their efforts to their direct perception of the visual world.

The path to artistic realism lies elsewhere. In fact, to create a veridical picture, one must *forget* or *suspend* many aspects of one's knowledge of what things are. Instead, one must experiment with various effects of line, form, shading, and the like in order eventually to produce equivalences that are more convincing. Elaborate tricks and complicated principles, like foreshadowing, chiaroscuro, and perspective, must be mastered if a convincing likeness is to result. A rectilinear table viewed from an angle cannot be drawn simply as a rectangle even though it is experienced as one; instead, it must be drawn as a trapezoid or some other irregular figure if it is to mimic how such an object at such an angle is actually perceived in the world. As Gombrich says of the great artist Turner, "he suppressed what he knew of the world and concentrated only on what he saw" (*Art and Illusion*, p. 296).

The nature and extent of the artist's achievement can be conveyed by comparing Constable's "Wivenhoe Park" with a rendering of the same scene by an eleven-year-old child (figure 7.6). Viewed at a suitable distance by an eye schooled in Western painting, the Constable painting gives a marvelous impression of the total pastoral scene, complete with fine details of texture and shading in the trees and clouds, delicate alterations of hue in the pond, subtle contrasts of motion in each of

Figure 7.6. A child's version of Constable's *Wivenhoe Park.*

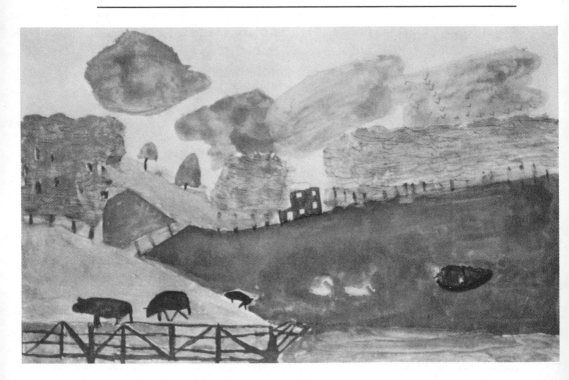

the cows, swans, and boatmen. One beholds a quite successful attempt to duplicate the visual experience of looking directly at the park. In sharp contrast, the child's far simpler rendering makes clear the precise identity of the elements in the scene—the cows, the house, the clouds, the boat—but at a severe cost. No longer can one discern the specific idiosyncratic features of each of these objects. One has instead "a tidy enumeration of the principal items of the picture, particularly those which would interest a child" (pp. 293–94).

To underscore this point, Gombrich suggests that one could readily decompose the child's drawing into a "cutout" and recreate the scene by propping up each of the component "puzzle parts" into a diorama. The Constable picture would resist such an exercise. The parts of the canvas flow smoothly into one another, for the artist has taken into account the numerous transformations undergone by shapes and color in light of the particular vantage point from which he elected to depict the scene. To capture their appearances at a given moment, he made their conventionalized identities less obvious, more ambiguous. Paradoxically, it may require more training to "read" the specific features of Constable's dense rendering than the child's "listlike" assemblage of elements.

Constable's achievement was no accident. Indeed, anticipating Gombrich's argument, Constable remarked: "Painting is a science and should be pursued as an inquiry into the laws of nature. Why, then, may not landscape painting be considered as a branch of natural philosophy, of which pictures are but the experiments?" (quoted in *Art and Illusion*, p. 33). As Gombrich details it, the progress that occurred in realistic art occurred over a considerable period of time, as one artist after another produced a schema, noted its deviation from the way objects actually looked, and then experimented with various effects until he arrived at a version somewhat closer to what was recorded on his retina. A number of historical factors culminated in this conquest of realism. These include the advent of geometry and science, mastery of principles of light, the introduction of the camera, and, perhaps most importantly, the constant embracing of methods of experimentation within the visual arts.

These factors happened to have come together in the West in the past several centuries, and that is why it was our culture, rather than another, that first mastered realism. That conquest came about only because many generations of artists had succeeded in suppressing their childlike knowledge of what things were and instead devised techniques for depicting objects as they appeared to the eye.

Thanks to Gombrich, we have gained an enhanced appreciation of the history of pictorial art from classical times to the twentieth century. At the same time, we can encounter clear affinities between the psychology of human artistic creation and the course of art history. A full consideration of art history, however, requires that we look beyond the framework that Gombrich has provided us. In particular, Gombrich leaves unilluminated the question of why artists eventually rejected realism in favor of cubism or expressionism; why there is a swing of the pendulum of taste, with realism emphasized at certain times while consigned to a minor role at other times; and, most enigmatically, why we come to value one work rather than another within a particular style or epoch.

A number of commentators have attempted to deal with these issues. One striking effort has been undertaken by the British artist and critic Suzi Gablik. In attempting to account for the same historical progression as that described by Gombrich, Gablik was drawn to Piaget's notions of the development of intellectual capacities. In her view, pre-Renaissance artists were proceeding in the manner of children who were not yet capable of performing logical operations. Renaissance artists were reminiscent of children capable of concrete logical operations. But only contemporary artists who indulge in computer or conceptual art exhibit the full panoply of intellectual operations. While this formulation is intriguing, I find it questionable in terms of the intellectual capacities it denies to artists of previous times and in its easy equation of traditional artists with children. Moreover, Gablik does not equip us to deal either with the question of artistic value or with the recent re-embracing of realism.

Several anthropologists and cultural historians, such as Alfred Kroeber, have embraced a contrasting framework. In Kroeber's view, artistic styles, like other fashion, inevitably involve a swing of the pendulum. Once one veers too far in one direction—say, in the direction of realism—one can confidently expect a reaction in the opposite direction—away from realism and toward stylization, schematism, or the breakdown of recognizable form. Kroeber's explanation accounts for certain trends in Western art, but again, it skirts issues of artistic value.

Still another approach, characteristic of intellectual historians like George Steiner, relates the art form of the period to the other events taking place within the culture. Thus, in examining the demise of realism in favor of such movements as cubism, these critics stress analogous events in other spheres—the breakdown of tonality in Western music, the rise of relativistic theories in physics, and the like. This approach, while descriptively compelling, evades exact explanations and risks becoming a circular route. Once one believes that artistic events of an era reflect other events, it is all too easy to corral evidence in favor of this claim.

Though these approaches offer valuable insights, I think we might gain additional perspective on the history of art by focusing instead on the topic we have so far ignored: why one work of art may be consistently valued over another in the same style and genre. Consider, for example, the two drawings reproduced here: "Group of Six Nude Figures" by the German master Dürer (figure 7.7), and "Studies of Men in Bondage," by Dürer's pupil Hans von Kulmbach (7.8), who may have been copying the Dürer work. Superficially, these drawings are highly similar. Yet nearly all students of art would instantly rate the Dürer above the von Kulmbach for reasons that can, at least partially, be articulated. Moreover, in this assessment, realism as usually defined would play little role: in certain ways von Kulmbach's drawing looks more like a photograph than does the Dürer. In attempting to justify the intuitive impressions of this pair of paintings, historians like Jakob Rosenberg have cited at least three factors.

First of all, Dürer's composition is much more interesting. The placement of figures, each assuming a different pose, sets up a dynamic tension among them, even as their gazes draw one repeatedly toward the central figure bound to the tree. In contrast, the von Kulmbach is a simple triangular arrangement in which the eye travels once or twice around the vertices without picking up any sense of direction or closure.

A second factor is the quality of line and texture in the painting. In the von Kulmbach, the line is regular, unvarying, and static, whereas in the Dürer it has "spring" and full-bodiedness. Similarly, the shading in the von Kulmbach is uniform throughout and rhythmically unrelated to the outline of the figure; in contrast, the elaboration of detail, the interior circular shading, and the attention given to heavy and light lines increase the vitality of the Dürer figures.

Finally, and perhaps most importantly, the Dürer picture contains a greater range and depth of expressive features. Each figure has a characteristic personal mien which allows us to read his mood, whereas the figures in von Kulmbach's drawing rival one another in dullness. Furthermore, the Dürer as a whole comes alive—the vitality of each

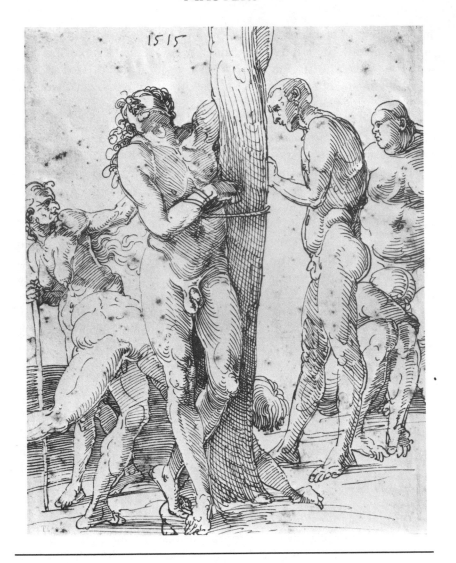

Figure 7.7. Dürer. *Group of Six Nude Figures*

figure leads to overall dramatic tension and invites further exploration.
The von Kulmbach seems to express no mood whatsoever.

This specimen of connoisseurial analysis adopted from Rosenberg's
remarks underscores the fact that we approach and evaluate artwork
in terms other than those of simple realism. Consideration of composition, expressivity, and the elaboration of detail and texture—those

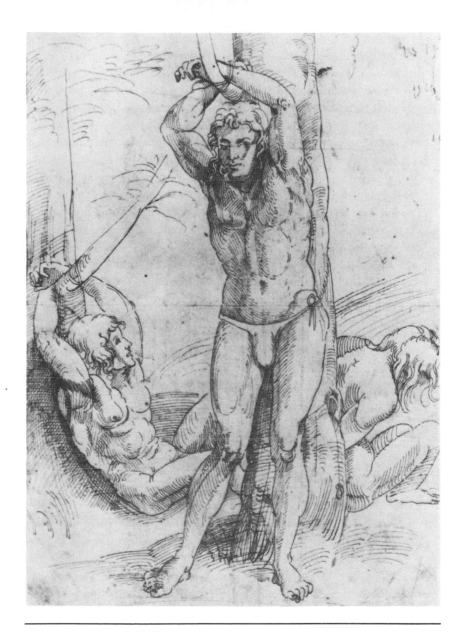

Figure 7.8. Kulmbach. *Studies of Men in Bondage*

symptoms of the aesthetic stressed by Nelson Goodman—contribute significantly to our assessment of the merits of the work. We may achieve greater understanding about art history and artistic value if we view its course as an interplay among these several factors, for in addition to being concerned with realism, artists have been perennially concerned with composition, details of texture, and expressiveness. What does change across artists, styles, and eras is the particular type of composition or expressivity that is valued and the amount of interest in realism.

How can this mode of analysis help to illuminate our central issues? First of all, it suggests that Western art became remarkable during a certain period (roughly 1500–1850) for its relatively single-minded emphasis on realism. During other times, a more pluralistic set of goals and factors held sway. Even so, given the emphasis on realism, at no time was this the only concern of artists and of artistic viewers. Instead, set against a sometimes excessive interest in realism was a perennial concern with other features of graphic depiction and a broad portfolio of preferences in the areas of composition, balance, and detailed texture.

For instance, as the art historian Heinrich Wölfflin has reminded us, Western art has oscillated over the centuries in the extent to which it embraced straight and uniform lines as opposed to shaded and irregular ones; balanced composition as opposed to dynamic and asymmetrical tension; the surface capturing of details as compared with the expression of underlying moods and feelings; the smooth changes of evolution as compared with the dramatic thrusts of revolutionary change.

The particular ratio obtaining among these factors can explain why, over and above concerns with realism, the pendulum has shifted in each of these aesthetic realms. For instance, during the late medieval and early Renaissance eras, the ideal in painting featured regular, balanced compositions; a century or two later, a preference developed for canvases that featured dynamic and asymmetric balance—and so painters like Delacroix and Goya came to the fore. Another moment of decisive change can be observed in the latter half of the nineteenth century. At that time the stately, posed, and highly realistic canvases favored by the French academicians gave way, often amidst great protest, to the more suggestive, informal, and fragmentary works by members of the impressionist school. A formula for ascertaining which works are treasured both within and across eras may have to incorporate shifting preferences on each of the aforementioned dimensions.

This line of analysis may also be extended to other forms of art.

Although factors of realism clearly play a minimal role in music, in examining the course of Western music over the past several centuries, one certainly encounters shifts in the standards for compositional form, ornamentation, and expressivity. Moreover, the combination of weightings on these different factors seems highly relevant to the determination of merit among several selections of music drawn from the same era. By the same token, in non-Western forms of graphic art, where realism has rarely been a major factor, other aspects of artistic symbolization may combine to determine judgments of merit.

Of course an attempt to account for the history of art and for aesthetic value at the same time is a herculean assignment. It is Gombrich's singular achievement to have provided a convincing account of one central element—realism—in this riddle. In addition, sensitive to the other issues raised in this discussion, Gombrich devoted a chapter in *Art and Illusion* to the problem of expressivity, and in his most recent book, *The Sense of Order*, he investigated issues of design and composition. If these latter efforts are less noteworthy, it may be because the issues are even more difficult to deal with and because the relevant psychological concepts have yet to be developed. Even so, Gombrich at least states his views with exemplary clarity. Thanks to his pioneering dissection of issues, future discussion can proceed at a more sophisticated level.

PART II

ARTISTIC

DEVELOPMENT

IN CHILDREN

INTRODUCTION

IN HIS *Critique of Practical Reason* Immanuel Kant cited two miracles as standing out above all others: the starry heaven above and the moral law we all carry within ourselves. I would dare to propose a third, which has long struck me as equally marvelous: the creative activity of the young child. I find both exhilarating and mysterious the rampant word play in which children engage, the many songs they echo and embroider, and the appealing figures of speech they devise. Perhaps above all I have always treasured that sequence of artful scribbles which includes ingenious compositions with a fanciful content all their own and ultimately culminates in acceptable representations of the external world.

In fact, for as long as I can remember, I have been fascinated by children's artistic activities, at first those in which I myself engaged and then, somewhat later, those I beheld in other youngsters. In high school I began to teach piano to other children and continued to do so, somewhat haphazardly, during college and graduate school. But it was only when I spent a semester teaching children aged five to seven in an open classroom that I became wholly convinced that their artistic activities constituted a miracle of Kantian proportions, one that deserved—no, required—a comprehensive explanation. Much of my research in the intervening years has been an attempt to understand better the nature of children's artistic activities—those of my own children, those of children I have taught or observed, and those of the handful of special children who have the talent to become artistic masters.

To pursue this effort, it has been necessary to locate artistic development with reference to other better-traveled trajectories of human growth. In most areas of development, the formula is simple: youngsters get better, more skilled, more sophisticated with age. But such a unilinear portrait does not do the arts justice. In some ways young children are especially intimate with the arts; and the story of artistic development is replete with declines, zigs, and zags, rather than following an automatic upward progression. It is crucial to understand what is distinctive about artistic development and to consider how its unusual trajectory may have implications for development writ large. My first publications probed that line of analysis.

But it would be a paltry examination of the arts which took its assignment uncritically from the rest of the field of developmental psychology—its heroes, its problems, its areas of ignorance. An equally important and far more pleasurable task is to immerse oneself in the phenomena of "child art"—the sorts of things children typically do (and fail to do), the nature and limitations of their understanding, their capacities to talk about art, the vast and instructive individual differences that obtain among young budding artists and across diverse artistic media.

The essays in the following section survey the field of children's artistic development as I have come to view it. The essays may be thought of as falling into three general classes.

The first several essays portray the general outlines of artistic development. We begin with a short informal survey to set forth the crucial issues of children's creative powers. There follows a more leisurely and somewhat more scholarly inquiry into the trajectory of artistic development, which touches on the development of picturing ability and of metaphoric competence. The next essay focuses on a neglected but intriguing area of artistic development: children's own understandings (and misunderstandings) of the artistic process. The discussion of general artistic development concludes with a description of the first phases of symbolic development. This essay focuses particularly on some unexpected but instructive individual differences among children which emerge early in life and which may well determine what artistic direction, if any, the child eventually pursues.

In the second group of essays we turn to particular art forms. There are of course numerous art forms in our culture (and many more in other cultures), and my colleagues and I have had the opportunity to survey only a few of them. We take a look at three artistic media: drawing, music, and literature. And within the area of literary development, we consider two contrasting facets: the specific capacities to produce and understand metaphor and the more general (and elusive) phenomenon of literary imagination.

In the final pair of essays we turn our attention to extreme populations: first we enter the world of the autistic child through a consideration of Nadia, who has electrified the clinical community (and befuddled scholars of artistic development) with her remarkable drawings. We conclude by considering prodigious children, whose speed and unerringness of accomplishment challenge those who aspire to explain all artistic and scientific accomplishment within a single framework.

8

EXPLORING THE MYSTERY

OF ARTISTIC CREATIVITY

THE PRESCHOOL YEARS are often described as a golden age of creativity, a time when every child sparkles with artistry. As those years pass, however, it seems that a kind of corruption takes over, so that ultimately most of us mature into artistically stunted adults. When we try to understand the development of creativity—asking why some people finally emerge as artists, while the vast majority do not—the evidence for some corrupting force is persuasive, at least on the surface.

Step into almost any nursery school and you enter a world graced with the imagination and inventiveness of children. Some youngsters are fashioning intricate structures out of blocks. Others are shaping people, animals, or household objects out of clay or Play-Doh. Listen to the singing: there are melodic fragments, familiar tunes, and other patterns composed of bits and snatches from many songs. As the children speak, you hear the narratives they weave and their charming figures of speech.

Beyond their obvious charm, some of these youthful creations are powerfully expressive. There is poetry: a youngster might characterize a streak of skywriting as "a scar in the sky"; a peer will describe her naked body as "barefoot all over." And, almost without exception, youngsters scarcely out of diapers will produce drawings and paintings that, in their use of color, richness of expression, and sense of composition, bear at least a superficial kinship to works by Paul Klee, Joan Miró, or Pablo Picasso.

But that kinship is nowhere to be found in an elementary schoolroom. The number of drawings drops precipitously and, in the opinion of many, so does their overall quality. At the same time, youthful language slowly sheds its poetry.

Noting this situation, parents, teachers, and educators have searched for a culprit. Schools, the banal taste of most adults, the undermining of cultural standards, the decline of Western civilization, the left half of the brain—these and other bugbears have been identified and vilified.

Yet it is possible to view this phenomenon in less pejorative terms. By attempting instead to understand fully just what has happened to the child, one can arrive at a more positive and, certainly, a more complex view. Three mysteries have to be solved: What is the nature of early childhood artistry? What happens to this golden age of artistic innocence? Is the activity of the young child-artist related to the practices of a mature artistic creator?

At Harvard Project Zero my colleagues and I have been observing children as they participate (or cease to participate) in a range of artistic activities. While neither we, nor our colleagues elsewhere, have come to definite conclusions, we have been moving toward an understanding of the drawings, songs, and metaphors created by young children. The key to children's artistry, we have come to feel, lies in understanding children's overall patterns of development. During the first year or two of life, the infant comes to know the world directly, through his senses and his actions. He learns about the world of physical objects—bottles and toys—and, of equal importance, he gains initial acquaintance with the social world. This knowledge is at first direct: the child's understanding is limited to actual encounters with the objects and persons of his world.

A revolution in knowledge, one crucial for artistry, marks the years following infancy. In the period from age two to seven, the child comes to know and begins to master the various symbols in his culture. Now, in addition to knowing the world directly, he can capture and communicate his knowledge of things and people through any number of symbolic forms, most notably linguistic ones. At this time virtually all children readily master the language (or languages) of their surroundings.

But language is by no means the only (and in many cases, not even the most important) route for making sense of the world. Children learn to use symbols, ranging from gestures of the hand or movements of the whole body to pictures, figures of clay, numbers, music, and the like. And, by the age of five or six, children not only can understand these various symbols but can often combine them in the ways adults find so striking.

Let a few years pass and everything has changed. The penchant for succumbing to convention, for conforming to one's peers, comes to permeate children's activities. Even as children at play are determined to follow the rules exactly and to tolerate no deviation, so, too, in their use of symbols they will brook neither experimentation nor novelty.

Children now typically limit their graphic efforts to the faithful copying of forms about them. Some stop drawing altogether. Their language also exhibits a conservative streak. No longer will they unite elements from disparate domains into a poetic figure—body scars and vapors from an airplane must forever be kept asunder.

Although artistic work by children appears impoverished during this period, the common disparagement of this "literal stage" seems to me misguided. Far from being the enemy of artistic progress, literalism may represent its advance guard. That concern with realism that pervades the literal stage may be a crucial phase of development—the time for mastering rules.

In fact, as youngsters move through the literal stage, most exhibit a gradual improvement in their ability to understand and to respond to works created by others. But it is not until the years preceding adolescence that they show a sensitivity to those qualities most central to the arts—style, expressiveness, balance, composition. Only at this time do the tastes of youths become more catholic, so that they will tolerate abstract or impressionistic works as well as ones that are realistic.

That sharpening of tastes and understanding, however, has few reverberations in the creative realm. Only a small minority of those who created freely as young children resume their efforts; middle-aged piano students notwithstanding, most of the rest of us seem content (or resigned) to participate in the arts as members of an audience.

This developmental picture has led some scholars to speak of a U-shaped curve in artistic development. The first part of the U refers to the apparently high level of creativity found among preschoolers; the trough of the U designates the period of literalness, when the child's artistic creations are less striking in the eyes of many observers; the triumphant resurgence of the U marks the attainment (on the part of at least some adolescents) of a new, higher level of artistic accomplishment. Debate has focused on whether each end of the U designates the same kind of competence or whether, instead, the kind of creativity exhibited by most preschoolers is of a fundamentally different order from that found in the minority of adolescents who are artistically accomplished.

In my own view, there are clear differences between child and adult artistic activity. While the child may be aware that he is doing things differently from others, he does not fully appreciate the rules and conventions of symbolic realms; his adventurousness holds little significance. In contrast, the adult artist is fully cognizant of the norms embraced by others; his willingness, his compulsion, to reject convention is purchased, at the very least, with full knowledge of what he is doing and often at considerable psychic cost to himself. As Picasso once remarked, "I used to draw like Raphael, but it has taken me a whole lifetime to learn to draw like a child."

In truth, no one knows for sure why most of us cease artistic activity or what distinguishes those few individuals who achieve greatness in the arts. Nonetheless, an examination of the biographies of major artists and a consideration of principles of human growth provide a few hints.

A *sine qua non* for ultimate artistic achievement is inborn talent. There is doubt on how to measure it, how to define it—even how to prove its existence—but it seems beyond dispute that certain youngsters possess a natural aptitude for accomplishment in the arts. Whatever their skills in athletics, interpersonal relations, or logical thinking, they demonstrate early on a fascination with and an ability to progress rapidly in the symbol systems of one or another art form. They sing in tune, play constantly with rhymes, and sketch people or animals with great facility.

A contributor of equal significance is the environment in which one develops. During the natural artistry of the preschool years, active intervention is unnecessary; simply equipping children with materials (paints or xylophones) and exposing them to works (stories or drawings) suffices. But with the onset of school and the preoccupation with rules and convention, the environment must assume a more active role. This is a time when children crave knowledge of how to do things: they want to know how to play an arpeggio, render a drawing of a building in perspective, or write a mystery (or even a parody of Sherlock

Holmes). Accordingly, teachers willing to instruct and models of how to do things become crucial.

Indeed, I suspect that there exists a kind of "sensitive period" during the years preceding adolescence. The future artist needs to acquire skills at a rapid rate so that by adolescence he is already accomplished in his craft. If he is, he can then withstand the rise in critical powers of his adolescent years and still conclude, "I'm not that bad."

If, however, his own efforts prove inadequate in comparison with the achievements of others, he is likely to despair and to abandon artistry altogether. Supporting this theory is the historical fact that gifted artists have all apparently passed through a literal stage. But they negotiated it with great rapidity so that, by adolescence, they were already creating works of extremely high quality.

Even the combination of native talent, appropriate pedagogy, and high skill does not suffice to yield the creative artist. The competent craftsman, yes—the innovative master, no.

It is here, I believe, that traits of personality and character come into play. One bent on achieving artistic greatness must harbor a heightened motivation to excel, to distinguish himself. Possessed of a powerful vision, he must feel compelled to express that vision, over and over again, within the symbolic medium of his choice. He must be willing to live with uncertainty, to risk failure and opprobrium, to return time and again to his project until he satisfies his own exacting standards, while speaking with potency to others.

All of that said, it is important to note that most of our knowledge of artistic development comes from studies in Western societies. We simply do not know whether, given another cultural setting, the same stages would be realized, the same number or variety of artists would emerge.

Ultimately, a lifetime of experience, skill, and dedication separates the young child "whose gift controls him" (in the words of André Malraux) from the adult artist "who controls his gift." And yet, in the enjoyment of incessant exploration and in the willingness to disregard what others may say, there exists a bond between each child and each gifted adult artist. Moreover, for both, an artistic medium provides the means for coming to grips with ideas and emotions of great significance, ones that cannot be articulated and mastered through ordinary conversational language.

"If I could say it, I wouldn't have to dance it," insisted Isadora Duncan, thereby capturing an important strand of similarity between the adult artist and the young child.

9

THE CHILD AS ARTIST

IN CENTURIES PAST, there would have been little dispute in Western societies about how an individual enters the arts: the route was well defined. Among those relatively few individuals blessed with talent, and readily distinguished from the rest at an early age, some would elect (or be selected) to follow a life in art. They would then begin an arduous process by first enrolling, formally or informally, in a school, workshop, or atelier. There they would work with individuals of undisputed artistic achievement and learn the basic principles of their craft—how to draw from life, how to mix colors, how to employ light, shading, and other effects. Over a period of time, and given the requisite effort, they would pass through a number of stages, ranked roughly as apprentice, journeyman, expert, and master. At the conclusion of this process, which might take years or even decades, they would be designated as artists by their community and would be allowed, in turn, to disseminate their hard-earned knowledge to others.

This picture is, of course, an idealization; probably at no time was the path from talented youth to acknowledged master artist that well defined—quite possibly risk and uncertainty have always marked the life (if not the very *definition*) of an artist. But such an ideal portrait does convey one very important feature: the attainment of artistry was acknowledged by virtually all individuals to be an arduous and time-consuming process, one that could be achieved only by a few after many years of training. Any thought that the attainment of artistry was easy, or that the young child might properly be viewed as an artist, would have been cursorily dismissed.

ARTISTIC DEVELOPMENT IN CHILDREN

No longer does the relationship between child and artist seem so remote. A century ago, when the Swiss pedagogue Rodolphe Töppfer and the French poet Charles Baudelaire made the first tentative suggestions of a relationship between the child and the artist, they were probably considered outrageous, but nowadays such comments barely elicit any reaction whatsoever. Our romantic tradition, remolded in terms of a modernist ethos, has made us responsive to the notion of the child as artist, and the child in every artist. The question is no longer when does an individual become an artist but rather, what are the similarities—and differences—between the artistry of children and the artistry of adult masters.

The reasons for this dramatic change in attitude are complex and cannot be fully treated here. It perhaps suffices to designate two powerful influences. First, we have learned in the past century to pay serious heed to all of the activities and products of the child—to observe them carefully and to search for ties to the more accomplished activities of the adult. As a complement, our ideas of what counts as artistry have also changed radically. The line between the fine arts and the activities of ordinary individuals was much more clearly defined in

Figure 9.1

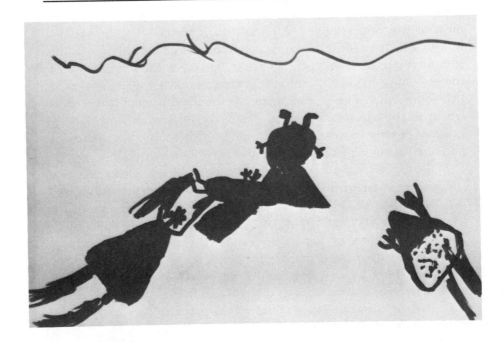

centuries past than it is today. And the kinds of works esteemed now have at least a superficial resemblance to those produced by children.

Consider, for example, the pair of drawings juxtaposed in the accompanying illustrations (figures 9.1 and 9.2). While the tadpole figures and the collection of scribbles would have been ignored in years gone by, a person who values the simple forms of Klee and Miró, as well as the abstract lines of Jackson Pollock and Franz Kline, cannot be so dismissive. And even as we look with increasing seriousness at the drawings made by children, often locating in them clear ties to the major movements of the twentieth century, so, too, we listen carefully to the sounds made by children. We hear the charming stories they repeat or relate, we listen with satisfaction to the little tunes they have devised, and, most dramatically, we are touched and sometimes even excited by the figures of speech such children make. When a three-year-old refers to the sensation of his feet falling asleep as "bubbling gingerale"; when a toddler describes a flashlight battery as "a sleeping bag all rolled up and ready to go to a friend's house," or refers to a group of nuns as "penguins," we are prompted to dub such youngsters as miniature (or, at the very least, future) poets.

Figure 9.2

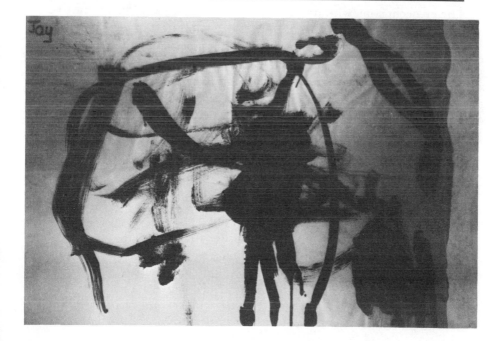

ARTISTIC DEVELOPMENT IN CHILDREN

The saga of the young child as artist gains in persuasiveness in the wake of events in children's lives in the years after early childhood. Following closely upon entrance into school, the charm, originality, and attractiveness of works by children are no longer as apparent. Nearly all who have studied the matter would agree on the decrease in quantity of works produced that might be considered art. Children aged eight, nine, or ten are far less likely than their younger counterparts to produce copious collections of drawings, paintings, clay figures, or three-dimensional constructions. Children of these ages are also far less likely to produce charming or intriguing figures of speech. Moreover, this decline in quantity is accompanied by decisive shifts in attitudes. These children reject the impressionistic or abstract works of art produced by others, even as they voice hostility to figures of speech: "You can't say a tie is loud, because ties don't make noise." This attraction to realism and literalism, this distaste for the fanciful and adventurous, has so impressed certain observers that they have defined a "literal stage" in artistic development during the early years of school.

Whether there is equal decline in the quality of artworks is somewhat more controversial. Relativity of standards proves crucial here. The shift toward realism at the age of seven or eight, which would have been esteemed a hundred years ago as aesthetic progress, is now regarded by some as a lamentable decline in adventurousness and flavorfulness. The preoccupation with precision in speech, which would have pleased schoolmasters in decades past, is now regretted, at least in certain circles. It seems fair to conclude that, measured against contemporary standards, the artistic productions of school-aged children are seen as less interesting than those of very young children.

Taken together, these various trends suggest that before children reach the literal stage they are very close to the wellsprings of creativity and that they share some similarities with gifted adults in both the processes and the products of artistry. Young children and the arts seem attuned to one another, but, at least in our culture, a wedge appears to be driven between them following the entry into school. But surely such an assertion, no matter how appealing, cannot simply be accepted at face value. If a genuine relation obtains between children and art, this must be demonstrated rather than asserted; and part of the exercise of demonstration must entail the possibility that the similarity is illusory rather than genuine. And so we must ask whether the activities of the young children described above are really artistic, and if not, in which ways they deviate from central aspects of the artistic process.

The Child as Artist

It need hardly be mentioned that these are complex questions which do not admit of simple and precise answers. Even to make a start, however, one clearly needs some definitions of what counts as artistry, some criteria by which to evaluate the processes and products of the child. Of crucial import in such an enterprise is a willingness to consider the child's performances in the context of his overall development: indeed, only in that context can the individual actions, attitudes, and preferences of the child be adequately and appropriately assessed. In tracing the development of the child's behaviors, then, and in assessing them against some rough-and-ready definitions of what counts as genuine artistic efforts, we hope to make progress toward assessing the significance of children's artistic activity. In the process we should glimpse those factors that appear regnant when the child can (legitimately) be said to be entering the arts.

Following upon the first year or two of life, during which children come to know persons and objects directly through their own actions upon them, a revolution occurs in their relationship with the world. At this time, children first become able to process the various symbol systems of the culture. Where, earlier, they could relate to personal or social objects only through direct interaction with them, they now become able to refer to such objects through a myriad of symbolic vehicles. During the period from age two to seven children learn to speak, to draw, to gesture, to handle systems of mime, number, and music. Moreover, they accomplish this feat of learning with such speed and efficacy that it seems reasonable to view them at their entry into school as fluent symbol-using creatures. By this time children have clearly achieved skill within various media: their drawings, stories, tunes, and gestural sequences are competently executed and can for the most part be "read" or decoded by others in the society. We may, then, speak at this time of a "first-draft"knowledge of certain procedures and norms of artistic practice. But is it legitimate to honor these productions with the epithet of "art"?

Such an enterprise is legitimate only if one is willing to adopt some definitions and to apply them judiciously to the products of youngsters. We have been aided in this task by the work of the philosopher Nelson Goodman, who has viewed artistic objects as symbols and has isolated those characteristics of symbols which make them function as works of art. While Goodman's position will not be fully laid out here (see essay 6), two of his "symptoms of the aesthetic" can at least be introduced in an informal manner.

ARTISTIC DEVELOPMENT IN CHILDREN

According to Goodman, a drawing functions as an aesthetic symbol to the extent that it exploits the *replete* and *expressive* properties of the graphic medium. When functioning in a replete manner, a drawing exhibits and highlights the various potentials of line—such as thickness, shading, and texture. Thus a line drawing of a trail of ants should exploit each of these features, while a stock-market chart of identical appearance would not, and hence, though symbolic, could not be functioning as an artistic symbol. As for the symptom of expressivity, a drawing will be viewed as an expressive symbol to the extent that it conveys specific moods, expressions, or emotions. If a drawing can be read consistently by individuals within a culture as "sad" or "happy," "angry" or "graceful," it is exploiting the expressive properties of the medium.

The appeal of these definitions lies in their potential for clarifying issues raised above. In theory, we might be able to judge the artistic status of children's works simply by rating representative drawings on their degree of repleteness or expressiveness. In fact, however, such a task would prove a monumental and, possibly, futile undertaking: the standards whereby such drawings would be evaluated would be difficult to determine (in the absence of knowledge of the children's thinking behind their drawings) and apparent expressiveness or repleteness might well be achieved by accident. In other words, the determination of repleteness or expressivity would be a completely subjective matter. Accordingly, my colleague Thomas Carothers and I arrived at a less direct but more reliable procedure for assessing the aesthetic sensitivity of young children.

Figure 9.3

Figure 9.4

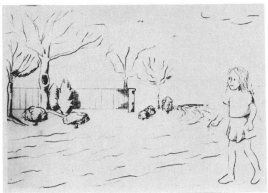
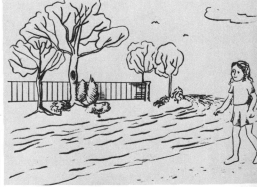

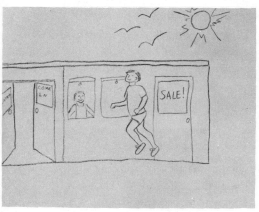 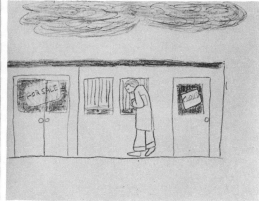

Figure 9.5   Figure 9.6

We presented school-aged children with drawings that were comparable to one another save in their repleteness or their expressiveness.
Drawings resembling those made by children were used so that they
would not intimidate the children. In a first test, children were shown
two scenes (figures 9.3 and 9.4), which are identical except in terms
of the thickness of line and type of shading. Children were told that
these incomplete drawings had been made by different artists and were
then asked to do two things: first, to complete the drawings in such
a way that they would look as if the original artist had finished them;
and second, as a control against the lack of technical drawing skills,
to choose from a second pair of drawings (not shown here) the complete
drawing that seemed appropriate.

On a second test children were shown the two drawings (figures
9.5 and 9.6), which were similar save in the mood they were expressing.
Referential clues such as the signs ("Sale!" versus "Closed") were
included in the drawings to aid the children in detecting the differences
in mood. Children were then asked to add drawings of trees and flowers
to the two scenes. By asking the children to depict these features in
the way they would have been done by the original artists, we hoped
that they would produce trees and flowers that were appropriately
"sad" or "happy." Again, as a control against lack of drawing skills,
youngsters were later asked to choose from two completed drawings
the one that was most appropriate.

The results of the two tests were quite direct and straightforward.
First graders could neither complete the drawings nor choose what

was deemed the appropriate finished drawing in either of the two tests. The one exception to this characterization was that the first graders did distinguish betweeen thick (dark) and thin (light) lines. Fourth graders could generally choose the appropriate completion from a pair of drawings but had difficulty in completing the unfinished drawings in a way that was adequate in regard to either repleteness or expressiveness. Finally, sixth graders showed considerable skill in both production and perception on both dimensions, although certain aspects of repleteness continued to elude them.

Such a study is open to many criticisms and its results will certainly have to be repeated. But when considered along with other studies of children's awareness of artistic properties, the findings caution us against assuming that the activities and attitudes of young children can readily be equated with those of older artistic practitioners.

Only during the middle school years do children seem to attend to the rendering of artistic works—only at this time does the *way* in which an effect is achieved or an object represented come under scrutiny. By the same token, only at this time do children seem able to vary their products in order to achieve diverse effects (for example, drawing a wrecked car differently from an intact car) or to aid others in recognizing them. We thus encounter a paradox: children become sensitive to the aesthetic aspects at the very time when their own work often seems to wane in interest. To this paradox we shall eventually return.

Another contrasting instance of artistic growth comes from the realm of literary language: the creation of metaphor. Preschool children exhibit a decided penchant for producing alluring figures of speech— metaphors, assonances, rhymes, and other rhythmic patterns—and, as was the case with drawing, there is a precipitous decline in the incidence of such figurative language once the school years begin. Again we confront the challenge of ascertaining whether the activities of young children "count" as genuine works of art.

Over the past several years my colleague and I have devoted considerable energies to the collection and analysis of figures of speech from young children. Some of these figures have been borrowed from protocols culled by other researchers; some have been taken from our own studies of general symbolic development; still others have been elicited in the course of experimental tasks, which include the completions of stories and the renaming of familiar and unfamiliar objects. In most cases these metaphors are instances in which an entity (like a splotch on an easel) is given a name that differs from its usual one and is drawn from a remote domain (like a case of the measles) but which is nonetheless judged appropriate in a given context.

To count as a figure of speech, rather than an overgeneralization, a category mistake, or some other kind of "error," a figure of speech must meet strict criteria. In our own studies, we have considered as candidate metaphors only those renamings where it can be established that the child demonstrably knows the literal name and the conventional uses of the object in question. While such a determination cannot be made with reliability in every case, it is possible, using a concerted set of methods and obtaining interjudge reliability, to receive a high degree of assurance about whether any instance in a child's linguistic corpus should count as genuine metaphor.

Our studies suggest that even among preschoolers it is valid to speak of metaphoric language. For one thing, the metaphoric language produced (and appreciated) by young children is almost exclusively of one of the following forms. Either the child engages in a renaming of an object based upon a perceptual resemblance (for example, a pencil is renamed a rocket ship); or the renaming is based upon a similarity in action (a pencil is used as a hairbrush and renamed a hairbrush); or the renaming is based on an amalgam of perception and action (a pencil is used as a toothbrush and renamed in this manner). Virtually never have we encountered a figure of speech that bears psychological connotations.

Further limitations characterize these early figures of speech. Particularly in the context of experiments, young children tend to produce responses that strike adult judges as anomalous. Thus, in one interesting set of results, preschoolers produced an absolutely higher number of appropriate metaphors than any other age group; but these same youngsters also produced a much higher proportion of anomalous or indecipherable (and presumably idiosyncratic) metaphors. Also, the metaphors produced by children appear to be accompanied by less tension or apparent disparity between the conventional meanings of the words, and thus seem less of an achievement than those produced by older children or adults. It remains to be shown that such tension is sensed, and then overridden, in the metaphors of young children. As was the case with drawing, children who have entered school produce fewer metaphors and take a dim view of them.

At least two factors must be taken into account before we conclude that the preschooler stands closer to the adult artist than does the youngster of elementary school. First, the decline in proclivity to produce metaphor may not signal any decline in competence. Our own studies suggest that, if pressed, children can produce metaphors just as they had earlier; it is only that they are less at ease doing so, quite possibly because they are more sensitive to the tension involved in transgressing category boundaries. Second, as in the case of drawing, the school years progressively see a marked rise in children's ability to understand metaphor. Not only does sensitivity to perceptual and functional metaphors increase with age, but children at that time also become able (for the first time) to understand those expressive and psychological metaphors that seem to completely elude the preschooler.

Again, then, we encounter the paradox that just when the incidence of artistry seems on the wane, superior insight into the nature and meanings of figurative language or graphic output comes about. School children seem able for the first time to appreciate a range of uses in an artistic medium, to appreciate the choices made by artists, to understand and, eventually, to value the various effects that can be produced.

It may be profitable to view these trends in another way. In the earliest years of development, children achieve initial command of symbol systems of the culture, but this mastery remains, in large measure, a private matter. To be sure, youngsters are exploring what the system can and cannot do, they are actively experimenting and toying with it, and in the process they often achieve effects that are quite pleasing to themselves and marvelous to others. Moreover, they do not execute these activities in total ignorance of the surrounding society. Certainly by the age of six or seven, children are sufficiently aware of the standards of the culture that they no longer produce works that are totally egocentric. Thus it seems reasonable to speak of a flowering of artistry or, as I have come to view it, of the achievement of a "first draft" of artistry.

However, an important shift occurs at about this time in the children's lives—one that reverberates across virtually every aspect of their existence. As children enter school (and possibly, in part, as a result of this entry) they gain a heightened awareness of, and concern with, the standards of their culture. Indeed, children become occupied, and preoccupied, with the rules and standards honored by those about them—how to dress, how to speak, how to play games, how to behave in a morally approved manner. They even become obsessed—they want to get these practices exactly right—and it becomes important for their psychological well-being that they not violate them.

Part of the burden of this involvement with, and immersion in, the practices of the society is that children become highly aware of the conventional boundaries between domains, the rewards in conforming, the risks of violation. And so the kinds of adventurous deviations or experiments, which are today so valued in the artistic realm and which younger counterparts undertake with little damage to their psyches, become virtually taboo. Until children are secure in just what the boundaries are, until they know in their bones that a violation will not unsettle them (and others), until they feel that the rules will remain as a comfortable point of departure, a background against which experimentation can take place, they will remain mired in the literal stage.

Nonetheless, if there is in fact a literal stage (and the biographies of great artists can provide ample documentation of its existence), there are various ways to pass through it. Quite likely something within our own society, perhaps its standards or its pedagogical practices, makes the literal stage a dénouement of artistic practice for most youngsters. And just as likely, there exist cultural milieux (for example, the land of Bali) where educational practices during the "literal years" leave open the possibility for an active later participation in artistic and other expressive kinds of behaviors. The way that we handle the educational challenge of the literal years—the kinds of aids we give to children, the pluralistic or monolithic models we propose—will determine how the children negotiate their way through the stage and what they will do once they have passed through it.

Our developmental journey has allotted to the preschool child a "first-draft" mastery of the artistic process. At the same time, we have seen both the necessity for, and the possible significance of, negotiation through the literal stage. We know, however, that the literal stage remains a last point of artistic productivity for most youngsters in our society. Adolescents who paint or adults who contrive novel metaphors are exceptional rather than commonplace occurrences.

The question thus arises: Who achieves artistic excellence in later life? In pondering this question, we necessarily revert to our original query about the relationship between the artistry of the young child and that of the acknowledged practitioner. If proven recipes for ultimate artistic achievement were ever widely available, they are certainly scarce today. Nonetheless, a few considerations seem worth mentioning.

As in days past, the signs of early talent—indices of special skills and rapid rate of development—are very important. While such talent can certainly be frustrated, it is difficult to see how children with meager signs of early talent will ever attain artistic heights. Here the milieu of the school years becomes vital. This is a time when children are willing, even eager, for training in the arts, and gifted teachers can help them to develop their skills.

It becomes crucial to achieve competence by the time of adolescence, for during the teenage years youths come to confront firsthand the full range of alternatives in an art form, as well as the peaks of excellence achieved by selected elders and peers. If their own work falls too far below this standard, they are very likely to despair and to cease their artistic activity altogether. If, on the other hand, youths have achieved sufficient skill during the preadolescent years so that their works basically "pass muster," the chance remains for a longer, and perhaps even a lifelong, engagement with the arts.

What happens in the years following adolescence remains a mystery: human sciences may never be able to furnish convincing accounts of impressive individual achievements. Generalizations about artistic mastery are rife with risk. Yet, the information available in biographies of artists, coupled with results of our own studies of artistic development, suggest that artists have certain characteristics which bear more than a superficial resemblance to those of young children.

While mature artists have much better developed skills, far more control of their gifts, and superior abilities to experiment systematically and to choose deliberately among alternatives, much in their processes of creation is reminiscent of children. Both young children and adult artists are willing, even eager, to explore their medium, to try out various alternatives, to permit unconscious processes of play to gain sway. Moreover, both are willing to suspend (for somewhat different reasons) their knowledge of what others do, to go their own way, to transcend the practices and boundaries that overwhelm and inhibit "literal-age" children (and, quite possibly, lesser artists). While the tension overridden in transgressing custom is incomparably greater for older artists, the capacity to resist usual practice belongs no less to young children.

But it is in the forms of expression allowed by the arts that the closest tie exists between the young child and the adult artist. For both, the arts provide a privileged and possibly unique avenue by which to express the ideas, feelings, and concepts of greatest moment to them. Only in this way can individuals come to grips with themselves and express in ways that are accessible to others their own vision of the world. In the end, the artistic achievement emerges as intensely personal *and* inherently social—an act that arises from the most profound levels of one's own person and yet is directed to others in one's culture.

10

CHILDREN'S CONCEPTIONS

(AND MISCONCEPTIONS)

OF THE ARTS

WITH ELLEN WINNER

WE WOULD NOT expect children to learn to understand computers by having them examine a terminal or a printout. Yet that is the way we expect the young to become sensitive to ballet, theater, and the visual arts. Schools bus them to plays and museums; Leonard Bernstein offers youth concerts on television; and somehow artistic understanding is supposed to result.

To find out what such activities might accomplish, we asked questions of the children themselves. We wanted to see how their understanding of different art forms, concepts, and processes develop. We did not have explicit "right" answers in mind, but we wanted to understand better the way children of different ages think about the arts. And we found that, irrespective of social class, children pass through three distinct stages in their understanding of art.

Very young ones, between four and seven, go through a mechanistic phase in which they concentrate on the concrete aspects of art. Ask a five-year-old boy where a painting by Goya came from, for example, and he is likely to say a factory. Children of this age view artistic production as a simple, mechanical activity, and they believe that all judgments of artistic quality are equally valid.

Children around the age of ten are quite literal-minded and think a painting should be a painstaking copy of reality. Unlike younger children, ten-year-olds believe that there are ways of deciding whether a work is good or bad: the criterion of judgment is the degree of realism achieved.

By adolescence, youths have a more complex view of art, and their attitudes are not as rigid as those of younger children. They recognize differences of opinion and values but, reminiscent of the preschoolers, they may also view all art evaluation as relative.

These stages emerged in extensive interviews with 121 children, who were drawn equally from middle- and working-class families and who ranged in age from four to sixteen. Our conversations—patterned after those conducted by Jean Piaget—were flexible and open-ended, and we seized any opportunity to probe for elaboration on a child's answer.

We showed each child a picture, or read a poem, or played some music. We said that we were interested in his or her reaction and had some questions to ask, but that there were no right or wrong answers. We posed questions in seven general areas:

The source of art: Where do you think this came from?

The production of art: Who could do it? Could you make it too? What does it take to make something like this? Could an animal make it?

The medium: What is the difference between a photograph and a painting? Is the sound of a waterfall music?

Style: How can you tell if two paintings were done by two different artists?

Art and the outside world: What is the difference between a real shell and a painting of a shell? Does an artist always need a model?

Formal properties of art: How can an artist tell if a painting is finished? Could part of the work be changed? Would it still be the same?

Evaluation: Do you like it? How can you decide if it is good?

Children of different ages favored certain kinds of answers. We indicate here the typical responses of three major age groups: four to seven years, ten years, and fourteen to sixteen years.

The youngest group had a concrete and mechanistic concept of paintings and emphasized their technical aspects and limitations, such as the size of the canvas or the amount of paint available. They had no notion of art as being different from other aspects of the world. Indeed, many of these children at first denied that paintings are made by people. "All pictures are made at the factory," they insisted. Some offered animistic explanations: stories have always existed, songs are "made by God," paintings "just begin." Others said that art comes from materials: a poem comes "out of a pen," a painting comes "from paper and paint," and music comes from an organ, piano, banjo, or clock radio. Under our persistent prodding, two thirds eventually conceded that people make art.

On the other hand, when asked whether anyone could create a work of art, most children readily agreed. One child, summarizing the mechanical bias of his peers, claimed that anyone can make a picture, but "machines make prints and this is better than people making things." Only a few said that artists, or a special group of people, make art. Some peculiar responses were also found. One child was under the impression that "only the richest man" can paint, and another thought that "only a young man" can make art.

None of these children had the slightest inkling that it takes talent and training to produce a great work of art. "You just pick up a crayon and draw," they said, or "you just trace another picture." If painting is easier for some people, it must be because they are older, have watched others, or have simply had more lessons. "How long does it take to become good?" we asked, and they told us precisely: "One hour." "Three days."

Because almost all of the five-year-olds defined painting and writing in mechanical terms, as the simple wielding of a brush or pen, they concluded that animals could create art if they have the physical ability. Half said animals *could* paint because they have feet, tails, or trunks to hold the proper objects: "A tiger puts a pen in his mouth," "an elephant uses his trunk." The other half said animals could *not* paint because they lacked the right appendages: "they don't have hands," "their claws get in the way," or "they can't hold a brush."

The children usually confused the work of art with the thing it represented: they identified a Goya equestrian painting as "a horse" rather than as "a painting of a horse." When we pressed, most of them conceded that the horse was also a picture, but the medium was always of secondary importance to them, a transparency through which they looked at the object.

Just as they confused art with object, the children did not respect the usual boundaries of art forms. Some saw no difference between a photograph and a painting. Others had no way of distinguishing music from any other sounds, such as rhythmic tapping or water falling. In a way reminiscent of certain avant-garde artists, they said you could consider the noise of a car going by as music "if people like it" or "if you want it to be."

The children had little sense of an artist's style. We showed them a traditional painting (by Goya) and an abstract one (by Kandinsky) and asked if both could have been painted by the same person. Yes, said almost half the children. No, said the others, because "the artist would have gotten too tired if he had painted both."

Children's ideas about art in general are often contradicted by their own actions. For instance, little children draw many pictures that do not represent actual objects they see, but those we questioned nonetheless assured us that painters need a model to copy or that you make a picture by "looking at another painting and making it a little like it." One preschooler carefully explained to us that "if you're writing about what you see on a nice day, you couldn't write about it in the middle of the night."

If models are necessary for painting, we asked, would it be possible to draw a picture of something that cannot be seen in the world? Oh yes, they said, contradicting themselves. You can paint "a house that isn't there," or a fairy-tale person, or things that can be seen "only if you have invisible glasses in your eye."

We were intrigued to find that the four- and five-year-olds often liked abstract paintings more than realistic ones because of their "pretty colors," "nice design," or some imagined subject. They were also more likely than older children to tell us what the abstract work was about, or to find a specific image in it (such as a toy).

But by the time formal education took over, the child's interest in the real world was becoming dominant. Six- and seven-year-olds preferred traditional paintings because they were more realistic and therefore more impressive. Photographs, they said, are better than paintings because they are more lifelike, just as real objects are better than photos because they are solid and can be played with. "A real shell has an inside," they said, but a picture of a shell is "flat" and "just a copy."

Perhaps because they lacked a sense of the formal properties of an artwork, four- to seven-year-olds held some peculiar notions. For example, physical limitations rather than aesthetic ones determine when a work is done: a painting is finished when the artist "fills up the paper" or when the paint is dry. And, when considering whether a work could be altered, these children showed no awareness of the work as an integral whole. Their preoccupations were either mechanistic (if you've got the right equipment, such as a "special eraser," of course you could change a painting) or legalistic ("if the artist had made it and he sees there's a difference he might kill the person who changed it").

In general, children did not make critical judgments about the quality of a work of art, and there was no agreement about how one decides what is good. Some thought that all opinions were equally valid. If two people disagree in their judgments, "both are right," or perhaps they should vote on who is right. Some of the children took the subjective view—a painting is good "because I love it," as one child announced. A few thought that art evaluations should come from the authorities—not art critics or teachers, but "mommies and daddies," or "the boss."

By the age of ten, however, children did recognize proper authorities. It was not just you or I who decided what was good or bad, but, as one child explained, "people who have thought longer have better opinions."

Children at this intermediate stage were beginning to define the properties of different art forms. They felt that the noise of a passing car or the sound of tapping were not music but that a waterfall was because it created a rhythmic pattern. They were learning to recognize style and knew that a landscape by Poussin and one by Corot were by two different artists, even though they had the same general content.

Yet children of this age were intractably literal, viewing art primarily as an attempt to copy the details of the external world; the more accurate you were at this task, the better. In fact, the ten-year-olds were less able than the five-year-olds to conjure up imaginary worlds. To be sure, they agreed that one can paint something "that can't be seen in this world." However, they cited visible things like the moon and stars as examples of such "unworldly" things.

Perhaps their preoccupation with meticulous realism in art is a stage en route to more complex forms of aesthetic understanding. Perhaps one must master visual reality before one can translate it into abstract forms. In language and literature, by analogy, children must learn to use words literally before they can use them figuratively.

Few children go on to appreciate abstract forms of art. The adolescents we interviewed clung to traditional, realistic works, preferring these to abstract ones. The teenagers, of course, were more knowledgeable and sophisticated than the younger children. They thus agreed that there are many different ways and occasions on which to create art, and they understood its distinctly human and symbolic features. They knew that it was not enough to have paper, paints, and a hand or claw; an artist also needs talent and imagination.

Like the younger children, however, adolescents were unconcerned with the aesthetic issues involved in tampering with a work of art. No one noted its integrity as a unit, its uniqueness. While the youngest children worried about changing a painting on legal or punitive grounds, the adolescents brought up ethical factors: it would not be fair to the artist, they said, and you certainly would not claim credit for changing someone's efforts.

When asked how to evaluate art, teenagers were also reminiscent of very young children; it was all relative, they insisted, all a matter of taste. The adolescents seemed to have lost what the ten-year-olds were beginning to acquire—a set of standards that could be applied to any work of art—and insisted instead that no one painting was intrinsically better than any other. "There is no correct way to play music," one explained. "Good" art is whatever you like, just as some people favor spicy foods and others prefer bland tastes.

Many of the children's impressions about art seemed a natural part of their cognitive development. Even without teaching, a child will, over time, learn that a painting is not literally the thing it represents. And with time children learn the difference between the mechanical wielding of a brush and painting, between animal and human art, and between a bird's song and a symphony.

But because they rarely encounter issues of this sort, many children may not achieve the most basic forms of artistic understanding. Little children do not learn what makes one form of art unlike another, in what ways music differs from the sound of rain, how a great painting surpasses a mediocre one. Instead, they insist that an artist needs a model, even as they paint happily without one. And they create countless sketches and rhymes, but believe that paintings and poems come from factories.

Teachers and parents can help show children, at the proper stages of their development, where these contradictions lie. If children at the start of school saw and talked to artists at work, art might become more real, less remote. If children in the early grades could follow the creation of a painting from beginning to end, they might better understand the difference between an object and its representation.

And if children in the middle years of school wrote poems in class and discussed together why one phrase or word was preferable to another, they could begin to appreciate the formal criteria for judgment. All works of art are not equally good; music is different from sheer noise, and paintings need not be photographic copies of reality. Children are being shortchanged if they are not exposed to these ways of thinking about the arts. Indeed, if children are left to acquire understanding on their own, the whole domain of the arts may remain for them as distant as a star, as mysterious as the speaker of a dead language.

11

MAX AND MOLLY:

INDIVIDUAL DIFFERENCES

IN EARLY ARTISTIC

SYMBOLIZATION

WITH DENNIE WOLF AND ANN SMITH

MAX AND MOLLY, both aged three and a half, made the drawings reproduced here (figures 11.1, 11.2, and 11.3). The drawings share certain commonalities, notably the simplicity of forms, disregard of fine detail, and freedom in rendering spatial relations, which make them recognizable as the work of very young artists. Yet the differences between them are equally pronounced and perhaps even more striking. Max's drawing is highly active, featuring the clash of forms in a dramatic and dense array. Molly's bold, large-scale outlines make for much simpler and "quieter" drawings. But as the accompanying commentary indicates, Molly activates those simple contours with a rich story line, filling out their simplicity with dramatic play and narrative. Whereas Max strives to have the lines "tell all," Molly uses her drawings chiefly as a backdrop for her narrative abilities.

The charm of children's drawings sometimes obscures the achievement they exemplify. Just twelve months before these drawings were

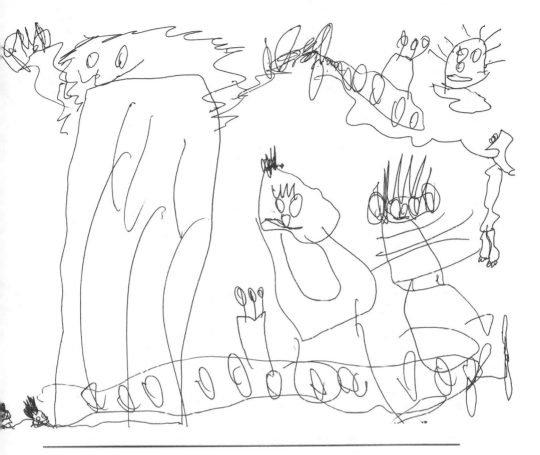

Figure 11.1. "Here, I'm done."—Max, age three and a half

made, neither child was constructing recognizable forms, let alone depicting events and experiences in the world. An additional year before that, the infants could hardly wield a marker at all. The swiftness and inexorableness with which children acquire the ability to use various artistic media is a formidable accomplishment that is only dimly understood at the present time. By the same token, the reasons for the characteristic differences obtaining among the works of children have yet to be unraveled. Recent research specifically focused on the child's creative use of symbols offers fresh hope that the puzzle of early child artistry may one day be resolved.

Appreciation of symbols is necessary for every aspect of life: whether

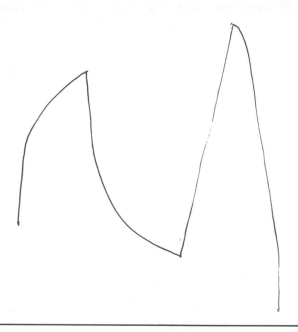

Figure 11.2. "An M . . . What does that spell? It spells M for Molly."

Figure 11.3. "And it could be a rabbit. See, it's got big ears. One, two. It's Flopsy, the talking rabbit. Flopsy, Mopsy, and Cottontail. . . . [holding up the paper, speaking in a tiny voice] Hello, I'm Flopsy, the talking rabbit, and I live with my brothers in a tiny house in the forest."—Molly, age three and a half

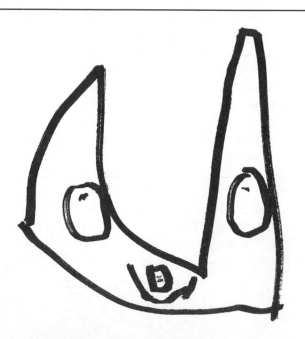

one is reading a map, computing change after a purchase, engaging in an argument, or simply contemplating a picture, one must recognize that a certain element, or set of elements, "stands for" some object or experience in the world. Indeed, so pervasive is symbol use in human culture that it is difficult to designate an area of human expression where symbols and symbolization are not entailed. Moreover, symbolization seems to play an especially important and prominent role in the arts. Not only do all art forms feature symbolization, but certain varieties of symbol use, among them the expression of emotion, exemplification of sensuous properties, and reference to the symbol itself are the particular province of the arts. Hence it is an outcome as happy as it is natural that much of the child's early symbol use centers about the media of the arts. Any effort to understand early symbol use must focus on the child's involvement with paints, clay, music, and literature; and any examination of the child's early visual and auditory products will inevitably invade the domain of the arts.

Philosophers, sociologists, anthropologists, and psychologists have at least paid lip service to the existence of symbols, referents, and systems of symbols. Some of the most insightful thinkers—among them Ernst Cassirer, Claude Lévi-Strauss, Clifford Geertz, Émile Durkheim, and Sigmund Freud—have deemed symbolization central to their inquiry into human activity. Within developmental psychology there has been a recognition that the opening two years of life are relatively devoid of symbol use, and that it is in the period between the ages of two and five that the child acquires an incipient mastery of the symbol systems of his culture. Indeed, whether one sees the child in the five-to-seven age group as relatively advanced or as a highly immature organism depends to a large extent on the assessment made of his symbolic competence and on a correlative judgment about the extent to which symbolization exemplifies the highest point of human intellectual activity.

There has, then, been considerable interest in symbol use. And yet earlier efforts in this domain have been marked by at least two crippling deficiencies. In the first place, there has been a strong tendency on the part of many commentators to lump together diverse forms of symbols and media. Perhaps when the very importance of symbolization was at issue, such a marshaling of forces was judicious; yet now that symbolization is generally acknowledged as central, the virtues of lumping together all aesthetic-symbolic systems evaporate. The fact is that symbol systems and media differ radically from one another in the nature of their elements, in the ways in which such elements are combined, in the kinds of reference of which they are capable, and in the psychological and neurological mechanisms that they invoke and evoke. Just contrast, for example, a natural language, which contains discrete words combinable according to a system of rules, with a pictorial symbol, devoid of isolable parts, resistant to syntactic analysis, and featuring innumerable untranslatable details. Or, to draw an example from the realm of media: contrast the potentials and the limitations of work with Play-Doh or clay with the "demand characteristics" governing such alternative media as collage, finger paint, or block-building.

Paired with the practice of merging all symbols has been an equally unproductive stance: an exclusive concentration on a single psychological aspect of symbol use. Both introspective evidence and empirical considerations suggest that a symbol is a complex, multifaceted element, and that symbolization is a correlatively intricate process. Indeed, even the youthful products glimpsed at the beginning of this essay clearly reflect potent intellectual operations, considerable neuromuscular control, and two highly individual personalities with implied variations in motivation, purpose, and self-assessment. Yet within the psychology of symbol use there has emerged an entrenched practice of considering symbolization in one, and only one, of two possible ways. We refer here to two traditional approaches.

The *cognitive approach,* exemplified by such researchers as Jean Piaget and Jerome Bruner, construes symbolic activity as pre-eminently an intellectual achievement. Only after the child has attained specific levels of general cognitive understanding will he possess the capacity to isolate various symbols, relate them appropriately to their referents in the world, and, eventually, infer the rules governing that system. And only after these milestones have been passed can he create full-fledged products *within that system.* Cognitivists, accordingly, focus on the intellectual underpinnings supporting competent symbol use, and they concern themselves with symbol use and art chiefly as evidence for mental growth.

The complementary approach, one centering on *affective* aspects of symbol use, is represented principally by students of personality, clinical psychology, and psychoanalysis. Taking for granted the child's ability to comprehend and produce symbols, investigators probe the uses to which symbolization is put, the reasons underlying these varied uses, and the role occupied by symbols in the emotional and affective life of the child.

114

Individual Differences in Early Artistic Symbolization

Peering at the drawings of Max and Molly, the cognitivist can make an assessment of the intellectual development of these children, for instance, by evaluating their mastery of spatial relations and their capacity to encode meaning. In contrast, the affectivist notes the *kind* of symbolization favored and, with the help of a clinical history, relates it to the child's relationship to his parents, the particular crises of past weeks, the goals and fears that presently occupy the child.

In counterpoising the cognitive and affective approaches to symbolization, we have sharpened the contrasts exceedingly. Yet even when sensitivity to the relation between cognitive and affective aspects exists, one point is clear: developmental psychologists have yet to devise an adequate means of characterizing all of symbolization—one doing justice to the wealth of influences and factors reflected in each symbolic product. In this essay we describe the modest beginnings and preliminary findings of one inquiry into early symbolic products. In so doing, we may able to suggest at least the faint outlines of a more comprehensive and accurate approach to early artistic activity.

Our discussion to this point has suggested three features of early symbol use: the great variety among children, as only hinted at by the works of Max and Molly; the need to investigate each symbolic medium separately in the wake of the telling differences among them; and the desirability of integrating in some manner the stances of the affectivist and the cognitivist, lest a misleading, one-sided view of symbolization result.

Such considerations led to our pilot study. A dozen children, ranging in age from two and a half to five, were drawn at random from a nursery school that enrolled the offspring of middle-class families. These youngsters were observed over several months as they engaged in daily preschool activities and as they played spontaneously with various symbolic media. Each child was also seen in more "controlled" surroundings by an experimenter who probed the child's approach and his responses to a number of experimental demands. Children worked individually with an observer in a series of approximately four sessions spread out over no more than a month.

Because of our interests in the child's performance with different symbols, and in the range of performance within a particular symbol system, these tasks varied along two dimensions. First of all, each child was asked to work with four separate symbolic media: language (storytelling); symbolic play (acting out a scene with geometric blocks that could "stand for" imaginary characters); two-dimensional depiction (drawing with Magic Markers); and three-dimensional depiction (molding or sculpting with Play-Doh). Then, within each of these four media, the child had to perform four tasks: produce a "work" or symbolic product spontaneously; complete a work which, though begun, had been left incomplete by the experimenter; assemble a work out of several parts or segments supplied by the experimenter; and copy or reproduce as faithfully as possible a work or performance exhibited by the experimenter.

The nature of these tasks is best conveyed by a few examples. To assess the ability of the child to produce a work "spontaneously" in the area of symbolic play, the experimenter provided the child with a set of ambiguously shaped wooden blocks. As a warm-up exercise, the experimenter asked the child to imagine what several of the shapes might be. Then the child was given the entire set of blocks and asked to "pretend whatever you want." To assess the ability to "copy" in the medium of clay, the experimenter showed the child a person molded out of clay and asked the child to "make one just the same." This task was repeated for two additional items—for instance, a car and a hat.

Analogous tasks were presented with other media. The ability to "complete" in the area of language involved playing with the puppet Steven Story-Teller, who loves to start stories but who never knows quite how to finish them. The puppet began by saying, "Once there was a cat who wanted to be a person. He thought that eating what people ate would help. So every day for lunch this cat had three sandwiches, four kinds of soup, six cookies, two marshmallows, and ten pickles." Steven Story-Teller then asked the child to finish the story. Finally, the ability to "assemble" in the area of drawing was assessed by inviting the child to play a game of "making things." The child was given a set of diverse geometric cutouts and shown how they could be assembled into patterns resembling simple objects. Subsequently the experimenter asked the child to assemble a man and two other items, such as a boat and a dog.

We hoped that through the use of several media we could obtain information about the way in which one child could handle different avenues of symbolization, and that the administration of several tasks would fix the limits of his competence with a medium. In one extreme case—the copy task—the form of the product was completely determined; while in the other extreme—the spontaneous task—the form of the product was determined by the child. Usual experimental procedures were employed; sessions were recorded and transcribed; the order of task presentation was counterbalanced across children; and the data were analyzed separately by, and then discussed among, three psychologically trained experimenters until a preliminary consensus on the findings had been reached.

Naturally, the administration of sixteen tasks to twelve children, and the accompanying accumulation of notes on informal classroom play and symbolization, yielded a literal closetful of data. Moreover, given the limited sample size, the crudity of data analysis for symbolic products, and, perhaps above all, the insistence on the part of many three- and four-year-olds on "redefining" our tasks, the results were suggestive at best and should not in any sense be regarded as conclusive. Yet, our results seem worth reporting for the light they shed on the three issues raised above: the variety of early symbol use in children; the distinction of symbol use in different media; and the integration of cognitive and affective aspects.

First, some general findings. We were astonished by the tremendous individual differences among the dozen participants in our study. Indeed, so singularly individual were our subjects that generalizations sometimes eluded us. Nonetheless, we did encounter some striking and recurrent patterns among our subjects. Some were inveterate *verbalizers;* in seeming indifference to the stated task, they produced copious amounts of language. Whether asked to tell a story, act out a scene, or fashion a clay figure, their response was likely to be an extensive narrative, perhaps featuring different voice parts, marked by only minimal action or visual-spatial operations. Other subjects were committed *visualizers;* though they certainly could talk, they did so reluctantly and minimally. Instead, they would plunge directly into drawing or building, exploring the possibilities with startling effectiveness, offering linguistic comments only sparingly, perhaps chiefly to silence the ever-inquisitive examiner. (In subsequent research, we have redescribed the two groups of children as "patterners" and "dramatists.")

Our subjects could also be classified as *self-starters* or as *completers.* The former group required but the barest stimulus to begin working with an aesthetic medium. And once such children commenced, they worked "fluidly" and effortlessly, fashioning one product after another. Other children, when confronted with an empty sheet or a formless wad of clay and an attentive observer, were quite reluctant to commence work. Such undefined situations appeared to evoke considerable anxiety. Yet given a product to finish, assemble, or copy, these completers took off; often they constructed a work more appropriate to the demands of the task and even more inventive than the abundant but often undisciplined productions of the self-starters. It is interesting to speculate about the end point of two such distinctive types of responses, asking if the self-starters are more likely to become creative artists and the completers to fill the ranks of critics, audience members, and editors.

Some other apparent dichotomies deserve passing mention. Certain of our subjects seemed quite *person-centered;* their characteristic forms of symbol use emphasized communication over creation. Their works often featured another individual, their antennae were constantly attuned to human feedback and intercourse. Sometimes, indeed, persons were added even when entirely superfluous, as in the case where a purse was completed by the addition of a mother and a child. Others in the group were much more *object-centered:* their works featured physical elements and machines; their efforts were more private and seldom modulated by another individual's presence.

Certain differences appeared to correlate with the child's gender. Girls were more likely than boys to sing, to employ an expressive voice, to excel with mixed media (as in symbolic play where gesture, narration, and three-dimensional forms can be blended) and with verbal tasks. Boys were more likely than girls to excel with clay and with single-medium tasks; they disliked and performed less competently with verbal tasks; and they evinced a perpetual fascination with the character of Batman. The predictable difference in subject-matter preferences could also be discerned (dolls versus trucks); but exceptions to this trend were sufficiently apparent to undermine the claims of "inborn" preferences for certain subject matters.

A final and somewhat unanticipated finding was the popularity with several children of certain fixed ideas, themes, or trademarks. Such schemes—they might be a character like Batman, an object like the Yellow Submarine, a medium preference like a blue Magic Marker, a little emblem like a bug, a recurrent motif like an "ant home"—not only occurred frequently within a single medium but were even discernible in the productions of some children across media. These fixed ideas among our population were prevalent enough to suggest that perhaps a return to a familiar theme or territory is a necessary element in artistic growth. Indeed, to secure cooperation, we sometimes had

118

to revise our tasks, bringing them in line with the child's treasured fixed theme. For instance, if a subject refused to complete a story about a cat, we would ask him to complete the same essential plot but featuring instead his favorite character—Oscar, the Grouch.

Close scrutiny of the "portfolio" of these preschoolers leads us to a rather complex notion of the role of fixed themes in children's art. Traditionally, return to a subject or repetitive use of single forms has been viewed as evidence of a persistent unresolved area of conflict in a child's emotional life or, conversely, as pointing out a kind of intellectual fixation, an inability to generate new solutions or approaches. Our study tentatively suggests that fixed themes serve different purposes for different children. For a majority, these recurrent motifs and ideas represent not fixation but a familiar territory in which variation, addition of new detail, and novel combinations can be readily explored. A good example comes from the child who drew a simple oval form for an animal body. Over a period of weeks he experimented with the differences that size, orientation, color, and articulation with a variety of detail could induce in his original scheme.

For a minority of children, fixed themes do appear to signal a less adaptive, more regressive function. An instance is provided by the child who, when faced with a request to copy a human figure or complete a boat, insisted on "making pizza," kneading the clay in a purely motoric fashion, thus avoiding the challenge presented by the requested forms. In addition, there were individuals who returned to themes in a compulsive and inflexible way, with hardly any variation discernible from one encounter to another. The child seemed to be gaining comfort from the mere ritualistic repetition of a certain motif. In fact, in the case of one three-year old, the recurrence of a rigidly drawn princess figure—learned from an older child—may have sheltered the child from struggling to render the variety of types of human figures engaged in a range of activities; and so the fixed theme in this case constituted an obstacle to experimentation and growth.

Because we analyzed the children's products along numerous dimensions, we were able to plot developmental trends and note differences among tasks. Not surprisingly, there was a host of areas in which children simply improved with age: older children were more likely to plan, to be flexible, to follow instructions faithfully; and they were less likely to be playful or to repeat themes without alteration. In general, we found regular developmental trends in those tasks that tapped understanding of a medium, command of the task situation, and overall adaptability. In contrast, we failed to find such sequences in a number of areas, such as the child's characteristic approach to a task, his preference for language as opposed to action, and his assessment of his own capabilities. These contrasting sets of findings suggested a moral to us. Might it not be that those facets of a child's behavior that prove relatively constant throughout early childhood are of an affective cast, while those that are marked by a systematic change over time belong, relatively speaking, to the cognitive camp?

The specific task types provided further illumination. As already mentioned, the spontaneous tasks proved inviting to certain youngsters, while markedly intimidating for others. The copying tasks usually disclosed the highest limits of a child's capabilities; and yet, because such a task furnished a specific model, it often provoked anxiety. In contrast, the assembly tasks were only minimally threatening. Since one was given the "parts," creation from scratch was unnecessary; yet in the absence of an explicit standard to copy, "anything went."

Finally, the completion task yielded particular insights into the child's own psychodynamics. When the child was confronted with the raw elements of a situation or composition and required to bring it to completion, his own personality, motivations, problems, and priorities seemed almost inevitably to emerge. For instance, in completing a symbolic play sequence where a feisty beetle attacks a small bug, children who were unabashed at displaying aggression often "fought it out," while others sought to resolve the conflict through talk and arbitration between bug and beetle. Indeed, so revealing of current pressures and preferences were the completion tasks that they might become useful diagnostic adjuncts or supplementary projective tests for the clinician.

The diverse performances evoked by these tasks were quite revealing. They indicated to us how insufficient it is to look only at a child's spontaneous creations or solely at his performance within a given structured task. Only through administration of several types of tasks, and through a judicious collation of the findings across these tasks, can comprehensive conclusions be reached about the child's relationship to a medium. Moreover, once the range of demands within a medium is taken into account, even greater consistency may be detected in children's performances at certain tasks (all the completions, or all the assembly tasks) than in their performances within a medium.

Even this brief look at a few representative findings should convey the richness and complexity of a child's early symbolic products. Many of these products virtually "cry out" for further explanation: when one hears a specific story (about the death of a policeman) or notices a recurrent theme (rabbit ears or ant homes), curiosity about the source of these motifs is heightened. It seems to us that the only way of resolving this curiosity is to interact intensively over a long period of time with specific youngsters. Only then can one assess with some certainty just how a particular product comes into being. And so we have undertaken with a group of nine youngsters a longitudinal study of this sort. By following these youngsters through early childhood, we expect to secure reliable information about the range of factors that culminate in specific symbolic products.

Even the preliminary results reviewed here may suggest an answer to the central enigma of early symbol use. We have seen that the works of young children can be assessed on a broad array of dimensions and that these dimensions generally divide the subjects into two or more recognizable groups. There are typical visualizers; average person-centered youngsters; representative self-starters. Moreover, consistent with many earlier studies in the literature, we have confirmed that the works of young children can readily be categorized according to their level of technical competence. Once one becomes familiar with children's stories, play sequences, or graphic representations, it is a relatively straightforward matter to assess the "mental age," or "developmental level," of the producer of the work.

The great individual differences among youngsters stem, then, not from any single dimension (for, after all, many children will realize a similar level on that dimension), nor from the particular level of symbolization reflected (for, by definition, this will prove parallel across children at the same developmental milestone). Rather, the distinctiveness of children's products and, indeed, of each child's product, reflects the interaction of several factors: the child's general command of symbolization; his propensity for verbalizing, self-starting, and person-centeredness; the particular task posed within the medium; the recent events and pervading traits and motivations that characterize his life—just to cite a few.

Far from representing a deterrent to decisive research, however, these individual differences may turn out to be thought-provoking. We have seen that the cognitivist is so preoccupied with grouping subjects according to developmental level that the enormous differences across children within each level have tended to elude him. For his part, the person concerned with affective development has been so struck by personal characteristics and idiosyncratic qualities of specific young-sters that he has often overlooked profound continuities across children in skills of production and comprehension. We believe that, in the last analysis, the fullest understanding of the young child's work will come from setting aside this dichotomy, from thinking instead in terms of the intersection of multiple factors. As a preliminary step, we propose appropriation into the aesthetic domain of the concept of "cognitive style"—the particular way in which each child realizes the universal properties of symbolization at his level of development.

Whereas all children come to explore the variety of symbolic forms made possible by a range of media, they do so in ways that are peculiarly their own. Here an illustration is immensely helpful. Let us look briefly at the way in which the two children cited earlier make use of the same medium—drawing. Max, a small but active child of three and a half, has long gravitated to the tables where markers and stacks of computer paper are stored. At school and at home, drawing has been a favored activity. As he uncovered, at a remarkable rate, the possibili-ties and conventions of representational drawing, he used his widening knowledge in the portrayal of a wonderfully elaborate world where Batman, Robin, and the Joker and Sesame Street's Oscar, Ernie, and Bert intermingled in a wild melee of high adventure. He used his control of line and spatial relations to caricature as well as to capture the frantic pace of these forays. As a result, his drawings are rich in detail and remarkable for their dynamism.

Interestingly enough, the impetus for making such drawings often sprang from his own dramatic playing out of television-inspired epi-sodes, wherein Max and his closest friend were inevitably Batman and Robin in hot pursuit of a third child cast in the role of the villain Joker. Max's drawings were often reports on or extensions of these exploits. Coming in from outdoors, Max would often seize marker and paper to continue a chase that coming in had cut short. Alterna-tively he would engineer on paper what was out of reach in play—a wild battle of all parties aboard the Yellow Submarine with a giant octopus in hot pursuit. As a consequence, Max's drawings were win-dows on an engaging play world; his works exploited the power of the graphic medium to encode interaction, motion, sequence of events. As a result, Max focused his attention less on the creation of a conscious design (he was rarely noted in careful appraisal of *this* figure or *that* line). Rather, his drawings spilled over and out of active play and unfolded in rapid fire onto the paper, deliberately preserving, in blue marker line that barely paused, the sequence and intensity of the events depicted. For Max, the distance between immediate experience and drawing was very short. Drawing needed no supplement, no linguistic elaboration, to "tell it how it was." It was remarkably autonomous and capable. Max was clearly a visualizer.

Astonishing as was Max's achievement in drawing, it represented but a segment of a much larger accomplishment. During the second and third years, as a child's intellectual and physical autonomy wins him the right to play with sand, crayons, blocks, and paints, he struggles toward a definition of what is possible, difficult, or impossible with specific materials. During the fourth and fifth years he converts this physical understanding into a comprehension of media potentials, coming to an acute understanding of how to render figures, buildings, even action in each. Max learned essential formulas for reducing the three-dimensional world to the two dimensions of graphic symbols, for portraying action with agitated line, for conveying emotion through caricature. But this learning was in no way restricted to drawing. He made these same realizations for a broad array of materials. Thus he could also fashion a Batmanlike form out of clay, enact a narrative sequence with a set of blocks, and also relate an entire Batman saga in words alone: "And this is Batman and he is really strong—stronger than anybody, even the Joker. And he gets this cape and he wears it all the time. . . ."

The fact that the "accurate variety" of medium-appropriate symbols occurs so rapidly and so assuredly signals how fundamental is the notion that words, pictures, and gestures neither capture nor convey meaning in identical ways. In developmental terms this should awaken us to the possibility of different trajectories and time schemes for the elaboration of various forms of representation. (For instance, the possibility of representation in clay, given its inherent correspondence to a three-dimensional world, occurs earlier than the identical discovery in drawing, which demands the reduction of an object with volume to a contoured line.) In educational terms, this same realization hints that individuals might well exhibit talents and predilections in one form of self-expression rather than another. Where art is concerned, this realization should inform appreciation, sensitizing us to the particular vocabularies of given media: evoking wonder when Rodin captures the halo of hair in so massive a medium as bronze; allowing us to delight in the Japanese woodcut's feathery wave as well as in the square, woven wave pattern in Indian textile design.

Molly realized in quite a different way the potentials of the various media at her disposal. Her symbolic play ranged more broadly than Max's; she exploited the reach and transformation of fantasy, playing at being a rabbit, a gypsy, a witch. Moreover, her dramatic play drew its images from children's literature and personal recollection rather than from television, and as a result its accents and contours were essentially those of narrative. Molly delighted in taking on a new identity, changing voices, wearing costumes, putting on exaggerated expressions, and trying out new gestures. More than being a draftsman, Molly was an actress and a narrator. Molly's love of play-acting and stories meant that she came to drawing later and more incidentally than Max. Even though the same years and comparable mental abilities seemed to be present, their drawings differ widely in sophistication. While Max was devising complex scenes, Molly produced simple outlines.

This difference in the emergence of picturing seemed to reflect the role that the children attributed to drawing rather than to sheer capacity at two-dimensional depiction. Where Max used drawings to engineer events beyond the limits of dramatic play, Molly employed dramatic play to fill out the simple contours of her drawings. Molly's drawings usually presented a single character or object, outlined directly and without ornamentation. Detail and action were contributed by language and gesture, which transformed the figure into the central character of a small drama. The drawing was not, as it was for Max, an entire scene from a drama: it was merely the scenery. Against this backdrop, Molly herself acted out the various parts, eagerly moving her fingers or torso about to signify the movements of the actors, deliberately changing the pitch and intonation of her voice in order to portray the wolf, the frightened little rabbit, the protective mother rabbit, even incorporating nearby objects as props to her stage-managing. The marker still in her hand, but quite stationary, Molly often incorporated songs and rhymes into the narrative fabric she spun around her drawing, exploring auditory patterns more than visual design. As opposed to Max, Molly is a narrator, entrusting her meanings and feelings to language more often than to the drawn image. Being more nearly a "verbalizer," Molly makes drawings that are simple, their bold contours occurring in response to a character description or recounted event.

Even so brief a comparison reveals that children of the same age and comparable capacity react to an identical medium in markedly different ways. Not only do they employ it to depict characteristic messages, but they make of it radically different instruments. For Max the drawing *is* the drama; for Molly the drama begins once the drawing is done. Consequently, Molly's drawing may rest at schematics, whereas Max wrestles with finding out how to portray a flying figure, a boat on water, a figure falling over backward. Were one to reverse the grounds of consideration and take a close look at these children's command of narrative forms, it might well be that Max would emerge the schematizer, Molly the sophisticated user.

Our intensive observations of individual children have underlined the multifaceted quality of early symbol use. While discussion of symbolization was occurring on a theoretical level, it was possible to lump all symbolic activities together, to speak exclusively of the child's symbolic level, or to see in the child's symbol simply an occasion for a personality diagnosis. Such one-dimensional treatments are clearly inadequate, however, for giving a holistic picture of the different achievements of children like Max and Molly. Indeed, the real challenge for this generation of researchers is not whether we can glimpse in rapid alteration the cognitive and affective faces of symbolization, but rather whether we can perceive the same object in light of these and other facets of symbolization simultaneously.

Let us return, in this context, to Molly's sequence of drawings presented earlier. She began by carefully forming a large M, the first letter of her own name, which she was diligently learning to write. Her relative unsophistication in the graphic medium left her open to suggestion, and she glimpsed quite another possibility in the large letter form. Closing the giant M at the bottom she created a "rabbit"—"Flopsy, the talking rabbit." Holding the paper so that the rabbit was upright like an actor, she remarked, in a tiny voice, "Hello, I am Flopsy, the talking rabbit. I live with my brothers in a tiny house in the woods."

Even in this incident of a few seconds, varied abilities surfaced and intertwined. From the affective angle, there was a sense of pleasure and power at being able to "put herself on paper," either in the form of the letters of her name or as the creator of Flopsy, a figure of line that genuinely resembles a rabbit. Making an M into a rabbit was doubly meaningful, as Molly's own stories and dramatic creations often have a rabbit as heroine, or Molly herself as a small adventurous rabbit. In this light the M and the rabbit face might both be construed as symbols for herself, her pleasure at their creation deriving from an assertion of her own identity through the graphic medium.

The same series of events in Molly's drawings has intellectual facets as well. The pleasure of making symbols for the self rests on the understanding that a graphic form can refer to a live event, formulating it for oneself and sharing it with others. The "joke" of making an M into a rabbit is not only amusing, it bespeaks appreciation of the "real-world" distances between animals and letters. Much as the joke may create a relatedness between the joker and her audience, it also binds them together in the understanding that the same element may have diverse meanings (the diagonal lines serving alternatively as a letter or the partial contour of the rabbit's face). Other elements of these drawings also require consideration: the eye and hand coordination required to trace the M in the first place; the perceptual matching (or "visual metaphor") entailed in seeing the M as a rabbit's ears; the social awareness signaled by M as Molly fleshes out the spare drawing with an impassioned narrative. She is keenly aware of her audience, holding up the drawing so that the observer can see it, unfolding her narrative so that it has a public meaning, in a style that signals cognizance of the rules for composing a story. We see that these (and other) facets of Molly's pictures never serve but one master: indeed, only if the various lines, shapes, and meaningful components are perceived both as expressions of significant feelings and as attempts to capture knowledge can the power of the symbol be fully grasped. If the sequential nature of language compels us to discuss these facets separately, one following another, we are challenged to create a picture image in which the various facets underlying symbolization are organically fused.

As different from one another as Max's and Molly's picture of the world may be, it is still possible to render this kind of account of their various symbolic products. A highly individual and readily recognizable set of identifying marks already seems to be manifest in the miniature artistic efforts of the preschool child. Just what factors give rise to an intense involvement with the visual properties of media in one case, and with their linguistic and dramatic properties in the other, remains to be determined. If our preliminary study is any guide, researchers will eventually have to take into account the child's native endowment and predilections (including the structure of his brain), the predominant practices of his culture, the particular demands and expectations of his family, the availability of various production media, the particular tasks posed, the interaction of the child's level of symbolization, and current preoccupations and motivations during the occasion of symbolization. This is an ambitious program, particularly in view of the still meager tools and analytic powers of researchers interested in these questions. Yet even the ability to define with some precision questions of early artistry and symbolization represents progress. And since the ultimate outcome of such inquiries will be a deeper understanding of the individual's most personal and most meaningful creations, this investigative course seems worthy of continued intensive exploration.

12

THE GOLDEN AGE OF DRAWING

BETWEEN THE AGES of five and seven most children in our society achieve notable expressiveness in their drawings. Having mastered the basic steps of drawing and learned to produce acceptable likenesses, they go on to produce works that are lively, organized, and almost unfailingly pleasing. One feels that the child is speaking directly through the drawings, that each line, shape, and form conveys the inner feelings as well as explicit themes in the young child's efforts to understand the world.

There is also at this age, perhaps for the first and sometimes the last time, an easy, natural commerce among various media. The child sings as he draws, dances as he sings, tells stories while at play in the bathtub or in the backyard. Rather than allow each art form to progress in relative isolation from the others, children move readily and even eagerly from one form to another, combine the forms, and play them off against one another. In fact, an age of synesthesia begins: a time when, more than any other, the child effects easy translations across sensory systems; when colors can readily evoke sounds and sounds can readily evoke colors; when motions of the hand suggest lines of poetry or lines of verse stimulate a dance or a song.

This eruption of artistry at the threshold of school represents for me the central fact—and enigma—of artistic development. One can speak without exaggeration of a flowering of capacities during this period. But must we therefore conclude that the child of five, six, or seven is a young artist?

Many people have chosen to answer the question in the affirmative, finding in children's art the essential antecedents of later creative mastery. Taking their lead from the educational views of Rousseau, art educators like Herbert Read have seen the years of early childhood as a golden period in artistic development—one that may rapidly fade and that teachers and parents are thus challenged to nourish.

But there is another, less romantic view, which many psychologists influenced by Jean Piaget would embrace. According to these scholars, youthful works, whatever their appeal to sophisticated audiences, may represent something quite different to the child. Perhaps the child is simply engrossed by the process of producing components—be they the lines of a drawing or the notes of a song—while having scant interest in the eventual product. Perhaps those forms that so please us are but happy accidents. Indeed, children may have no choice in the matter but may feel compelled to produce what they do—in which case it would be, at best, misleading to attribute artistic significance to the final product.

To resolve these issues, which are central to any discussion of children's art, we must first examine some drawings by children of average gifts in this age group and demonstrate their special spirit and life.

Like nearly all boys (and many girls) who spend their Saturday mornings sprawled in front of the television, my son Jerry (as I will refer to him here) became fascinated by superheroes when he was on the verge of entering school. After a particularly exciting episode of "Batman," he made his first effort to draw one of his heroes. When he was younger he had a limited repertoire, consisting mainly of sticklike or tadpole-shaped human figures. Now barely four and a half years old, Jerry drew Batman with a pentagonal body, two protruding legs, a wide cape extending on either side, and the familiar pointy-eared head.

In the following days he was literally obsessed with drawing Batman. Every day after school he would rush home and undertake additional efforts—in color or black and white, in marker or in pencil, on lengthy galley proofs or napkins—to get Batman straight. By the second day, copying from a bubble-gum card, he had already gotten the shape of the cape under better control, attempted its fringelike bottom, separated it from the hero's body, and sought to capture the identifying emblem

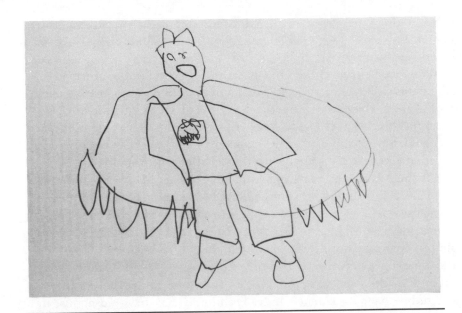

Figure 12.1

Figure 12.2

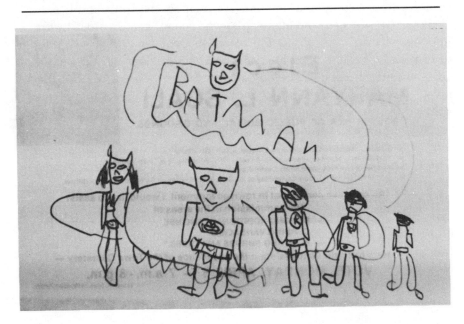

on Batman's chest and the distinctive boots and pants (see figure 12.1). Two days later he produced a whole cast of superheroes, each one sporting a characteristic emblem, a piece of headgear, and clothing (see figure 12.2).

Jerry's command of the forms was now well enough established so that he could produce each figure with a relatively small set of recognizable strokes; like a commercial artist, he had hit upon a formula, a kind of notation, a way of limning the superheroes so that they were readily recognizable. Excitement and adventure were suggested by the bright colors of their costumes and, in one case, by the dynamic linear patterns with which the costumes were rendered. Yet for the most part Jerry remained content to align the heroes alongside one another, like suspects in a police lineup.

The obsession with Batman continued for several months. Then along came the space extravaganza *Star Wars*, which caught the imagination of children all over the world, Jerry included. This time the task of depiction was more daunting, for *Star Wars* included a large number of characters that were not human or even humanoid. Before even seeing the movie, Jerry tried to draw—and to master—specific characters. Then, while drawing an exploding rocket ship, he made an initial attempt to include a spaceship from *Star Wars*. The following week he created his first full *Star Wars* composition. Beneath the title he portrayed the "ship of the good guys," the robot Artoo Detoo, the spaceship, the hero Luke Skywalker, and, as if to balance the forces

Figure 12.3

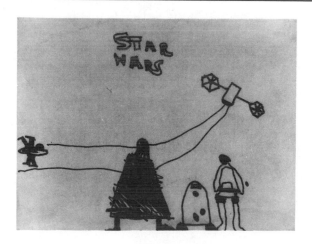

of good, the villain Darth Vader and the "ship of the bad guys" (figure 12.3). He had already mastered the iconography of the dramatis personae well enough so that he could make each recognizable.

The basic features of all characters having been mastered, Jerry was ready within a month for the next challenge: action scenes involving a number of protagonists. Sometimes these scenes were taken directly from the movie, which Jerry had heard all about but saw only later; sometimes they involved liberal invention from his own imagination, or a merger between characters from *Star Wars* and other media heroes.

Jerry turned his attention next to creating an organized scene. The first effort, reminiscent of the earlier lineups, featured Darth Vader strangling a rebel, ringed by the trash compactor on his right and a storm trooper and Artoo Detoo on the left. Up above floated a good ship as well as the ubiquitous *Star Wars* logo. Greater success was achieved in the final scene: a fight to explode the death star, the base of Darth Vader (figure 12.4). Here the death star is surrounded by a series of black circular explosions, a set of good-guy ships and a number of bad-guy ships, each hosting its own explosion. Though the final product is still static, a clear attempt has been made to capture the *Star Wars* conflict within a single frame.

One more illustration is worth noting. On a tiny piece of scrap paper, Jerry drew some paraphernalia from the *Star Wars* saga (figure 12.5). As he described it, "One ship is shooting at a rocket. On the other side is the blood explosion—that's because of the war." In this little episode we can see glimmerings of what will later become the norm in Jerry's and in other children's symbolic expression. The verbal story line is beginning to dominate: the drawings function increasingly as notations to supplement the story rather than as accurate or even fanciful graphic depictions of a scene that has been viewed "in the mind's eye."

Figure 12.4

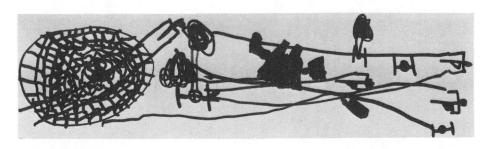

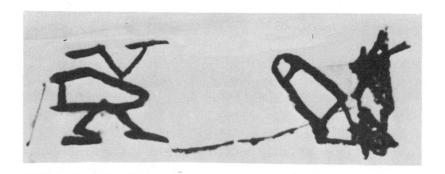

Figure 12.5

Just what is going on in these drawings? At times they seemed inspired primarily by a reportorial function: Jerry seemed simply to want to describe to someone how something looked or how it occurred. Much more frequently, however, the drawing seemed to be in itself an important expression, an act essential for the psychological well-being of the child. In describing this act, we may perhaps come to understand why children of this age draw so much, and with such passion, tension, and expressiveness.

We have viewed Jerry at an age when, like so many other youngsters, he was preoccupied with issues of action, power, and violence. No need to invoke Oedipal complexes or male aggressive drives here, though one may certainly do so. At a descriptive level, these themes are simply ones that rivet his attention, even as the process of baking cookies came to intrigue him some months later. Jerry did not have a vocabulary to discourse on the psychological themes of power and conflict; nor, indeed, did he seem to exhibit much inclination to converse at all about his drawings. They were not for the dinner table. Yet they were clearly important to him, as evidenced by his attraction to books, comics, and television shows that presented them. Jerry's *Star Wars* drawings portrayed his general passion and enthusiasm. But the vast majority of sketches also prominently featured violence, maiming, and conflict.

By the age of four, five, or six, children have made an initial cut at understanding the behavior and feelings that are being enacted, talked about, and worried about in their world. Some of these themes can be quite disturbing, and some of the fears they evoke can be almost disabling. Accordingly, it becomes very important for a child to try to make sense of them in his own way, to make peace, if at all possible, with powerful forces in the environment. Such "settling" and "understanding" activity is most likely to take place with those characters and forces that have already made a strong impression, are becoming increasingly familiar, and are slowly yielding their meanings. They are often likely to be characters that loom larger than life, characters whose traits and features prove unmistakably charged.

Given the preoccupation of children like Jerry with such fantastic characters, be they the mythic or fairy-tale heroes of old or the spacemen of tomorrow, the question arises about the degree to which these characters possess real-life potency. When questioned directly, most children will concede that they think *Star Wars* could not really have happened and that the characters they are drawing are "just pretend" or "not real." Their own behavior, however, indicates just as clearly that the characters possess vast power: the stories tend to induce real fears, such as those associated with robbers, parental punishments, or ghosts that might live in their own houses.

It is not really so much that the child expects Ben (Obi-Wan) Kenobi or the Jawa to enter his house one afternoon and sit down at the dining room table; indeed, should that happen, the child would probably be as amazed as his parents. It is rather that the child does not know for sure which aspects of *Star Wars* are likely to occur in the real world and which are purely fantastic, and so the criteria for whether one should be amused or frightened are much less certain.

Similarly, a child may not live in constant fear that Darth Vader will one day invade his room. But he knows that there are other villains and bullies (or parents) who can tyrannize him, and he knows the terror of unalloyed fear or anxiety. It is because the adventure stories remind him of these instances that they sometimes frighten him, even as they captivate his attention and interest. And it is through drawing, I submit, that the child makes his initial efforts to gain some control of his feelings about these powerful themes.

Even as Jerry's days and nights came to be dominated by the odd characters of *Star Wars*, his sister Kay (as I will call her here) developed a preoccupation that is common among many young girls: she became completely devoted to the world of horses. In this case the inspiration did not come from mass media, though Kay did collect numerous books about horses, but rather from her own experiences—initially during her visits to farms and, soon after, during her own attempts to ride.

At first, when she was six, Kay drew lone horses, which were graphically as well as thematically simple. They were elaborated out of a simple rectangular schema, with initially two, and then four, appendages for legs. The horses were, indeed, little more than elongated tadpole forms.

It soon became apparent, however, that the horse was more than just another schema in Kay's growing graphic armamentarium. She took special care in the elaboration of its form, and she began to weave her drawings of horses into stories, poems, and play scenes that were assuming an increasingly important niche in her daily imaginative life.

Shortly after returning home from a trip to a farm, Kay produced one of her simple schematic horses and captioned it with a poem that we helped her to transcribe (figure 12.6). In its disarming simplicity of both word and form, the verse captures a feeling she strongly endorsed:

A horse is a wild animal
A horse should be free
A horse should be left like it was built to be.

Two months later she depicted two of the horses on which she had ridden the previous summer (figure 12.7). The body schema was still elementary, but this time each horse was composed of a single amoebalike contoured line, and instead of standing squarely on the ground, the horses were shown heading toward a little girl—presumably Kay—who, we may assume, was waiting eagerly for them underneath

Figure 12.6

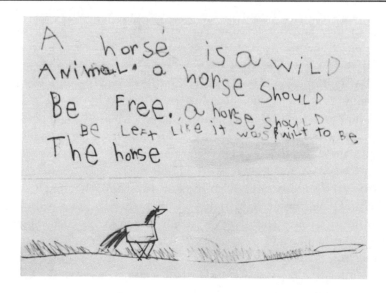

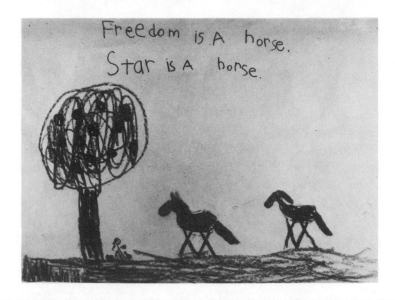

Freedom is A horse.
Star is A horse.

Figure 12.7

an apple tree. Other efforts of this period revealed that Kay was also experimenting with depiction of a riding habit and was placing horses in other simple compositions—for example, in a floral pattern.

Even during this early period it was evident that Kay's vision was practically the opposite in tone to Jerry's: a quiet pastoral life where one could love horses, a desire for a setting devoid of loud and harsh activity, a time for contemplation and for the exercise of the deep feelings of love and tender care. Yet one can also see at work many of the motifs and forms that characterized Jerry's involvement with *Star Wars:* deeply felt emotions; an emerging sense of compositional form in which the various elements of the canvas join to yield an overall expressive effect; use of color in which the orthodox hues of objects were sometimes sacrificed either in order to produce heightened emotional expression or to yield a canvas replete with pleasing blends.

Despite these converging signs of preoccupation with horses, I was not prepared for a remarkable work produced by Kay at the end of her sixth year—an illustrated account of an adventure that had befallen her the previous summer (see figures 12.8 and 12.9). The little book Kay fashioned relates the story in seven drawings, a single abstract design, and nine pages of narration. We learn that Kay and her friends had gone for a ride, when "suddenly a girl's horse stepped out of the trail for a second and stepped into a yellow-jacket nest. All the horses were stung." Thereupon, the other horses panicked; the youngsters were thrown; Kay and a friend were discovered by her mother; the owner of the stable was relieved that none of the girls had been hurt; and Kay remembered well her refreshing reward at the end of that day—a Coke.

In this story Kay deliberately simplified the various forms so that she could communicate a considerable amount of information in both words and pictures. She soon became able to concentrate much more fully on purely visual aspects of the horse. One drawing featured smoother, more contoured bodies and bent legs, as well as an effort to show one animal physically dominating another.

By the time Kay had turned seven, a subtle change began to mark her drawings. The horses themselves became more stylized. They tended to appear in a graceful walking or jumping position, their profiles now regularly arrayed to their right; their manes and tails were smoothly groomed; and they exhibited carefully placed features—every hair and limb seemed precisely in place. Sometimes they were placed in a scene with a rider; sometimes they were depicted alone; sometimes they oc-

Figure 12.8

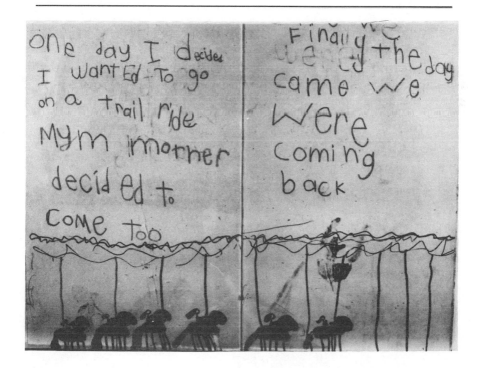

One day I decided
I wanted to go
on a trail ride
Mym mother
decided to
come too

Finally the day
came we
were
coming
back

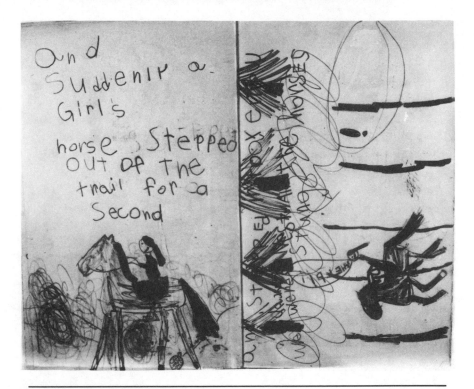

And
Suddenly a
Girl's
horse Stepped
out of The
trail for a
Second

Figure 12.9

curred in an organized composition, surrounded by carefully colored flowers and a sun with numerous rays of different hues (see figure 12.10). Another of her drawings, at age eight, was a concentrated attempt to produce a convincing likeness of a few particular aspects of the horse: its head, its facial features, and its neck (see figure 12.11).

But even as this increase in precision and, if you will, photographic realism can be discerned, a muting of creative originality also seems evident. Dramatic scenes give way to bucolic compositions: adventurousness in depiction gives rise to an elegant but essentially static composition that becomes wholly predictable. Kay herself lamented that her drawings were not as good as they had been two years before, and, at least in certain respects, I agreed with her. As she once put it, "I used to draw much better. My drawings were more interesting, but my perspective is three thousand times better now." The age of artistic expressiveness, or at least its original flowering, seemed to have come to an end.

138

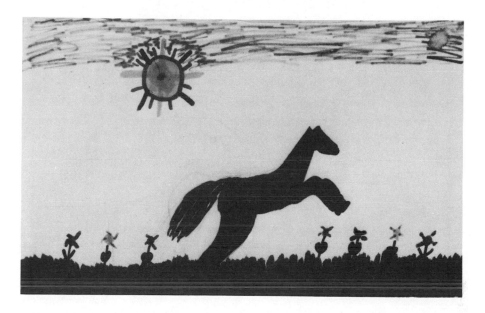

Figure 12.10

We have now observed some representative efforts of children's art—works that, I must stress, are in no way remarkable for children of that age. There is little doubt that the works have a certain power and charm, but we must now return to the original question and assess the extent to which they can be characterized as art.

Certainly, the care taken by children in making the drawings, their own pleasure in producing them, and the fascination the drawings sometimes have for others make it difficult to dismiss them out of hand. Surely the drawings are not just happy accidents. Before we can assess them as art, however, we need some working definitions of the word.

One criterion, much honored in the psychological literature, might be the degree of realism in the work. The history of art in the twentieth century, however, so clearly refutes this point of view that it is difficult to take it seriously any longer, except perhaps for certain limited experimental purposes. A second criterion is also flawed: the criterion of excellence. Not only is it extremely difficult to find standards of judgment that represent a genuine consensus over a significant period of time, but it is also quite possible that a work judged as excellent was

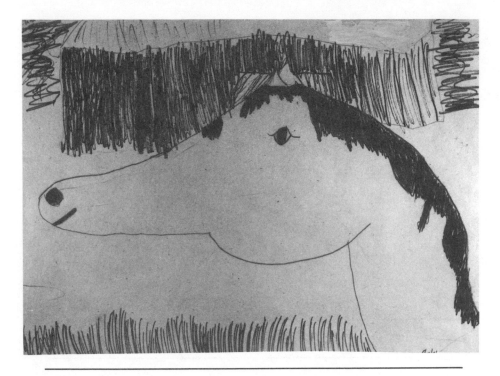

Figure 12.11

an accident (for example, the random marks of a chimp that happened to resemble a highly valued abstract work).

Some less chimerical and less fragile aesthetic criteria have been proposed by Nelson Goodman. He proceeds from the observation that artworks are symbols that function in certain kinds of ways—for example, by calling attention to their own detailed construction or expressing certain identifiable moods. Goodman has suggested that a work's artistic status depends on the extent to which it exhibits those properties of symbols that are considered aesthetic. Despite appearances, the definition is not circular, for Goodman has specified what he means by aesthetic.

As we noted in earlier essays, Goodman stresses two criteria. The first is the *expressiveness* of the symbols in a drawing. If a child uses the materials of a medium in such a way as to make a drawing that is lively, sad, angry, or powerful, that is one sign that he can fashion a work of art. A second criterion is *repleteness*, or full use of the medium's potential. If the child can use the material in a way that exploits several of its characteristics significantly, he is again demonstrating a capacity to use symbols in an artistic way. For instance, if the thickness, shape, shading, and uniformity of line all contribute to the work's effect, the child is exhibiting a command over repleteness.

While such definitions are a useful starting point, any individual assessment of these qualities remains highly subjective. Nonetheless, a promising method of determining whether drawings exhibit such aesthetic properties can be found in an ingenious study conducted by Thomas Carothers, who worked with me some years ago when he was at Harvard. As already described in essay 9, "The Child as Artist," Carothers exposed youngsters to drawings that were identical to one another save in the kind of artistic quality they displayed. He did this in order to determine whether the children would notice such properties as expressiveness and repleteness and whether they could in their own drawings exploit these "symptoms of the aesthetic."

Carothers found a remarkably regular sequence of behavior in his studies. First graders showed little or no artistic sensitivity on any of his tests. Fourth graders exhibited some limited sensitivity, particularly when they were given the opportunity to select the correct items from multiple choices, and sixth graders exhibited a fullblown set of aesthetic symptoms. Thus when measured by this relatively conservative set of instruments, children only gradually become able to produce symbols that qualify for the epithet of "works of art."

Additional support for the claim that children's aesthetic awareness increases with age comes from a dissertation by Diana Korzenik, an educator currently at the Massachusetts College of Art. Korzenik reasoned that if a child is to be considered in control of his capacities, he must possess some awareness of how a work looks to others. She asked some children to draw a specified subject so that a child seated in an isolated chamber, who was allowed to see only the drawing, would be able to recognize that subject—say, a figure jumping. The child doing the drawing was allowed to hear the guesses made by the isolated viewer and then to revise his drawing in order to make it more recognizable. If the child proved able to alter the drawing so that it could be identified, this flexibility would suggest the "dissolution of egocentrism" which figures crucially in any artist's repertoire.

Once again the youngest subjects—this time about five years old—proved quite oblivious to the reactions of others. They rarely altered their drawings from one trial to another, blithely expecting that the drawings would "speak for themselves." They confused intent for achievement, blaming the other child when he failed to guess correctly. By the age of seven or eight, however, subjects became quite sensitive to the demands of the other child; they sought to make drawings that were identifiable and, more important, altered each revision until the viewer could guess what was intended.

Nonetheless, the experimental evidence casts doubt on the easy assumption that the young child is an artist, at least in the sense that we apply the term to an adult artist. Certainly the artists honored in our culture can use line expressively and repletely; certainly they are aware of how things might look to others and are constantly making adjustments so that their vision can be apprehended.

In fact, works by Klee, Picasso (see figure 12.12), or Miró may seem ingenuous but are not, in any simple sense, copies of children's creations. What these notable twentieth-century painters are doing, I think, is reducing their artwork to the simplest forms possible—to lines, triangles, enclosures—and exploring the numerous ways in which those forms can be combined for specific expressive ends. If they embody a certain expression—say, that of calm or lightheartedness—it is because that is what the painter sought to express and not because the property happens to recur in children's drawings. If they perseverate with a single thickness of line, it is because they want that uniformity to come through.

While children of five or six have already mastered the basic vocabulary that enables them to portray the world, they may or may not attempt to apply it in a given work; such children simply do not care that much if they fail. Or to put it another way, they may indeed seek to achieve these goals and yet regularly fall short of them. In striving for precise symmetry, they achieve instead a sense of balance. In attempting to place the right number of objects on a page and to give each its own boundary and base line, they achieve harmonious composition; in striving for realism, they produce charming, recognizable deviations from a photograph.

To our eyes, these deviations produce a kind of delightful approximation, a near hit, a kind of "first draft" of higher art forms. We cannot forget that adult artists achieve these results by quite different means. They may purposefully turn their backs on all the intricate forms they can produce and the variety of moods they can convey in favor of self-consciously and deliberately capturing forms and sensibilities that are often associated with children. Part of what we admire in such work is, indeed, a fresh simplicity. But in this very opting for elements, the artist is making a far more complex statement—one confronting the possibility of innocence despite one's maturity, the use of great powers in the service of simplicity.

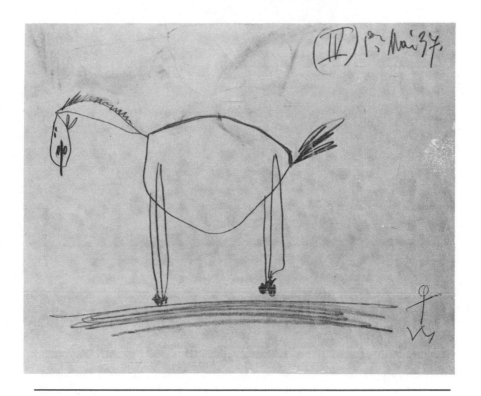

Figure 12.12. Picasso. *Study for the Horse,* study for *Guernica.* © SPADEM, Paris/VAGA, New York, 1982.

It is possible that I have done an injustice to the child. Children know of a range of moods, and overall they may be capable of more expressiveness and repleteness than I have suggested. Moreover—and herein lies the lesson of Kay's and Jerry's drawings—an artistic medium provides a special, even unique, avenue for grappling with important and complex issues that do not, however, lend themselves to verbal discussion at an early age. It is too simple to say, with Malraux, that "[the child's] gift controls him; not he his gift."

Indeed it may be this paradoxical, ambiguous quality that, more than anything else, conveys the special power and fascination in the drawings of the young child. Were the child as aware of the potentials of the medium and the range of alternatives as the adult artist is, he would *be* that adult—he would have already passed beyond the special world of childhood.

13

IN SEARCH OF THE

UR-SONG

FOR A LONG TIME people have wondered about the original language of the Bible. Was it Hebrew or another Semitic language? Or was it some other yet unidentified tongue? Many of a less theological bent, including linguists and philologists, have searched for a basic or original language, a pre-Babel tongue that all individuals spoke.

In fact, there have even been bizarre experiments on this topic. On a number of occasions individuals with the power to test their own pet theories of language have isolated hapless infants to see whether, without exposure to any language, they would begin to speak a particular identifiable language. The most famous experiment was conducted in the thirteenth century by Frederick II of the Holy Roman Empire. He isolated two children and let them grow up without hearing any tongue. But the history of such heartless experimentation goes back as far as the seventh century B.C. when, according to Herodotus, the Egyptian Pharaoh Psamtik I conducted a similar experiment. And the impulse traveled to such remote corners as Mogul India, where the same kind of experiment was made by Akbar the Great in the sixteenth century.

Unfortunately, these experiments—at least to judge by the records of them—did not realize the hopes of the original fashioners. None of the subjects seems to have uttered the magic words. From our present vantage point, we know that there is a genetic predisposition for language, and indeed even deaf children who have had no exposure to speech begin to babble at the normal age. Unless a child is raised in a linguistic community, however, he will not show evidence of language. He may utter bizarre sounds that no one else can understand; he may remain mute; or he may even perish as a consequence of this cruel isolation.

A parallel quest has been made for an original melody, a so-called *ur*-song (*ur* is a German prefix meaning "original, primeval"). Students of music have questioned whether there is, indeed, a basic human song or chant—one that hunters, fishermen, or Volga boatmen might, on their own, come to sing. If so, what is the nature of this song? Where does it come from? How will people sing it? What will prevent them from singing it? And how do we go from the *ur*-song to the vast variety of tunes and larger musical entities that are now sung or played across the world? Indeed, since music seems much less tied than language to the events and objects of a specific culture, the chances of finding a single *ur*-song, rather than a babble of basic melodies, may be considerable.

Opposing views can be adduced on this puzzle. No less an authority than the composer and conductor Leonard Bernstein asserts that indeed there is a basic melody which children all over the world first chant. He even identifies this *ur*-song. It consists of a repetitive, descending minor third, often elaborated by an additional step of a fourth. An example of a simple, repetitive, descending third would be the way children call "San-dy" or "Thom-as." An example of the descending third with the additional fourth would be such children's chants as "Little Sally Water" or "Ollie, ollie, in free." Taking his cue from the linguist Noam Chomsky, Bernstein claims that this basic song is a joint product of our human genetic predisposition and the physical laws that govern musical harmony. As he put it with typical flair in his Charles Eliot Norton lectures: "These three universal notes (that is, G, E, and A) are handed to us by nature on a silver platter" (p. 27).

Other scholars—for example, the noted ethnomusicologist Bruno Nettl—express some sympathy for the notion of a set of basic chants from which the diverse melodies of the world are eventually spawned. But in a time of cultural relativism, the belief that the harmonic system that happens to be favored by the West has furnished a universal *ur*-song has been challenged by many observers. A less ethnocentric con-

145

sensus claims that even the initial songs of children reflect the predominant melodic, harmonic, and rhythmic practices of a specific culture. No individual is normally raised in an acoustic vacuum. The tunes that he sings, no less than the words that he initially repeats, will reflect the sounds that envelop his society, rather than some universal tonal signal.

In truth, however, little has actually been established about the early course of singing. And in the absence of data, speculation has necessarily carried the day. Recently, however, some investigators have listened to the sounds produced by young children and from them have traced musical development within our own cultural setting. Their findings, combined with some suggestive cues from the world of bird song and some additional hints from development with other symbolic systems, offer a preliminary picture of the development of musical competence in youngsters.

Charles Darwin was puzzled by the existence of music. Why should a system whose evolutionary significance and whose functions were so obscure continue to exist and proliferate around the world? Darwin, however, may have been unnecessarily skeptical. After all, at least among some species, the production of musical or pseudomusical elements has clear adaptive value. The chief examples clearly are birds, who use their songs for mating and for territorial purposes. Perhaps we can gain some initial perspective on human song by listening to bird song.

A survey of bird song reveals a phenomenon of bewildering variety. Some species have one song, others more than a thousand. Some species exhibit great individual differences among "singers," whereas in other species variation is minute. Some species learn songs, including new songs, throughout life, while others seem capable of learning only during the first year. But is there an avian *ur*-song?

Fortunately, one can conduct experiments relevant to this issue. One can raise birds in isolation or even deafen them and see what happens to their songs in such circumstances. And one can experiment with those areas of the bird brain involved in song production and chart the effects on the usual patterns of development.

Such studies have been done over the past few decades by several imaginative investigators, including Peter Marler, Fernando Nottebohm, and W. H. Thorpe. Their findings, of enormous complexity, are constantly being revised and refined. Yet, according to Nottebohm, who has summarized this literature, experimenters have observed three major trajectories in the development of bird song.

In some species—for example, the ring dove—there is apparently a single song that eventually comes to be produced by every male member of the species. Here in nature is the equivalent of our *ur*-song. More surprisingly, no feedback or external stimulation is needed to learn the song. Essentially every ring dove will produce the same song even if no auditory feedback is available during the so-called critical period when the bird song is typically acquired.

In the case of most birds, however, there is a less direct route governing the acquisition of bird song. Typically, birds begin with a period of *sub-song*—a rambling, low-amplitude kind of vocalization, which apparently serves no communicative purposes and lasts only a few weeks. This "babble" is followed for a somewhat longer period of time by *plastic song*, a lengthier segment in which syllables are repeated until they constitute short phrases. The syllables and phrases are delivered variably for a period of several months. Finally, usually within a year, the "drill" of plastic song gives way to *stereotyped song*, or songs that will be similar to those produced by all other adult male members of the species.

Against this background of normal song development, scientists can examine the effects of various deprivations. Canaries represent one instructive pattern. These birds require auditory feedback for normal development, but otherwise they can go it alone. They prove able to produce a well-structured song even in the absence of hearing the vocalizations of others in their species. However, if they are deafened before the period of vocal learning, they will produce a song that is highly abnormal. It is more crucial for such birds to hear themselves than to monitor other members of the species.

A third developmental pattern, at the opposite extreme from that of the ring dove, is found in the chaffinch, a bird much studied in England. The chaffinch needs both auditory feedback *and* exposure to conspecifics if it is to produce a full, normal song. If deafened within the first three months of life, it will produce an extremely abnormal song, which may prove little more than a continuous screech. However, if it is deafened after it has learned its full song, there is no discernible deterioration in performance.

A further line of study relevant to our inquiry concerns the biological substrate of song. Bird song turns out to be one of the very few instances of brain lateralization in the entire animal kingdom. Just as the left hemisphere of the brain of human beings is critical for language production and comprehension, so the left hypoglossal nerve in the bird proves crucial for its production of song. As for the hormonal substrate, we know that the production or the suppression of testosterone in both males and females is intimately connected to song production. Given sufficient testosterone, the female, who usually does not sing, will be able to master the repertoire of songs in the same manner as the male. Further research on these biological aspects of one variety of music should eventually illuminate just what song consists of and how its development comes about.

Yet the variety of developmental patterns in bird song is slightly disappointing in regard to our inquiry. Even in this apparently simple organism there is no single, approved course for the development of song. The ring doves provide comfort for those in search of an *ur-song*, whereas the canaries and chaffinches exhibit a pattern that is closer to that propounded by the cultural relativists. Nevertheless, the basic sequence—a babbling sub-song; a plastic song punctuated with experimentation, variation, and a large set of fragments; and the final pruning into the more stereotyped song at about the time of maturity— serves as a highly suggestive model for the development of human musical skills, the processes that lead to musical competence.

While bird song is both exotic and fascinating, skeptics might well find it more prudent to examine instead the development of other symbol systems in human beings in the search for a basic song. Probably the chief candidates for consideration are human language and human drawing. Fortunately, both of these systems have been studied a great deal in recent years, and we are able with some confidence to indicate the developmental milestones in each of these domains.

In the case of language, there is of course a period of babbling that is found throughout the world, even in children who are deaf or blind. Production of sounds from all languages is common early in the first year, but eventually production is increasingly restricted to those sounds encountered in the individual's own cultural milieu. Following a period of relative quiet, children go on to produce their first meaningful words of communication—"doggie," "cookie," "mine." By the age of two they are stringing together two or three words in meaningful utterances; and by the age of three they can produce sentences of some complexity. Syntactic efflorescence occurs in the third and fourth years of life, giving rise to a great variety of grammatical structures as well as considerable expressive power. And by the age of four or

148

five most children are able to produce simple stories, including ones displaying some originality and considerable vigor.

Surveying with equal brevity the area of drawing, we find an instructively analogous picture. In the second year of life children begin to make marks on pieces of paper and to gain enjoyment from this activity. At first the scribbles are apparently unorganized, though they tend to reflect those circular and jabbing motor activities that are readily carried out by a pencil grasped in the hand. In their third year children become able to produce a variety of geometric forms, such as squares, circles, crosses, and mandalas: these seem to serve for mastering different shapes but are not marshaled for simple representation of objects in the world.

A dramatic watershed occurs around the age of three or four, when children become able to combine geometrical forms into coherent and recognizable shapes and to associate them deliberately with objects in the world. We now encounter "tadpole" figures of human beings as well as simple graphic representations of dogs, horses, tables, houses, birds, suns, and the other staples of childhood art everywhere. By the age of five or six children can produce organized compositions of some complexity and interest. In fact, this period has been deemed the "flowering" of artistic activity by observers of the infant painting scene.

While drawings are easier to preserve than children's songs, and children's first words somewhat easier to record or notate than children's pitch configurations, there is certainly no reason why children's early musical productions cannot be subjected to the same scrutiny as productions in other symbol systems. And, in fact, more than sixty years ago at least one scholar, the German genetic psychologist Heinz Werner, did collect some instances of children's early songs. Werner's work has generally been neglected, however, and for many years there was a virtual conspiracy of silence about the development of children's musical abilities.

That has changed. An active exploration of early singing is now being conducted at Harvard Project Zero (as well as in some other laboratories around the world). As part of a more comprehensive study of the development of competence across diverse symbolic domains, my colleagues Lyle Davidson, Patricia McKernon, and Dennie Wolf have been observing on a regular basis the development of musical abilities in a group of nine children during their first five years of life. This study has provided a fine-grained picture of the steps involved in early musical mastery among a group of firstborn youngsters in a

Western middle-class milieu. It does not solve the riddle of the *ur-song*, but it suggests, perhaps for the first time, some dimensions of the acquisition of early singing competence.

We begin with the observation that during the first year of life children's babbling includes melodic and intonational as well as phonological experimentation. Indeed, it may be inappropriate to isolate early language from early musical chanting—the two are indissolubly linked.

Nonetheless, two events of potential musical significance stand out during the first year of life. First, children prove capable of imitating the intonational patterns of the linguistic structures they hear about them. Indeed, imitation of the "song qualities" of speech and of singing seems more prominent during the first year than more focused aspects of communication. Second, many children seem able to match specific pitches at far greater than chance rates. According to William Kessen and Janice Levine of Yale University, when an experimenter sings particular pitches, the infant will sing them back with some accuracy. While there may not be a direct link from matching intonation and pitch to ultimate singing mastery, no doubt such "computational" capacities constitute a kind of basic skill on which ultimate musical achievement will be constructed.

What about the specific steps in mastery of song beyond the first year of life? The story, or perhaps we should say the melody, is long and complex, but it is worth indicating at least some of the highlights.

The first melodic fragments produced by children around the age of a year or fifteen months have no strong musical identity. Their undulating patterns, going up and down over a very brief interval or ambitus, are more reminiscent of waves than of particular pitch attacks. Indeed, a quantum leap, in an almost literal sense, occurs at about the age of a year and a half, when for the first time children can intentionally produce discrete pitches. It is as if diffuse babbling had been supplanted by stressed words.

The course for the next year is quite regular and, therefore, readily described. The first intervals sung by children tend to be seconds, minor thirds, and major thirds. In the second and third years of life, children embark on a seemingly systematic drill of each of these intervals as they appear in fragments, as well as a continuing expansion of the intervals from the tiny seconds and thirds of Bernstein fame to larger intervals, including fourths and fifths.

We may speak at this time of *spontaneous song,* the production of numerous fragments consisting of these seconds, thirds, and occasion-

150

ally fourths. Like the early sub-song of the bird, however, these patterns are distinctly unmemorable. They appear to lack organization, having little sense of tonality or harmony, and are rhythmically irregular; to jot them down accurately poses a notational challenge even for the musically trained ear.

By the age of two or two and a half, a new phenomenon emerges. For the first time, children exhibit explicit awareness of the tunes sung by others in their environment. The familiar nursery rhymes from our own cultural envelope—"A B C," "Old MacDonald," "Happy Birthday," "Twinkle, Twinkle"—now are noticed by the two-year-olds. The children make their own fledgling efforts to reproduce these songs, and thus commence the transition from spontaneous song to *learned song*. But children's first efforts at learned song are little more than fragments that they have been producing in their own spontaneous song. The only way in which we can confirm that the child is actually attempting to produce a song from his culture is when he repeats some telltale lyric, such as "H-I-J-K-LMNOP" or "an oink-oink-here, an oink-oink-there." At this point in development, the lyrics and the spontaneous song carry the day.

Toward the end of the third year of life, however, the spontaneous song begins to give way to the learned song. This occurs because the child has now acquired a sense of the rhythmic structure of the song; thus his efforts at learned song bear not only a lyrical but also a rhythmic resemblance to the model learned from his culture.

It would be misleading to suggest that the child already knows the songs of his culture or even that he has a skeletal frame for a particular song. Rather, the child now knows characteristic bits or embryonic tune segments, which he can repeat over and over again. Here, again, one is reminded of bird song, particularly the period of phrase song. This is a time when the child is apparently working with the building blocks of song: exploring small segments, practicing with them, combining them in diverse ways so that they now bear a kind of family resemblance to the target song but do not yet reveal its general structure. One is reminded of an orchestra as it tunes up for a performance—a time when the keen ear can pick out all the important fragments but not the shape of the piece to be performed.

Resorting to our other analogies, we may compare this period to the time when a child can produce short phrases or sentences which do not, however, combine into a comprehensible story; or to the time when a youngster can produce sets of geometric figures which do not yet combine into an organized drawing. The building blocks are there, but the skeleton of the building cannot yet be discerned.

A sea change occurs at about the age of three or four. Now for the first time the child goes beyond the characteristic bits of a phrase song and attempts to reproduce the entire learned song that he has heard emitted from the larynxes and record players of those around him. Whereas earlier the spontaneous song overwhelmed the learned song, the ratio is now reversed, as the learned song comes to dominate the child's vocal efforts. Furthermore, the learned song now exhibits those regular intervals and rhythms which remain difficult to discern in the simpler and less organized spontaneous songs. In fact, the child has a sense of the overall structure of the song and can even subordinate particular parts of the song to the overall song structure. From here on, children seem to represent songs in terms of their global "holistic" properties. Nonetheless, at this age the lyrics and the rhythm are still carrying the day as far as song production is concerned. Not yet in possession of a well-developed sense of key and tonality, the child is generally restricted to the overall contour of the song and to an approximate sense of tonal values.

The sea change also reflects similar dramatic changes occurring at approximately the same time in other symbolic media. Our three- or four-year-old tunesmith is also producing simple stories whose structure reflects the stories of those he has heard, and he is fashioning representational drawings, which capture aspects of the appearance of individual objects and the relationships among objects in a scene. Analogous breakthroughs can be observed in other domains, ranging from modeling with clay to creating a simple dance sequence.

While it is instructive to attend to the development of songs within the child's natural (and cultural) milieu, there are problems involved in figuring out the precise developmental steps. There is little control over the input to the child and little opportunity to observe his overall practice. We are at a loss to describe the components that culminate in the mastery of a given tune from the culture.

For this reason we have found it helpful in our own studies to teach the children a song they have not heard before and to observe on a regular basis the steps through which they pass in mastering this song. Lyle Davidson and Patricia McKernon taught our subjects an old folk song called the "Charlie Song," which is reproduced here. It is a deceptively simple melody. It resembles ones that children readily acquire at this age but exhibits sufficient melodic, rhythmic, and lyrical com-

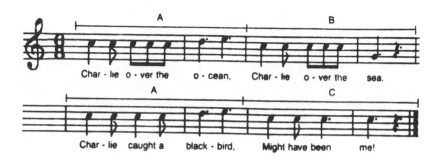

Figure 13.1. The Charlie Song

plexity to reveal the kinds of problems youngsters encounter (and the strategies they evolve) in proceeding from a skeletal to a fleshed-out version of a song.

Happily, our children, aged four to five, were able to learn the "Charlie Song." Equally happily, they did not learn it right away. Through their initial failures and their early successes, they clarified some of the later steps in the initial song mastery.

Our four-year-olds readily learn the words to the song. Indeed, one might say that the meaning of the song first inheres in its words. Shortly afterward, the children are able to acquire the surface rhythm of the song, which of course is closely yoked to the actual linguistic phrases.

The next major step involves mastering the contour of the song. The child at age four, or a little thereafter, has a sense of when the song goes up, when it goes down, how often it goes up and down, and the approximate sizes of the leaps in either direction. What is clearly lacking is an accurate sense of interval mapping (the ability to produce a fourth versus a fifth reliably) and a key sense that remains stable across phrases (for example, remaining in the key of C rather than shifting inadvertently to the key of D or G). The child may well remain within the same key during a short phrase and be able to reproduce a large leap (as opposed to a small leap), but the precision needed for accurate song rendition is not yet available.

We may note, parenthetically, another parallel with other symbol systems. Throughout the range of symbol systems that we have observed we find the same trends between the ages of three and five.

At the early end of this age period, children exhibit a kind of approximate or "topological" mapping, where general size relationships and spatial relationships are captured. For example, in drawing a person, they will get the relation between body parts or the number of toes and fingers approximately but not exactly correct. At the later end of this age span, children exhibit digital or numerical mapping, where specific distances, proportions, and numbers are mastered and retained. Nowhere is this more clearly manifest than in song development during the period from age four to five.

After a year of considerable practice with the song, the average child has passed two major milestones. The first involves the ability to extract the *underlying pulse* from the *surface rhythm*. Initially, the child's sensitivity to rhythm derives strictly from the placement of accents in the surface lyrics of the song; ultimately the child comes to appreciate that, underlying these surface rhythms, there is a regular repeated pulse, a metronomic drumbeat if you will, which organizes the way that the various rhythmic structures should be articulated. To put it pragmatically, the child can now beat time at regular intervals throughout the song rather than simply be carried along by the stress patterns of the particular syllables.

The second, possibly more complex, acquisition involves mastery of the tonal elements of the "Charlie Song." The child advances a long way toward the digital precision described above. On the one hand he has attained sufficient mastery to enable him to produce particular intervals with increasing precision: a third is a third, a fifth is a fifth, and they can be heard as such even by someone unfamiliar with the tonal intervals of the song. On the other hand, and of equal importance, the child now acquires the knowledge (and the appreciation) that there is a single organizing key that pervades the entire song. If the song is in the key of C, it means, as indicated above, that it should begin in C and remain in C, in the absence of an explicit modulation to another key, and should in general return at the end of the song to the tonic of the key in which it has been realized. This task is largely accomplished by the age of five by most normal children.

Certainly individual differences are vast in this area of human achievement, possibly greater than in any other symbolic domain that we have studied. There are some children who can learn new songs with surprising accuracy by the age of two or three, including a few who prove retarded in other symbolic realms. There are other children, even those of quite high general intelligence, who display selective problems with musical mastery and for whom a precise sense of interval and key will be extremely difficult to attain. (Such amusia is less likely to occur in connection with lyrics or rhythms.) Nonetheless, as it is based on the careful study of a small group of youngsters, the picture we describe should have some generality.

What, then, characterizes our young musician at the age of five? The child has gone from the kind of "outline sense" of a song, available at the age of three or three and a half, to what we might call a "first-draft" mastery. Not every detail is in hand (or mouth!), but the song is clearly recognizable. Moreover, major milestones in the areas of underlying pulse, key stability, and interval reproduction have been successfully negotiated.

How close is the typical five-year-old to adult competence in song? Some intriguing clues can be obtained from a recent study by Davidson. This researcher asked beginning vocal students at the New England Conservatory of Music to learn our "Charlie Song." The aspiring professional singers of course displayed less difficulty in learning the song, and some in fact exhibited "one-trial learning." But many of the same errors exhibited by the children could also be found in the imperfect renditions by these young and gifted adults. For example, both groups of subjects regularized the rather unusual ABAC plan of the song to a more canonical ABAB form. The same kinds of pitch mistakes were also made—intervals of seconds were inappropriately transformed to the more predictable intervals of thirds or fifths.

Perhaps the principal difference came from the fact that the older subjects already knew numerous folk songs of the "Charlie" ilk. Accordingly, they tried to fit this new tune into song structures, or "schemas," that they had already mastered and solidified—sometimes to their advantage, sometimes not. In contrast, the young children were still in the process of forming initial schemas, and so they were less likely to distort the "Charlie Song" to fit into a pre-established mold of the "This Old Man" or "Greensleeves" variety.

Even as we were intrigued by parallels in the acquisition of song at various ages, so too we have been struck by the commonalities across diverse symbolic domains. Whether it be music, language, or drawing, the child begins in infancy with a period of free exploration, using elements devoid of significance, such as individual tones, phonemic bundles, or discrete line. This is followed by a longer period in which the child explores somewhat larger units, or building blocks, such as melodic bits, words, or geometric forms. Only in the third or fourth year of life does the child come to combine these building blocks into such culturally approved products as learned songs, simple stories, or representational drawings.

It is at this point in development that the forms favored by the culture come to exert increasing influence over, and eventually to dominate, the characteristic bits that the children have been producing with relatively little instruction from the culture. In terms of our original discussion, we might say that any impulses toward the development of a universal *ur*-song, *ur*-story, or *ur*-sketch are permanently squelched at this time, as the meanings and forms donated by the culture impose themselves on the motifs or fragments that the child has been spontaneously generating. Whether, left to their own devices, children would nonetheless arrive at a common *ur*-form seems highly doubtful. Contrary to what Rousseau would have preferred, children seem to be predisposed at a certain point in development to acquire the forms of the culture, and it seems likely that in their continuing absence development would cease altogether.

But if the search for an *ur*-song seems doomed to failure, an interest in origins of diverse symbol systems may be crowned with greater success. Our exploration of early production of song, when viewed in light of discoveries about first drawings and first stories, suggests that there may well be common processes that govern all early symbolic activity. The course from autistic production of single elements to free exploration of characteristic bits and on to the first tentative combinations into meaningful symbolic products seems to move across a range of symbol systems and, at least in the case of drawing and language, can be observed across diverse cultures as well. While there may be no *ur*-song, there may well be *ur*-processes that lead to competence in singing.

Our discussion so far has implied that development in music bears strong parallels to growth in other symbolic domains. We must point out, therefore, that certain challenges in music—for example, learning the relations of pitch and harmony—have no strong analogies in other domains. The variety of ways in which music can be expressed—using voice, body, or instruments—and the ability to generate countless expressive forms without reference to external meaning are other features that distinguish that domain from, say, language or drawing. Some parts of the story of musical development resonate with other media, but others prove unique.

Musical development is scarcely completed at age five. Though five-year-olds can sing us a good tune, only exceptional youngsters play an instrument, use musical notation, or appreciate the various interpretations available for a given song or score. Knowledge about music and music theory is also absent. And it may well be that the ways in which children think about music or the way that they "think musically" continue to change. About these matters we know very little.

Most of these aspects of musical mastery await instruction, and unless the child's own family already has this knowledge and is willing to share it with the child, it is necessary to seek recourse (or courses) in the larger society. The rewards of such formal musical instruction, be it at the hands of a Suzuki master, a regular classroom teacher, or a friend, can be rich—equally for the child himself and for the society. As one who was a pianist as a child and who continues to gain his greatest personal sustenance from musical activity, I know in my bones the unique niche that music can occupy in human experience. Yet it would be derelict to pass over the fact that for so many individuals the onset of formal musical instruction marks the beginning of the end of musical development. The atomistic focus in most musical instruction—the individual pitch, its name, its notation—and the measure-by-measure methods of instruction and analysis run counter to the holistic way in which most children have come to think of, react to, and live with music. Often the clash of these musical-world views proves too jarring, and the child's musical flair becomes dimmer or even withers away. In fact, the challenge of musical education is to respect and build upon the young child's own skills and understanding of music, rather than simply to impose a curriculum that was designed principally to ensure competent adult musical performances. The ready exploration of bits and the intuitive sense of the form and contour of a piece are precious experiences, which should not—must not—be scuttled if a full flowering of musical talent is to occur in later life.

14

THE CHILD IS FATHER

TO THE METAPHOR

WITH ELLEN WINNER

NOT LONG AGO, one of us was conducting a Seder, the ritual Jewish meal commemorating the flight of the Hebrew people from Egypt. In relating to a group of children gathered around the table the events that culminated in the Exodus, he described how, after one of the plagues, Pharaoh's heart had hardened to stone. Noticing a look of bewilderment on several of the youngsters' faces, he momentarily assumed his role as a developmental psychologist and asked the children what they thought that meant. A five-year-old promptly replied that God had come down "and turned Pharaoh's heart into a stone." Another five-year-old protested that it was not God but rather a witch who had turned the heart into a stone. A six-year-old disagreed with both those "magical" interpretations, insisting that hearts cannot really turn into stones and that, instead, "the Pharaoh might have lived in a castle that was made out of hard stone."

"I don't think so," suggested his eight-year-old sister. "I think it means that the Pharaoh had very big muscles; they were hard like a rock."

Eventually, an adult suggested that it was the Pharaoh's mood, rather

than his heart or his muscles, that had changed. Some of the eight-
and nine-year-olds seemed to understand. But it was clear that the
figure of speech, in which the psychological process of becoming inflexible was described in terms of physical petrification, did not automatically speak to children. Moreover, the youngsters were quite inventive
in constructing their own explanations of that figure of speech and
in resisting the kinds of explanation that adults almost automatically
impose.

We discovered in our studies that such misinterpretations are a general phenomenon. Following a line of research begun by the social
psychologist Solomon Asch in 1960, we have asked several hundred
children of varying ages and social classes to interpret such figures of
speech. Despite variations in content and wording, we have encountered a surprisingly consistent pattern.

Let us consider what happens when children are presented with a
metaphor based on the same relationship we saw in our Biblical reference to Pharaoh: *After many years of working at the jail, the prison
guard had become a hard rock that could not be moved.*

Here, a link is made between the physical universe (hard rocks)
and the universe of psychological traits (stubborn lack of feeling).
To make sense of the statement, one must perceive the similarity between physical and psychological inflexibility. But that capacity is remote from the youngest children, who often supply magical explanations for such metaphors. Asked to explain a literally impossible
statement, they simply invoke a higher power as the "prime cause"—
for example, a king came and turned the guard into a rock. Most often,
however, children in the five-to-seven age range solve the problem
by altering the relationship between the two terms of the metaphor.
Instead of equating two elements, which to them seems nonsensical,
they associate the two terms (for example, the guard piled hard rocks
all day long).

Sometimes children in that age group realize that the statement cannot be interpreted literally, and that it is also inappropriate to alter
the relation between the two terms from one of "equation" (guard-
is-rock) to one of association (guard-acts-upon-rocks). So they try to
devise a way in which a person might be *like* a rock. But because
they are unable to understand how a hard rock might bear any resemblance to a psychological condition, they explain the figure of speech
in physical terms, perhaps commenting that the guard had hard muscles. Even though children from five to seven possess the vocabulary

needed to discuss psychological states, they avoid any crossing of domains from the physical to the psychological.

Only in the middle years of elementary school, between the ages of eight and nine, do children begin to appreciate that a psychological process is being discussed. At that point they have made a decisive leap: they recognize the basic intent behind the figure of speech. But the paraphrase may remain incorrect because the child does not appreciate the specific psychological dimension at issue. And so one hears of prison guards who are angry, or stupid, or fussy—descriptions that preserve the intended negative connotation of the metaphor but fail to zero in on the precise psychological condition. Not until children are near adolescence do they offer a consistently accurate account of stone-hearted Pharaohs and prison guards.

These findings suggest that children may be missing the point of much of the prose and poetry they encounter. In the area of poetic or metaphoric language, we appear to have encountered yet another developmental progression—the same kind of orderly series of stages that Jean Piaget discovered in many areas of mental development and that Erik Erikson has charted in the domain of personality. It is not entirely a surprise that children's performance in dealing with an artistic task improves with age. What makes the study of metaphoric language so fascinating, however, is that when one looks at the kinds of metaphors children produce, it becomes clear that they do not simply get better with age. In fact, closer examination of the figures of speech produced by very young children—those phrases that flow "out of the mouths of babes"—reveals that they are often strikingly inventive.

One does not have to search far to discover early metaphors that delight the adult ear. Every parent, every teacher, and every psychologist who has listened to children can supply examples. One of Piaget's own children, at the age of three and a half, saw some small waves on a beach pushing little ridges of sand back and forth and remarked: "It's like a little girl's hair being combed." At four and a half, the same little girl likened a bent twig to "a machine for putting in petrol." Kornei Chukovsky, a Russian short-story writer, collated hundreds of such spontaneous children's metaphors. A bald man was described by one child as having a "barefoot" head; another, seeing an elephant for the first time, declared, "This is not an elephant—this is a gas mask."

Chukovsky called the years from two to five a period of linguistic genius. In our own work, we have heard a two-year-old call a yellow plastic baseball bat "corn"; a three-year-old call a folded-over potato chip a "cowboy hat" and a red-and-white stop sign a "candy cane." Studies by psychologist Richard Billow show that preschool children are especially likely to produce inventive figures of speech. After the age of six or so, such novel usage appears to decline in spontaneous speech. We should pause to note, however, that those figures of speech do not include every type of comparison. Almost all early metaphors are based on a physical resemblance between elements, rather than on a conceptual, expressive, or psychological link. But the metaphors are often as striking and novel as those created by adults, including gifted poets.

Here we have a paradox worthy of closer examination. When one simply asks children to interpret or paraphrase metaphors, they perform poorly at first and improve only gradually as they grow older. But when one looks at their own speech patterns, one discovers nearly the opposite picture. It is in the earliest years of life that the most striking figures of speech are found; and it is during the very years when their comprehension of other people's metaphors improves that children's spontaneous output seems to wane. In the last few years, we have attempted to gain additional insight into this paradox, to determine whether it is more apparent than real. In our search we have carefully examined what children say and what they appear to mean when they say it. But data collection alone cannot answer the question of the significance of children's early metaphors. One can assess the significance of a child's comparison only after one has decided what a metaphor is—and is not—and which criteria to use in judging whether the child has in fact created one.

Metaphor as a figure of speech has intrigued and stimulated scholars for thousands of years. Aristotle considered metaphor a sign of genius, believing that the individual who could make unusual connections was a person of special gifts. From that ancient tradition has emerged a working definition of metaphor: the capacity to perceive a resemblance between elements from two separate domains or areas of experience and to link them together in linguistic form.

It is not enough just to yoke any two disparate elements. When T. S. Eliot compared the evening spread out against the sky to "a patient etherized upon a table," he created a powerful metaphor by linking two totally different elements. But had he written that the stars in the sky were like the prostrate patient, the metaphor would have failed dismally. Only in the first case is there any convincing ground momentarily linking the two terms; in the second case, no striking resemblance can be discerned between the two elements.

When, then, do we give a child credit for having produced a metaphor? If a child crosses the boundaries of a domain without realizing it, it makes little sense to award credit for the production of a metaphor. Similarly, if a three-year-old produces a painting that strikes us as artistically pleasing, we must ask whether the painting was a happy (but nonrepeatable) accident or an intentional creation. Suppose that the child who said that the bald man had a "barefoot head" thought that "barefoot" simply meant "bare"; or that the child who called the baseball bat an "ear of corn" thought that "corn" referred equally to all cylinders. In those cases, we could not speak legitimately of the creation of a metaphor. If, on the other hand, the child has roughly the same understanding of "barefoot" or "corn" as does an adult, and if, moreover, the child has available the literally appropriate words ("bald" and "bat") but elects not to use them, then it makes some sense to speak of the actual creation of a metaphor.

In making that claim, we do not seek to deny, or even to minimize, the differences between a child's and an adult's metaphoric achievements. For, to equate a yellow baseball bat with corn on the cob, a potato chip with a cowboy hat, or an elephant's head and trunk with a gas mask does not represent the ultimate height of metaphoric achievement. Shakespeare compared his love to a summer's day, and thereby enriched our conceptions of both phenomena; the children's metaphors are limited to physical comparisons and consist of simply ascribing new names to discrete physical objects. But if the essence of metaphor lies in giving one thing the name of another, the children's statements certainly qualify. However, the crucial question remains: Are such instances of unconventional naming mere mistakes disguised as metaphors, or do they represent intentional boundary crossings?

One way to get at the question is to examine very carefully the words, phrases, and actions produced by young children in the course of their spontaneous speech and play. It is a lengthy procedure, requiring the taping of children's conversations over a period of days, months, and even years. Fortunately for us, the psycholinguist Roger Brown had collected samples of spontaneous speech (gathered at two-week intervals over a three-year period) produced by three children between the ages of two and five. We looked through all of the recorded speech of a boy named Adam to see whether, in fact, we could find instances of metaphor.

162

The Child is Father to the Metaphor

The challenge in such an analysis was to avoid giving Adam metaphoric credit for namings that were merely overextensions or misuses of words, while at the same time crediting him properly for genuine metaphors. Consequently, when Adam, looking at a picture of a train, called the cowcatcher on the front a "sweep broom," he did not receive credit for metaphor because we had no evidence that he knew the word "cowcatcher"; he may well have believed the name "sweep broom" to be literally correct. But when Adam called a red balloon an "apple," he *did* receive metaphoric credit because he had used the word "balloon" correctly in the past. Similarly, when Adam held a pencil as if it were corn on the cob and, pretending to eat it, called it "corn," he also received credit for metaphor because he had *used* pencils appropriately in the past and the new name was accompanied by a nonliteral gesture.

Our study revealed surprisingly clear and systematic results. Between the ages of two and five, Adam produced 185 phrases that were rated as genuine metaphors. Nearly all of those were new names for ordinary objects in his environment. The resemblances that motivated the new names did not, at first, stem solely from the objects themselves but were *constructed* out of the pretend action of symbolic play, as in the "corn" example just described. Thus Adam put a pen inside the slot of a wagon handle and said he was "mailing" a letter; he put his foot in a wastebasket and called it a "boot"; and, hanging a yo-yo from his chin, he called attention to his "beard." While those metaphors may be based on perceptual properties of objects, the critical feature is that the transformation occurs on both a verbal and gestural level. In fact, the spoken word often strikes an observer as incidental to the symbolic gesture.

Such action-based metaphors declined sharply, giving way to a different kind of metaphor, one based solely on the physical properties of objects. For example, Adam likened a wheel to the letter "Q," and his mother's hair to "dark woods." By the time he reached the age of four, the predominant type of metaphor in Adam's speech no longer fed off the gestural transformation of an object but stood alone without the support of action. At all ages sampled, however, Adam's metaphors were grounded either on how an object could be handled, or on its shape, or on both. Not one of his metaphors was conceptual or expressive; never was he overheard calling a broken pencil "sad," "angry," or "a loser."

From the record of Adam's speech, it is clear that at least one child is quite capable of producing metaphors and of displaying metaphoric thought processes. The study of one child, however, is a rather risky data base from which to make generalizations about early metaphor. In the hope of reinforcing our initial findings, we undertook two additional steps.

The first thing we did was to examine speech transcripts of two other preschool children who were engaged in spontaneous play over a similar period of time. The two children also produced frequent metaphors, but they showed a remarkable difference in the kinds of metaphors they came up with. While almost all the metaphors produced by one child were gesturally based, the second child's were based on perceptual similarities, largely independent of gestural support. That finding suggests that the two different kinds of metaphor found in early language may be the result of individual differences (either in capacity or preference) rather than the product of a stage in mental development. Moreover, we have reason to think that the different patterns of making metaphors may reflect fundamentally different ways of processing information. Children who base their metaphors on visual resemblances may approach experience largely in terms of the physical qualities of objects. On the other hand, children who base their metaphors on action sequences may view the world in terms of the way events unfold over time. We believe that the difference may continue into adulthood, underlying diverse styles in the creation and appreciation of artistic forms.

A number of questions still faced us. We wondered, for example, whether additional differences would show up if we used a larger pool of subjects representing a wider age span. Can children produce metaphors when they are not at play or when they are not permitted to touch objects at all? Are metaphoric renamings more likely to occur in cases of objects with conventionally defined functions and striking names (cups, pens), or with more loosely defined functions and vaguer names (wooden blocks, shapes cut out of paper)? In the latter case, with such "abstract" objects, the child's metaphor does not have to counter established functions, and the ascription of a new name may be an easier task.

In an effort to answer those questions, we carried out, in collaboration with our colleague Margaret McCarthy, a large-scale cross-sectional study with preschool children. Rather than relying on spontaneous speech in free play, we tested all children in the same way so that we could compare the results. Since once cannot simply ask a child to produce a metaphor, we devised a puppet game in which child and experimenter took turns giving "pretend" names to a set of objects, such as a potato masher and a plastic flower. The seventy-seven children involved were sometimes allowed to handle the objects. At other times they watched the experimenter use the object in a way that suggested a pretend identity—using a cup as a hat, for example—but were not allowed to touch it; or they were asked to rename untouched static objects.

By and large, this large-scale study supported the findings of our more intensive longitudinal studies. Most three-year-olds and nearly all four- and five-year-olds had little difficulty in coming up with appropriate metaphors for objects. Once again, their metaphors were based primarily on the appearance, particularly the shape, of the objects. For the youngest children, the situation in which the experimenter manipulated the objects proved slightly easier, but overall the children showed a surprising ability to produce metaphoric renamings (and to select them in a multiple-choice condition) even when they were required to rename the objects without the experimenter's support.

As in the earlier studies, there were limitations in the metaphors produced by the youngsters. Metaphoric renamings almost never drew upon psychological or expressive possibilities; the physical qualities of the object to be named always dominated the child's renamings. However, when youngsters of school age and adults were given the same test, they too focused on the physical.

Although a greater flair for metaphor was not found among the older children and the adults—in fact, on this task, adult-level competence is apparently achieved in early childhood—neither did we uncover any decrease with age. We were somewhat surprised by this finding because in earlier studies there have been strong hints of a *literal stage* in the middle of childhood—a time during the early years of school when children produce few metaphors on their own, and when they seem to be troubled by, and actively to reject, figures of speech produced by others. Our own view is that there is, indeed, a decline in the *spontaneous* incidence of metaphor during the school years. The decline may reflect two factors: first, once the child has mastered a basic vocabulary, he is under less pressure to stretch the resources of language to express new meanings; second, a general bent toward conformity and rule-guided behavior discourages the school child from violating those categorical boundaries he has just finished constructing. Such a literal cast to language is reminiscent of the strong desire on the part of children of that age group to produce drawings that are highly realistic, and of their disdain for abstract works of art. Yet they appear to retain the potential to produce metaphors as part of a game— or part of the *rules.*

What picture of children's metaphoric competence emerges from these studies? From one perspective, it seems that the production and the comprehension of metaphor reflect separate streams of development. The evidence indicates that, in the case of production, metaphor is a basic capacity. It is discernible in the play and talk of the preschooler, and it may even decline somewhat with the coming of rule-governed and conventionalized behavior.

At the same time, we have evidence indicating that comprehension develops slowly in the course of childhood, that the young school child is beset with uncertainty about the meaning of simple figures of speech, and that only in the preadolescent years can children be credited with genuine metaphoric comprehension. In that area of development, as opposed to most others, it would appear that production outflanks comprehension.

But a closer examination of our data suggests a more consistent view of the origins of metaphoric thought. It seems that the difference among age groups derives less from the kind of metaphoric capacity than from the kind of metaphor that is at issue. Preschoolers are not only able to produce metaphors based on a physical ground, but they are also beginning to understand metaphors based on physical grounds when, for example, they are asked to select the correct metaphor from a set of choices.

For children, the main difficulty lies in dealing with more psychological and less physically grounded metaphors. We know that children have difficulty in talking or thinking about emotional or psychological properties. Moreover, even when they are able to describe psychological traits in literal terms, they still have difficulty in mapping the physical onto the psychological domain. So it is not surprising that the metaphoric competence that requires this ability does not ordinarily emerge until the preadolescent years.

As we continue our investigations of figurative language, we are becoming increasingly convinced of the importance of metaphoric processes in the life of the individual. We can discern metaphor in the very first forms of learning, in which the child searches out commonalities in objects or situations known to be different, and then proceeds to behave in a similar fashion toward comparable elements. We also encounter metaphor in the highest reaches of creativity, where someone is articulating a scientific theory or describing a subtle mood. Both situations feature the perception of a resemblance between elements (as well as an awareness that the elements belong to different domains) that constitutes the hallmark of all genuine metaphoric thinking. And we see repeatedly the important role played by metaphoric thought and by metaphoric examples in a teacher's efforts to convey a novel concept to a student.

Educational efforts might be concentrated on developing metaphoric capacities that begin to evolve at an early age. For instance, parents of literally oriented school children might try more often to use figures of speech in situations that freshly illuminate topics of interest to the child—in describing, say, baseball players, rocket ships, or television programs. Or teachers, when working with children who find it difficult to produce expressive metaphors, might provide inviting linguistic frames—for instance, fill-in sentences such as, "The brightly colored dress seemed as noisy as _____."

The need for special practice with metaphor was brought home to us sharply when we came across a new "translation" of Shakespeare, prepared especially for high-school students. Among the rewordings in "The Shakespeare Parallel Text Series" are the following:

Original	Translation
Stand and unfold yourself	Stand still and tell me who you are
Lend me your ear	Listen to me
Tomorrow and tomorrow and tomorrow	Tomorrow follows tomorrow and is followed by tomorrow

The motivation behind such an endeavor is obvious. Instructors fear that their students cannot understand figurative language and so, rather than dispense with the Bard altogether, they have sought to purchase clarity even at the price of barrenness. Here our studies acquire a certain timeliness. If, as we have shown, students of this age have the potential to deal with complex metaphors, there is no necessity to rewrite Shakespeare. But as the clamor for basic skills continues to grow, it seems high time for the fourth R—rhetoric—to re-enter the classroom.

15

THE BIRTH OF

LITERARY IMAGINATION

INFANTS playing with the sound of language, toddlers grasping a stick and hopping about the room as if astride the speediest steed, youngsters building castles with moats in the sand, preschoolers launching missiles to Mars, school children garbing themselves as scary monsters or beguiling princesses—these are the stuff of childhood imagination, the worlds invented by young children. No one who has been around children would question these phenomena (and many could add to this list), but these play activities prove no easier to explain than to explain away. Perhaps for this reason such childhood pretense and imaginative activities have intrigued clinicians, artists, psychologists, teachers, and, not least, parents and peers. Still we have very little understanding of the nature of these early imaginative activities—the reasons for their existence and, equally mysterious, the reason they blossom in some children while they wither away in so many others.

One can discern two contrasting views on the child's imagination. One group of commentators rejoices, enthuses, and is even overwhelmed. For instance, the Russian writer of children's books, Kornei Chukovsky, speaks of a period of childhood "genius" in language, when every young child is a gifted poet. The New York educator Richard Lewis collects the poems children recite or write down and presents them to the world as youthful examples of art. And many scholars concerned with children's behavior claim that children gain deep suste-nance from encountering works of literary imagination, such as fairy tales. In fact, no less an authority than the psychoanalyst Bruno Bettel-heim claims in *The Uses of Enchantment* that children appreciate fairy tales at a very profound, if unconscious, level. In his view, such tales prove of inestimable value at times when children confront central conflicts in their lives.

But more skeptical voices can be heard to ask: How can you credit a child with imaginative powers if the child does not already have a well-articulated sense of reality? Certainly children can be seen as ex-ploratory creatures, playful experimenters, but not as having genuine creative imaginations. For, such critics contend, imaginative activity presupposes control, deliberate intention, and the ability to select among alternatives—and it is just such "executive functions" that the young child does not, *cannot,* have. From this point of view, children's *apparently* imaginative activities are best written off as happy accidents. Individuals with this point of view would applaud Piaget's response when asked whether the child at play was aware that he was operating only in the pretend mode. Piaget shrewdly commented that the child would never think to ask that question.

One way to replace speculation with evidence is to look specifically at the natural development of children's literary imagination, to adopt the lens of the ethologist and secure a natural history of what children do, say, and think in the area of the literary imagination. In this essay we will search for relevant evidence in the child's earliest pretend play with household objects, toys, and people. We will observe the crucial transition whereby imagination comes to inhere increasingly in words rather than in actions, as we eavesdrop on the child's initial attempts at storytelling. We will look on with admiration at the gradual flowering of narrative around the beginning of school. And, finally, we will test whether children's literary flair is reflected in their compre-hension of literary works drawn from the community in which they live.

By such an examination we can gain perspective on whether imagina-tion is better thought of as present from the first or as a higher stage in human development; we will consider whether imagination might be considered an "individual difference," characterizing some children more so than others. To be sure, we will find truth in each of these characterizations. But ultimately more insight can be gained by treating imagination as a fact of every developmental epoch, one having its peculiar embodiments at each stage of the child's intellectual and affective growth, but one that becomes fragile at certain key points in a child's life.

Our first line of evidence comes from children's play in the second year of life. At this time, the child begins to imitate the simple actions of adults—for instance, following a mother around while she is vacuuming or joining her as she cooks a meal in the kitchen. Even this initial mimicry has structure. Children first enact the role of "agent" as they push the sweeper or stir the soup. But soon enough they become able to use other implements, such as dolls, either as recipients of actions, as when they serve the doll dinner, or as agents in their own right, as when the doll is treated like the mother, a teacher, or even the child himself.

Such behaviors by children still in diapers are immensely charming. It is not surprising that many adults already confer upon these activities the label of imaginative play. And yet dispassionate examination reveals that these early enactments are simple, mundane, and extremely down to earth. The child is carrying out our activities as best he can, in the way that he observes them, with scant amplification or modification, let alone invention. The tea party unfolds in the same stereotyped way each time, as do scenes of doctor and nurse or of putting a baby to sleep. We have here selective imitation, not productive imagination.

This is not to deny the amazing constructive power involved in such activities. Unlike other animals and unlike the infant during the first year of life, the child of two has clearly entered the realm of symbolic activity. No longer carrying out an action (like feeding himself) just for practical ends, he can use other objects or elements *including himself* to enact various roles, produce various actions, secure various consequences. He may eat symbolically, using pretense gestures and pretend food. Moreover, such symbolic enactments are carried out seemingly for the sheer enjoyment of representational activity. There is no ulterior motive—unless one wants to count increased knowledge of the world and more effective communication about it. Needless to stress, this achievement of symbolic activity is enormous— in a sense, the greatest imaginative leap of all. Upon it will be constructed all subsequent forms of play, including the play of literary imagination. And yet it would be misleading to characterize this activity as imaginative in the usual sense, for it involves only the most straightforward play and replay of elementary schemas or scripts.

But soon, children's play departs increasingly from mundane reality. This sequence can readily be seen in the child's play with physical objects. Only at the beginning is the child's play restricted to materials that closely resemble the actual objects used by his elders. As Greta Fein of the University of Maryland has indicated, children soon become able to accept a wide range of substitutes for these objects, substitutes that deviate along predictable lines from sheer replicas.

Fein singles out four symbolic milestones, or transformations, that occur during the second and third years of life. In one transformation the child becomes capable of *decontextualization:* he can imitate a sequence in a context other than that in which it customarily occurs. For example, the child's vacuuming of the house no longer need occur during cleaning time: instead, the child may pull out a toy vacuum, or suitable substitute, whenever he spies (or posits) some imaginary dust.

A second kind of transformation involves *object substitution.* By the age of two and a half or three, children become able to use a wide range of objects or blocks to stand for an absent object—for example, a stick, a pencil, or any other lengthy rectangular object will serve equally well as a vacuum cleaner. And within another six months the child can use objects that bear no evident physical resemblance to the object being depicted (a truck for a Hoover) or even objects that are purely imaginative.

Transformations also occur with individual actors. In *self-other transformations* the child first becomes capable of using realistic objects (like dolls) to stand for the role of agent. Soon he can also use a non-realistic object as an agent: the block can become either the doll that does the feeding or the doll that is itself fed. And so by age three or four, our young player can use almost any entity to symbolize almost any agent or object in almost any situation.

This brings us to the last, or *collective symbolization,* transformation. Here a set of objects can stand for disparate elements. The only prerequisite is that all the players understand the substitutions, roles, and themes involved and together negotiate the arrangements satisfactorily. So we can have a bunch of objects—or a group of children—represent the members of a family as they plan a meal, take a trip, or settle a dispute. We have come a long way from baby pretending to drink milk in its mother's arms.

Onto this impressive developmental sequence we must graft an equally instructive "individual difference." As Dennie Wolf and Sharon Grollman at Project Zero have recently documented, young children differ revealingly from one another in the extent to which they are willing to accept various substitutes for the objects with which they are playing. Children who are "object-dependent" pay very careful attention to the physical attributes of an object and insist upon having objects present throughout their pretend play. If they want to portray a pie, they look for a round object; if they want to launch a rocket ship, they seek a long rectangular piece. Other children have been dubbed "object-independent." These youngsters are willing from an early stage to use just about any block or object to stand for what they want to suggest, granting little importance to actual physical resemblances. Even more significantly, these children will often simply use the object as a point of departure and then go on to confer a set of meanings upon the object or even to ignore the object entirely as they fashion entities in their mind.

In the light of our earlier discussion, this apparent "individual difference" might seem a "crypto-developmental difference." Perhaps our object-independent children are simply brighter: perhaps they have negotiated the stage where objects must resemble their referents and simply moved on to a later stage, where substitutes suffice, willy-nilly. Wolf and Grollman have examined their data with this hypothesis in mind and they find it wanting. To be sure, with age all children become more accepting of a grab bag of objects as substitutes for particular referents. Nonetheless, children continue to differ throughout early childhood in their relative willingness to override the manifest physical properties of an object. Whether one looks at one-year-olds in the earliest forms of symbolic play or four-year-olds with quite elaborate play sequences, one can expect to encounter one group relatively dependent upon (and comfortable with) the existence and physical features of objects, and another group relatively carefree with regard to these objects. It may well be that adults in our society are more willing to treat as "truly imaginative" those youngsters who can disregard the physical dimensions of objects. Yet such a judgment must be seen as inhering in the eye of the beholder, for if one examines the structural sophistication and complexity of play sequences, the object-dependent and object-independent children actually turn out to be indistinguishable from one another.

One other feature of this early pretend play should be noted. Even though children shift easily in and out of play, and from one script to another, they are not totally oblivious to what they are doing. If an adult insists on taking the pretense too seriously—for instance, eating a pretend hot dog or not getting up after having been shot dead—the child may get very upset. Clearly, at one level at least, the child does honor nascent distinctions between pretend play and reality.

While the development of imagination proceeds apace during childhood, its locus undergoes a revealing and pivotal change in the third and fourth years of life. In the early part of this period imagination is almost exclusively realized in pretend play with objects and other individuals. Children need to have these real-world "props" in order to sustain their flights of fantasy. By the fourth year, however, much of the "action" in play is picked up by language, and, indeed, in children four to five years of age it is narrative language rather than props and persons which carry the day as far as imaginative activity is concerned. And so imagination literally becomes *literary imagination*, with words becoming the chief participants in imaginative sequences—the entities which make things happen.

The shift from playful action to linguistic play is accompanied by an equally central development—the discovery and realization of *narrative structures*. The earlier play sequences of children are simply that—collections of actions which may (or may not) follow upon one another in daily life but which in any case do not constitute a narrative or story. What is missing from these sequences is the central aspect of a story—the identifying feature, some kind of problem or conflict that is recognized and confronted by a protagonist and eventually brought to some kind of resolution, preferably a successful one. Such a recognition of narrative conflicts and solutions constitutes the heart of fiction, at least in the West.

Relating a story is in itself no mean task. The child must "control" one or more characters as they encounter and deal with a central problem. At Project Zero, researchers Dennie Wolf, Shelley Rubin, George Scarlett, and Sharon Grollman have sought to reveal and trace this process by presenting children with the outline of a narrative problem and monitoring how they attempt to solve it, first in action and words and then increasingly through words alone. For example, in a typical problem a little girl is trapped by a ferocious lion from which she wants to escape. By age three, children are aware of the centrality of these problems and the need to resolve them. The three-year-old, however, does not have sufficient command of resources to solve the problem within the limits set by the narrative—for example, by facilitating a change of heart in the ferocious lion. Therefore he will typically resort to *deus ex machina* solutions. Faced by the little girl trapped by the lion, a three-year-old will simply pick the little girl up and take her away from the lion, declaring "she's safe now." Another child of the same or slightly older age, who relies more exclusively on words, will mimic this solution on the purely verbal level. He will simply say, "Little girl go home, safe now." The formidable task confronting the child is to recognize that, yes, the little girl must be rescued but that only certain solutions are acceptable within a story. Only the young school child appreciates that he has the power to defang the lion by changing him into a different kind of creature or by conferring upon the girl new powers, ones that should, however, be appropriate to the other implications in this particular narrative.

At first the boundary between the fictional world and the real world is highly—excessively—permeable. The child of three shows little reluctance simply to invade the problem area with actions or words and impose a solution on that basis. At an intermediate stage, the child realizes that optimally the problem had to be solved within the confines of the story, but does not know exactly how to do it and so is likely to fudge—to announce a change of heart or the acquisition of new powers but not be able to motivate them sufficiently. Only at school age does the child have sufficient command of narrative resources so that he can solve the problem entailed in the story in an appropriate way. Only then can he take into account the actual powers and limitations of the principal characters and the enveloping situation.

The impulse to express the solution in words, as opposed to gestures or actions on objects, entails a whole raft of additional problems. In the absence of the more accessible (and less abstract) materials and gestures, the child must select words that capture the intended meanings, are appropriate to each of the characters, have the desired effects upon the other characters, and communicate effectively to listeners. These are hardly straightforward assignments. To make matters yet more complex, the child must honor rules governing what is permitted in a verbal narrative—when do you say "he said"? how do you say "meanwhile"? how do you assume the voice of the narrator as opposed to that of a protagonist? Much of the problem, and hence much of the development, of story competence in the preschool years involves a mastery of what can and cannot be said in words, and how to do things with words: how one describes characters; how one narrates sequences of activities; how one acknowledges a problem; how one anticipates what is going to happen and describes what has happened; how one handles dialogues, narration, knowledge of the audience, and the like. It is a daunting assignment, to say the least, and one that we researchers are just beginning to know how to describe, let alone explain to anyone's satisfaction.

In negotiating this territory, the child is helped greatly by his new-found knowledge of particular genres. Rather than simply dealing with the common activities of daily life, the child is now able to draw upon certain schemas or conventional patterns in the narrative realm. There is the monster schema, for example, where a victim is pursued relentlessly by a heartless (if sometimes ludicrous) monster; or the fairy-tale schema, where supernatural forces intervene to make a once hapless character into one who lives happily ever after. Mastery of these frames proves of tremendous help to the child, for now he gains formulas for solving a whole set of problems. Of course mastering the genre takes time, and knowing when it can be properly invoked poses yet a further challenge for the child.

To some extent the child who is assimilating these genres resembles the much younger child who is imitating his mother: there is often rote imitation of phrases ("and they lived happily ever after" or "I'm going to get you") without comparable understanding. But there are also highly instructive simplifications and distortions. We learn about insensitivity to role change when the child fails to motivate the new freedom that has been granted to a trapped character. We encounter inability to mobilize resources when the child allows the monster to annihilate his victims rather than to receive his just punishment.

Sometimes the very difficulties encountered by the child in honoring the fictive boundary or in adapting a story frame contribute to the charm of the child's imaginative activities. After all, when a purely stock approach is used, it is hardly noticed. But when a child, thrown upon his own resources, confuses the monster frame with the fairy-tale frame (thereby having the monster live happily ever after) or embraces a physical solution when a psychological one is wanted (thereby making the prince taller rather than happier), he may end up producing a more surprising story and therefore may appear more imaginative to those of us in search of charm and novelty. However, it is clearly different to come up with such a contrived solution when one is actually trying to come up with the proper solution than to devise such a solution, Barthelme-style, just for the effect.

Even as appreciation of the "core" problems of narrative is increasing, children's mastery of the structure of narrative is undergoing vast strides. The child of two or two and a half can handle but a single episode—an agent carrying out one action, such as a nurse giving a shot to a patient. A three-year-old can concatenate a couple of episodes, generally in the appropriate order. By the age of four most children have command over a sheaf of episodes: they can combine them into sets and order them in diverse ways to achieve contrasting effects. The more skillful child can also move back and forth within the narrative time line, anticipating what is going to happen and reflecting back on what did happen. Using the proper neutral tone of voice, the child is able to comment, in sophisticated "meta-linguistic" fashion, about the narrator's role or about characters within the story.

In fact, it seems fair to say that by the age of five the child has acquired a "first-draft" knowledge of the literary realm. The child understands the centrality of problems in stories and generally solves at least simple problems by exploiting the resources of the story itself. Nor is the child tied to repetition of the same one or two tired old scripts. He now has enough real world knowledge, sufficient familiarity with different genres, and adequate control of the linguistic resources of narrative so that he can produce an assortment of appealing literary narratives.

Perhaps at this age the term "flowering" of literary imagination can more appropriately be invoked. The child can now conjure up lengthy and complex narratives involving a number of characters who carry out different sequences of behavior—sometimes consistent, sometimes inconsistent with one another, but always filled with spirit and life. I have referred to this phase as a picaresque period, the time when the child's characters, like protagonists of eighteenth-century novels, embark upon a never-ending series of adventures, and where the fun inheres in following each of the adventures rather than in searching for an underlying moral or principle of closure. Consider, for example, the shades of *Tom Jones* in this extract from a five-year-old's effort, which actually goes on for several pages:

Once there was a skunk and he didn't have a home. And he made a home and was going to visit someone and someone chipped [*sic*] down his home. And he went and called up the police and you know what the police did? The police killed the bear because the bear ate up the house 'cause it was made out of honey. And suddenly the bear—there was another bear—and he made a home for the skunk. Then he went out for a walk and a horse came and put a bag of food at the door. And then he came back and ate all the food. He went to bed and then he went and chopped some trees for the fire. And he got a hose and he filled up a pail of water. And he put crane in the chimney and then he went out for a walk. Then he took a long string with him and sometime he pulled the string and suddenly all the waters went out of the pail with the big crane and put the fire out.

Then he found a friend and they went for a walk and they had supper at a little restaurant. . . . (Pitcher and Prelinger, p. 126)

One should not conclude, however, that the child is incapable of coming up with a more rounded story. Many youngsters at this age can create stories that exhibit a genuine sense of composition, rather than simply being a sausage link of disparate segments. Here is a tale told by four-year-old Lila:

Once there was a fish named Flower. She went down in the water and said, "Oh, my gosh, where's my lover?" She went down in the cellar where my house is. She saw a big father fish which had a sword in his nose. She ran away from the house and hid in another house. She ran up the water and flapped out. She swam away. She went to another house in a deep, deep river. She saw her own home which had her lover in it. They kissed each other. That's the end. (p. 101)

The age of five represents a watershed in the development of literary imagination. As we have noted with respect to drawing skills, literary imagination spawns multiple lines of growth during the school years. Some children tell few stories and engage in little imaginative play. Other children continue to tell stories but become increasingly bound by rules: they want to tell only stories that follow the strict rules of a genre. Like the school child who embraces literal language and who spurns metaphor, many children aged eight or nine like to tell stories but only those that adhere faithfully to the schemas of the culture. Children also differ in whether their narratives tend to be matter-of-fact and historical, or whether, though faithful to the genre, their stories are of a more fantastic sort, as in science fiction, adventure, or the wholly invented worlds of the Oz or Narnia variety. Not infrequently the child of this age becomes attracted to "formula stories" which are readily available in the popular media. At the age of seven, two of my children fell in love with the "Encyclopedia Brown" tales (a junior version of "Sherlock Holmes," in which one is invited to solve the mystery by oneself before discovering the author's preferred solution). And at age ten my son became totally enamored of the "Choose Your Own Adventure" series, where one has the opportunity, by ordering and reordering parts of a story, to devise an indefinite number of variations of the same plot constituents.

Only with the advent of the preadolescent years do children exhibit sufficient mastery of genres, however, to be able to attempt parodies—self-conscious deviations from established genres designed to evoke humorous response from one's audience. The twelve- or thirteen-year-old can spoof an "Encyclopedia Brown" story or a fairy tale and can also appreciate parodies, ironies, and other literary experiments that feature a twist on the established genre.

We know more about the stories children tell than about the stories children understand. That is because it is easier to collect children's narratives than it is to probe their understanding. Yet if we want to determine whether, as Bettelheim implies, youngsters respond at an unconscious level to the many latent themes in children's literature, we must attempt to assess how these stories are actually apprehended.

Our own studies and those of other investigators have suggested that Bettelheim's claims about preschool youngsters are exaggerated. Children clearly enjoy stories and love the word-play as well as the bizarre characters and exotic actions. Dr. Seuss would probably have won popularity in many cultures during many eras. Moreover, children clearly appreciate the struggles between good and evil in the story. As the creators of *Star Wars* well knew, even the youngest tot can tell which characters are good and which are bad. Still, there are clear limitations. Preschoolers do not appreciate the possibility that characters can change: they regard them as fixed entities. They are not aware of the fact that if two characters are in conflict, only one of them can have his way. Moreover, they tend to focus much more on surface accouterments (what characters wear, own, and want to have) than on underlying motivations and intentions (how they feel, what they seek). To be sure, when tales are stripped down to bare essentials so that all deceptive material has been eliminated, children can be shown to have some sensitivity to intention and motivation. But most stories in real life are not so stripped down, and so they feature ample misleading surface materials which can lure and even dominate the child's attention.

To support this characterization, let me cite a study conducted a number of years ago by Shelley Rubin, Jane Hanenberg, and me. We were interested in whether, in listening to familiar stories like fairy tales, children were sensitive to the underlying motivations and goals of characters—the reasons evil characters behaved as they did, the struggle between good and evil, the eventual resolution of conflict in favor of the benign force. Given our druthers, we would have liked to have asked children these questions directly, using stories they had often heard before. But equipped with the stern super-ego of the experimental psychologist, we knew that our conclusions would be reliable only if we used materials the children had not yet encountered, and only if we measured their understanding by less direct but more reliable sources of inquiry.

We reasoned as follows. If a child genuinely understands the motivation embedded in a typical fairy tale, he should be on the alert for such motivation; and if adequate motivation is for some reason lacking, the child should find some way to transport or import it to the story. Therefore we contrived a tale afresh, but one that was in many ways similar to the numerous fairy tales all children in our culture have heard. In this particular case, we related "The Princess and the Queen": the tale of a king whose good wife had died, leaving him with a beautiful and clever daughter whom he loved very much. However, the king remarried a new and evil queen, who proved to be insanely jealous of the beautiful rival for her new husband's affections. The queen posed a trio of very difficult tasks to the daughter and made her survival dependent upon the execution of these tasks. Of the children we studied, half at each of several age groups heard the story told in a simple, matter-of-fact way without any motivation supplied; the other half heard the story told with all the motivations (jealousy, love) graphically spelled out. All the children heard the story without an ending. Their job was to finish the story, answer various questions about it, and return some days later to relate the story to us once again.

As we had expected, this unfamiliar fairy tale posed great difficulties for first and third graders. Even when motivations were clearly described, the children seemed unable to appreciate just what made the various characters tick, the nature of their goals, and the extent to which queen and daughter were engaged in irreconcilable conflict. The third graders were in fact completely immobilized by the nefarious queen. Her powers were so overwhelming that they could find no way to defeat her. And so the youngsters simply assumed, contrary to the dictates of the fairy-tale genre, that she would carry the day: the princess was made to fail on the final task and simply faded away thereafter.

The sixth graders provided a different and highly instructive picture. They were able to end the story in a manner appropriate to a fairy tale: the princess solved the final, most difficult task, she was rescued by a Prince Charming, and the queen was so angry that she whirled herself (in Disney fashion) into a mad frenzy before disappearing into the night. Moreover, the sixth graders revealed to us, by their retellings some days later, that they had mastered the genre of fairy tales. Those children who had heard a version without any motivation actually provided considerable rationale for the characters' actions. And the longer the distance from the original time of telling, the more motivation inveigled its way into the stories. This finding indicated to us that sixth graders, unlike the younger subjects, have a firm grasp on how fairy tales work. In retelling the story, they (either deliberately or unconsciously) wove into the story the feelings and motives that would make it intelligible to others and to themselves. As if to drive home this point, the sixth graders were also the only individuals who had sufficient mastery of the fairy-tale genre to enable them, if they chose, to provide parodies, either in their completions or in their retellings of the story.

To be sure, this study encourages a conservative interpretation. It may well be that younger children have greater sensitivity to motivation than this rather formidable task elicited, and that they routinely gain more information from oft-repeated fairy tales than they did from "The Princess and the Queen" heard for the first time. Yet even if our age estimates are off, the study at least gives us pause before we accept claims that the young child is privy to the latent themes of literary works. Though young children may love to hear fairy tales and may be attracted to the dramatic clashes in the stories, they seem unable to understand the motivations of each character and the ways in which they interact in the plot.

Such insensitivity to psychological aspects of a story has been echoed in several other investigations of literary imagination. In our studies of children's comprehension of metaphor, described in the previous essay, we found that when the metaphor was based strictly on surface similarities (for example, "the prison guard was like a tall tree") the children could readily understand it. There only the recognition of perceptual similarities was required, and children are quite discerning in recognizing such parallels. But when the metaphoric characterization required psychological understanding ("the prison guard was like a hard rock"), the essential insight escaped children below the age of middle childhood. By the same token, when we asked children about the reality or fictive status of characters on television, they could discuss this question in terms of superficial traits: they indicated whether the individual could fly or deflect bullets, and they placed great weight on whether he was depicted in a realistic photograph or in a cartoon.

What the children failed to appreciate was the psychological reality, the underlying personality of the personage. And so they would indicate that Superman was more genuine than Charlie Brown. In this case the "cartoon" factor dominated: the child completely overlooked the fact that, as an individual, Charlie Brown displayed plausible psychological traits, while Superman was "out of this world."

In each of the major phases of literary development, then, certain aspects of imagination are brought to the fore even as others lie relatively dormant. But over and above this developmental sequence, which may well characterize all normal children within our society, we must take into account revealing individual differences. We have noted that from the very first children differ in the extent to which they embrace the realm of fiction and in their willingness to disregard the dimensions of physical objects. We have every reason to expect—though we have not yet amassed the evidence to prove—that such individual differences endure throughout childhood. And we would expect that those children who in early life are relatively independent of objects would be far more likely to engage in fantasy or imaginative activities in the literary domain than those who show a strong dependence upon objects. (It is not surprising that many creative adults remember that during their childhood they conjured up imaginary companions, or even imaginary worlds.) From those who seem tied to the objects of physical reality, we would expect a preference for more purely narrative forms, such as history or journalism, or perhaps even an avoidance of the literary realm. These individual differences may well arise from deep psychological differences between children, such as their willingness to lose themselves in play, to relinquish control of impulses, to take risks in their acts with other individuals. However, these individual differences should not be confused with developmental differences: we have noted that the structural complexities of narratives devised by object-dependent children proved comparable to those of object-independent children.

Other factors also color the child's imaginative output. One obvious component is motivation: the extent to which the child is driven to try out new things, to engage in literary exploration, to play with words and scenes, to create fictive worlds. Sometimes this motivation is beneficent, as when the child secures considerable pleasure out of creating and exploring worlds of his imagination. However, this inventiveness could also have a more defensive origin. In such cases the child's satisfaction with his own experience might be sufficiently meagre to force him to resort to inventions, to imaginary friends, to imaginary worlds, in order to gain sustenance and maintain his equilibrium.

Environment also counts. Children raised in households where such play of the imagination is encouraged, where parents invent stories every night, are far more likely to regard this as an "approved" activity and to engage in it than are those children raised in environments in which such fantasy is absent or actively discouraged, perhaps as inimical to personal values, religious tenets, or aesthetic standards.

Even given appropriate motivation, personal style, and supporting environment, the advent and maturing of literary imagination is not a foregone conclusion. Just as the child's logical understanding of the world must be constructed, so must his ability to engage in pretense and fantasy. There may well be natural inclination toward this activity, but in order to carry it out comprehensively and with proper control, the child must attain considerable sophistication. This "constructive" characterization is borne out both by the recurrent difficulties that young children have in keeping the fictive realm separate from the rest of their lives and by the problems that even more sophisticated adults encounter in the willing suspension of disbelief.

Further evidence for the constructive aspects of literary imagination come from a totally separate population. There is now an impressive amount of evidence that, as a consequence of brain damage to the right hemisphere, individuals lose the ability (which they had carefully constructed during the childhood years) to honor the conventions of the fictive realm. Like preschool children, they fail to appreciate the rules embedded in a particular script or narrative: they intersperse and interject themselves at will; they argue with premises in the story. In their behavior with narrative materials they signal their failure to appreciate that a separate realm of experience with its own principles and boundaries has been constructed. In still other pathological populations—for example, alcoholics suffering from Korsakoff's disease—one can encounter an instructively contrasting set of symptoms: an inability to stop confabulating, an inveterate tendency to create narratives—rather as if the "fabulating faculty" has been given leave to go off at will.

Through a further study of the natural development of literary imagination in children's play and storytelling, we will doubtless learn more about our opening conundrum: the extent to which it is valid to speak of the young child as a creative genius or, alternatively, as an immature individual ignorant of his activity and therefore not worthy of the epithet of a literary imaginer. And yet a central mystery is likely to remain. Whatever their individual style or cultural milieu, nearly all children find it natural and enjoyable to play in the sand, to enact cops and robbers, to engage in verbal play, to listen to stories from the lips of their parents or the screen of their television. These aspects of literary imagination seem to be universal. But it is an entirely separate matter to determine which of the millions of children who engage in these activities will later in life somehow be impelled, on their own, once again to create new worlds, to invent realms of fictions into which other people can be invited and about whose reality they may become convinced, as they have been persuaded in earlier times by the worlds of a Charles Dickens, a Marcel Proust, a William Faulkner. We all can invent our own story and many of us can pen the novel of our own lives, but very few of us are given to devise new worlds which carry conviction for others and for ourselves. The features that distinguish Faulkner or Dickens from the rest of us lie somewhere in the individual development of each child. But just where they lie and whether they can be fostered in individuals is a question that has so far eluded scientific study.

16

NADIA'S CHALLENGE

PHILOSOPHERS of science are fond of claiming that a theory, or model, can never be disproved by a new fact or even a set of facts, but only by a new and more comprehensive theory. While this may be a useful rule of thumb, it suggests, misleadingly, that individual findings cannot have revolutionary reverberations. In fact, when a solar eclipse in 1919 showed that certain predictions by Einstein of the way light would be deflected were correct, the theory of relativity gained immeasurably in stature. Conversely, proponents of the theory that intelligence is inherited suffered a severe blow when data presented by Sir Cyril Burt were shown to be fraudulent.

A well-entrenched field of study—the psychology of children's art— has recently been put on trial, thanks to a handful of drawings produced by a single autistic girl named Nadia. A century ago, when scientists and educators turned their attention to the study of children, they frequently began by collecting children's drawings. After all, nearly every child draws, and most draw enthusiastically for several years. Drawings are fun to look at, easy to store, and lend themselves to systematic (though not necessarily penetrating) analysis.

The drawings have usually been interpreted—and even distorted— to support one psychological perspective or another. Consider, for instance, the way various authorities would analyze a child's drawing of a gorilla that shows the contents of the animal's stomach, as if in an X-ray view. Those of a psychodynamic persuasion focus on the symbolism of a picture and might see such a drawing as an expression of oral fears—being devoured by a monster—or of sexual or aggressive drives. Those in the cognitive tradition of psychology overlook the symbolic implications of the subject matter and attend, instead, to information about the child's thinking processes as evidenced in the drawings. In their view, the child draws what he knows instead of what he sees; thus, he includes what he knows belongs to an animal— the stomach and its contents. Some cognitivists even consider the drawing an index of the child's intelligence.

Whatever their particular slant, psychologists have agreed about the general evolutionary course of children's drawings. According to the orthodoxy, children pick up markers for the first time at the age of twelve to eighteen months. They scribble for perhaps a year, then go on to make discrete geometrical forms, such as circles, squares, triangles, and crosses. These forms are gradually combined, and by the age of three to three and a half the child displays a rich repertoire of geometric patterns.

At that time the first genuine, spontaneous representations emerge. Circles with two lines radiating downward become human beings (called "tadpoles" in the literature on children's drawings); circles with four lines extending below serve as dogs or horses; circles with eight radiating lines represent suns. Soon the child can create more complex representational figures—again constructing them by combining geometric forms. By the age of five or six, he can group figures into scenes that exhibit a sense of balance and color.

While these primitive compositions often possess considerable charm, children of this age lack the ability to portray distance relationships, to capture objects at unusual angles, or to control such aesthetic essentials as quality of line. These more sophisticated aspects of drawing appear only in the years before adolescence, if they ever appear.

Enter Nadia, born in Nottingham, England, of Ukrainian *émigré* parents, in October 1967. According to Lorna Selfe's book, *Nadia*, this youngster seemed at first to develop in a relatively normal way. The second of three children, Nadia said her first few words at the end of her first year but thereafter became increasingly autistic. By the age of three, her developmental profile was already markedly impaired: motor development was slow; she neither understood the words of others nor was able to communicate through language, gesture, or pretend play.

A lethargic child, Nadia nevertheless displayed, at the age of three and a half, an extraordinary capacity to draw. Using her favored left hand, she began to draw animals, particularly horses, in a way reminiscent of a highly talented adolescent or adult artist. Unlike any young child known to psychologists, she had reportedly skipped the various scribbling, schematic, and tadpole stages. When producing representational figures, she did not juxtapose the usual rigid schemata on one another. Rather, her drawings showed a remarkable fidelity to the contours of the object itself, as if they were being slavishly traced, and soon came to feature perspective, foreshortening, and other tricks of the artist's trade.

Figure 16.1. Drawing of a rooster in Nadia's picture book.

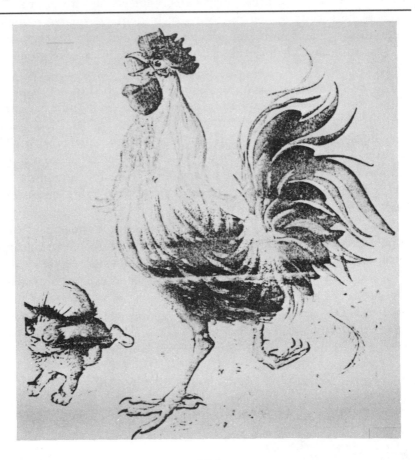

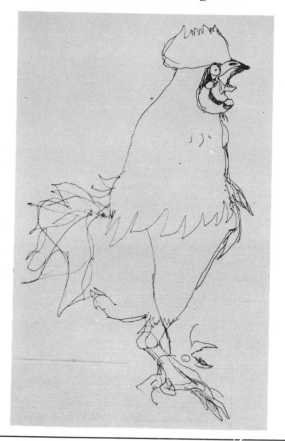

Figure 16.2. Nadia's rendition of a rooster.

How Nadia drew is as amazing as what she drew. Her drawings were usually inspired by pictures that she had once seen; yet she did not draw with the model in front of her, nor in most cases had she even recently seen the model. The pictures were mere points of departure; she varied her versions, experimenting with different forms until she hit upon an approach that satisfied her own exacting, if mysterious, standards. (See the reproduction of the rooster that served as a model for Nadia, and her version of it.) More tellingly, she did not need to draw details in any particular order; Nadia was so in command of the medium that she was able to place one detail in one location on the paper, another detail in another, and then join them at a later point, serenely confident that the composite parts would fit.

187

Clearly, then, Nadia was an anomaly—so much so that publication of Lorna Selfe's account of her talents threw into question the entire collected wisdom of earlier students of children's drawings. If one English girl with severe cognitive and emotional deficits could draw like a master from the first, then the stages painstakingly described by scholars (and painstakingly passed through by preschoolers) turn out to be only typical occurrences rather than necessary developmental milestones.

Even as the experts have shaken their heads in disbelief at Nadia's drawings (no one has yet, to my knowledge, pronounced them fraudulent), they have wondered if the classic portrait of children's drawings can be salvaged. Perhaps Nadia is a freak: in that case, we should not have to revise our theories, because it is *she,* and not our model, that is at fault. Perhaps she has a unique degree of eidetic imagery—that "photographic" ability to retain in one's mind's eye an exact image of elements that have disappeared from sight. But if that were the only necessity, then why don't other people with eidetic imagery draw as well as Nadia—and why can't all of us draw as superlatively when we have a model in front of us?

Perhaps Nadia is a throwback to an earlier time, drawing in the same way as the cave artists of Lascaux, who were able to capture the contours of animals in a single flowing line. But the cave artists were presumably normal, though gifted, adults, not aberrant five-year-olds, and recent evidence suggests they had to practice their craft for a long time. Perhaps Nadia is a genius—like Rembrandt, Raphael, or Picasso—but an examination of Picasso's childhood drawings confirms that not even he could draw like Nadia until his preadolescent years.

One especially prevalent explanation of Nadia's precocity stresses the absence of language. Perhaps drawing, in normal individuals, is strongly influenced by the ability to speak and to form concepts. These factors of cognition, so vital to most human activities, may interfere with depicting the world in a visually faithful manner. Only someone like Nadia, bereft of language, can look directly at the world and draw it the way it appears—or so the argument goes.

Evidence to support this line of reasoning comes from the fact that when Nadia did begin to talk around age nine, her drawings declined sharply in quantity and, according to her therapists, in quality as well. Nor is this an isolated observation: other gifted autistic children have also relinquished their talents in the process of shedding their more virulent symptoms. One critic has gone so far as to suggest that those who taught Nadia to speak were guilty of a crime, since they undermined the one genuine talent she had.

I cannot accept the "linguistic" interpretation of Nadia's giftedness. Other autistic children do not draw as well as she does, and most children cease to draw imaginatively after the age of six or seven, even when they are not autistic. Still, I feel comfortable with one implication of this theory. Assume that the human mind consists of a series of highly tuned computational devices whose location and structure we have not yet identified, and that we differ vastly from one another in the extent to which each of these devices is "primed" to go off. We know that certain individuals—both normal and brain-damaged—can execute prodigious feats of mind at an early age. Such children have, during their early years, played chess, sung operas, performed

Figure 16.3. Nadia's drawing of a horse and rider, executed at age five and a half.

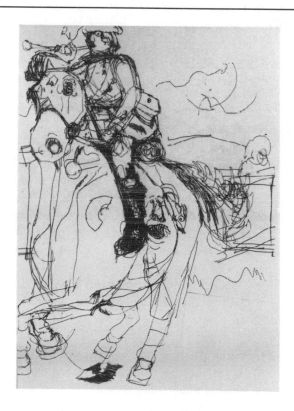

mathematics, read fluently, and learned foreign languages, all with little help from the outside—even when they have been woefully lacking in other skills.

Though most such prodigies seem to be "computers" in the traditional sense—that is, their skills are of a calculating variety—there is, in principle, no reason why a similar faculty could not exist for graphic skills. Such a computational device would study the way in which objects are depicted in pictures (Nadia did that for months at a time), direct the movement of eyes back and forth along the appropriate contours, and then reproduce forms manually on a separate sheet of paper. With repeated practice, the once-faithful copies would eventually achieve more of an individual identity; a person possessing numerous schemata for a given object (say, a horse like Nadia's, reproduced here) could travel freely from one to another and eventually calculate many of the possible forms in between. This is what Nadia, like preadolescent artists who are able to draw the full gallery of televised superheroes, became able to do.

If we assume that Nadia possessed such a computer, one worthy of an artistic genius, and if we further assume that she had no other way of capturing her experience, we can at least conceive how she could have progressed so rapidly within a few years: by concentrating all of her time and all of her effort on drawing, she was able to activate her computer in the fullest possible way. And it is indeed proper to speak of progress, for her drawings at age five and six were far more remarkable than those done at the age of three or four. Furthermore, the only drawing of hers saved from the age of three and a half is far simpler than later drawings. In fact, to my eyes, it is the only one that might, conceivably, have been done by a precocious preschool child.

The scientists may be able to refurbish their theory enough to accommodate Nadia. In my view, she may well have passed through the earliest stages of drawing just like every other child, but with unparalleled rapidity—perhaps in a matter of weeks or even days. Her natural talent (in my terms, possession of a computer) combined with an uncanny capacity to analyze the pictures and the tenacity to drill for hours on end enabled her to achieve, by the age of five, the level of a skilled adolescent.

When she was seven and a half, Nadia entered a school for autistic children. She soon became more sociable, engaged in games with other children, improved steadily in language comprehension, and even began to say a few single-word utterances. Within two years, she was handling simple addition, subtraction, reading, and writing. By the age of nine (in 1977) she would still make a drawing of good quality upon request, but she seldom drew spontaneously. Now enrolled in an autistic unit for adolescents, Nadia is once again being encouraged to draw. And according to Lorna Selfe, the psychologist who once worked with Nadia, her most recent drawings are reminiscent of her childhood works, evidencing the same fine lines and vivid action.

Whatever the aesthetic status of her current and future work, however, Nadia's early drawing activity differed from the practices of serious artists. Nadia displayed no interest in capturing her ideas, feelings, and concepts in a medium that might convey meaning to others. Rather, she sought to work out her own visual experiences in the sole vehicle of expression available to her (even when it meant ignoring the edge of the paper and scribbling on the table, or superimposing a new drawing on a previous one).

In this way, if in no other, this autistic child resembled her five-year-old peers. For no matter how charming and expressive their drawings may be to our eyes, children in this age group are not fully engaged in artistry. Like Nadia, the scribbling five-year-olds are simply exercising their more modest talents at visual depiction in a way that seems pleasing. The ultimate flowering of artistry may require a society that has a genuine interest in its budding artists and values their creations.

17

THE PRODIGIES' PROGRESS

IMAGINE a musical audition where the contestants are barred from the view of the judges. The first candidate plays a Bach *partita* for violin in a way reminiscent of the legendary master Fritz Kreisler. The second contestant sings an aria with exquisite pitch, rhythm, and verbal articulation. The third plays a simple but elegant piano sonata that he has himself composed.

The curtain is raised to reveal two surprises: first, the contestants are all four-year-old preschoolers—youthful musical prodigies; second, the youngsters represent three entirely different populations. The first is a Japanese child who has been enrolled since the age of two in an intensive Suzuki Talent Education program. The second child is a victim of infantile autism, a youngster incapable of normal communication or the simplest problem-solving, yet able to reproduce entire operatic compositions perfectly upon a single hearing. The third auditioner is a child-prodigy composer, belonging to the succession that includes Mozart in the eighteenth century and Felix Mendelssohn in the nineteenth century. Three dazzling musical achievements, presumably attained by disparate musical routes in three distinctive youngsters.

Though such achievements can perhaps be made most readily (and dramatically) in music, an analogous trio of individuals could be assembled in other domains of competence. For example, in the area of visual arts one could cite an autistic child like the gifted artist Nadia (see previous essay); or a child growing up in an intensive "hothouse" artistic atmosphere, such as that reputedly found in Bali; or a young prodigy who will one day become a major master like Picasso or Klee. In fact, even outside the arts, in domains such as mathematics, chess, or expository writing, one may find a comparable range of gifts, perhaps emanating from an equally wide array of sources.

As a starting point, we may dub all of these children "prodigies": they are performing at a far higher level than others of their age, thereby defying developmental norms and theories. It would be convenient for psychologists if we could ignore these youngsters altogether, or if we could simply absorb them into mainstream developmental psychology. But as we saw in the case of Nadia, such solutions will not work. Certain youngsters simply become too skilled too rapidly for them to be treated as though they were "just like other children." Their precocity is often restricted to a single area, thus challenging "structural" accounts of development, such as those favored by Piaget. The fates of such children are also varied: some (like Mozart and Picasso) go on to become acknowledged geniuses; many others slip away into oblivion or become mediocre practitioners of their chosen specialty. And, of course, precocity is not a requisite for high attainment. Individuals as diverse as Charles Darwin, William Wordsworth, Winston Churchill, and Vincent van Gogh showed little or no sign of precocity and yet eventually attained the heights of their fields. Clearly, the problem of the prodigy is too broad and pervasive to be slipped under the rug of "acceptable statistical deviations."

Extraordinary achievement has long captivated scientists. The pioneering psychologist Francis Galton assembled lists of the most "eminent people" of his time (some of whom, like Charles Darwin, were his relatives) in order to show that "genius" was largely inherited. Proceeding in a more systematic way, the noted Stanford educational psychologist Lewis Terman followed the youths with the highest IQ's in California throughout their adult lives. And in an effort to study the children who are the brightest of all, Leta Hollingworth, one of Terman's students, collected portraits of a handful of children with IQ's over 180.

Well motivated as these studies were, they told us little about prodigiousness—not, I think, because they failed to address the issue directly but rather because they proceeded from a misleading notion of talent. Galton did not study children at all. Terman and Hollingworth, both sold on intelligence testing, equated achievement with a high score on an IQ test. In the light of our current understanding, it seems clear that a high score on an IQ test reveals little about genuine prodigiousness. In fact, the kind of factual knowledge and versatile problem-solving ability that seems to produce a high IQ may even be antithetical to the rapid progress within a given field of expertise, which is the hallmark of prodigiousness. Moreover, and interestingly, even though many of the high-IQ individuals did well by societal standards, none of them, to my knowledge, made creative breakthroughs of a truly noteworthy sort.

Basic to this "IQ mentality" is a belief that individuals are born with a certain amount of ability—a "fixed-trait" view of mental powers. Though it may be impossible to eliminate talk of a general component or components of intelligence (it seems entrenched in our language), an increasing number of psychologists now reject that way of thinking about intellect. The view of the mind put forth by the Genevan psychologist Jean Piaget seems an advance over former views.

Rather than thinking of individuals as being born with "more" or "less" intelligence, Piaget views the growth of the mind as a process wherein all individuals must pass through the same course of interactions with the world. It is essential to experience these interactions if one is to attain the mark of full-fledged intellect—the higher levels of operational thinking. Individuals may differ in the rapidity with which they pass through these stages, and there may be some correlation between such speed and scores on IQ tests. But the Piagetian view focuses on the attainment over a period of time of thinking skills rather than on the mastery of factual information, the ability to memorize strings of numbers, or an individual's vocabulary—all mainstays of the IQ test.

There are limitations in Piaget's views as well, particularly with respect to the issue of prodigious behavior. First of all, like the IQ inventors with whom he studied, Piaget viewed intellect as a single, highly organized capacity that cuts across all domains of knowledge. In other words, if one knows an individual's "operational level," one can predict his performance on all tasks. Secondly, Piaget showed little interest in the differences among individuals, especially differences between the average individual and the individual with special gifts. He would have had little, if anything, to say about the young Bobby Fischer or Pablo Picasso as a child.

A scholar much influenced by Piaget's thinking, David Feldman, of Tufts University, has developed several Piagetian notions in ways that make them applicable to the enigma of prodigiousness. In addition to developing a useful framework, Feldman has also worked intensively with a small group of prodigies and has illuminated the nature and extent of their talents. In the light of Feldman's work, it proves possible to frame a tentative answer to the question: Which prodigies succeed and why?

Rather than viewing all intellect as one seamless piece, Feldman distinguishes among different uses of the mind. Certain abilities, such as the mental operations studied by Piaget, are within the ken of every normal human being: hence they are *universals* of intellect. Others are ubiquitous within a given culture but may not be practiced at all elsewhere—for example, literacy is a universal capacity in *our* culture, while swimming is universal in some South Sea islands.

Still others are considered *special, disciplinary,* or *idiosyncratic* domains within a given society: for example, in our society some individuals are highly skilled in music, mathematics, or chess, but a high degree of proficiency in these domains is not expected (or found) in the average individual. Finally, at the opposite end of the continuum from universal is *unique* knowledge—that form of intellect within a domain that is initially pursued by just one individual but may ultimately lead to the founding of a field. Examples would include the mode of thinking invented by Isaac Newton or Charles Darwin. The striking thing about such accomplishments is that if they happen to prove adaptive within a cultural setting, they may eventually become dispersed throughout that culture. The once unique accomplishments of Isaac Newton and Charles Darwin have become attainable by many individuals living in Western society.

According to Feldman, the range of human accomplishments can be usefully catalogued in terms of their location within the continuum from *universal* to *unique.* As it happens, most intelligence testers and Piagetian researchers have been interested primarily in the universal end of the continuum: those skills (like language or logical thinking) of which we are all presumably capable. On the other hand, the areas where prodigies tend to occur are the disciplinary or idiosyncratic domains—deployments of mind where a few people do amazingly well, perhaps from a very early age, while most do not ever attain appreciable levels of expertise.

Having constructed this continuum, Feldman then makes a crucial proposal. Rather than being entirely different from the rest of us, prodigies are best viewed as individuals who move through certain "special" domains at a very rapid rate. According to this analysis, which injects Piagetian thinking into "non-universal" domains, every individual necessarily starts out in a domain as a novice; then, as in a medieval guild, individuals have the opportunity to become an apprentice, a journeyman, and eventually an expert or master. Perhaps all of us have the potential to become a journeyman, if not a master, should we work very diligently in one of these domains. The prodigy is the individual who passes with lightning speed through the entire developmental progression.

Of course speed of development during the early years does not necessarily culminate in greatness. One can be highly gifted at an early age without ever attaining mastery in adulthood. As a practical matter, however, it turns out that nearly all individuals who eventually achieved a dominant position in their fields were, in fact, prodigies. The psychologist John R. Hayes has documented that the achievement of mastery in diverse fields of competence involves at least ten years of steady work, even in the case of the most superbly gifted individuals, like a Mozart or a Rembrandt. It may simply be too difficult to cover the same terrain between the ages of twenty and thirty that prodigious children traverse during their preadolescent decade. No less than in swimming or tennis, the early years may be decisive in the creative realm.

Beyond question, individuals differ markedly from one another in the extent to which they can negotiate their way through a domain. In all likelihood, hereditary factors play their part: certain people seem specially "prepared" to grasp the regularities in specific domains of knowledge, as prepared as *all* of us are to grasp the rules that operate in the realm of language.

But individual gifts and tenacity are not the only variables. In order to understand the origins and ultimate fate of prodigious behaviors, one must take into account other factors as well. First, there is the nature of the domain itself. Some domains require very little interaction with the outside world, little knowledge about one's own psychology or about other individuals' personalities: they are relatively *self-contained*. It is in these domains—such as chess or mathematics, and also certain aspects of music—that an individual can progress very quickly with relatively little direct tutelage. In contrast, in such domains of knowledge as literature, philosophy, or history, one is much more dependent upon years of experience in the world. Not infrequently, supreme achievements in these fields do not emerge until one's mature years, as happened, for example, in the cases of the philosopher Kant and the poet Yeats.

Another factor of importance, one often overlooked, is the maturity of the domain itself within a given society. Sometimes a domain, like mathematics, has been highly developed, in which case progress at a rapid rate becomes possible. Moreover, the fact that a domain is situated in a locale which cares about that field can engender prodigious behaviors. Upwards of 50 percent of the chess prodigies in the United States come from three metropolitan areas—New York, San Francisco, and Los Angeles—which, taken together, have but 10 percent of the population. One can find similarly high percentages of youthful violinists in families of Russian-Jewish extraction. But when a domain may have developed only to a slight degree in a society, or perhaps not have been invented at all, there can be poignant results. The potentially greatest chess player in the world cannot even become a "hack" if the game has not yet spread to his locale. And even the most gifted mathematician cannot make genuine innovations if he lives in a culture where mathematics has been little developed. What is innovative within his culture will be "old hat" elsewhere.

This fate in fact befell the Indian mathematician Ramanujan, said to be the most talented natural mathematician of this century. Working virtually on his own in India, Ramanujan matched the accomplishments of several centuries of mathematics. However, this work had already been performed in the West, and so when he finally arrived in England it was too late for him to join the forefront of his profession. Mozart's musical talent might have shone through in any age and culture: yet there may have been a special fit between his particular flair and the style of classical music he heard in his home and which he was later to recast in such innovative ways.

Through a consideration of these factors, Feldman arrived at an interesting recipe for the geneses of prodigies. In his view, prodigiousness is due to a set of events that he termed "coincidence." As Feldman explained in his book *Beyond Universals in Cognitive Development:*

I see early prodigious achievement as the occurrence in time and space of a remarkable preorganized human being, born and educated during perhaps the optimal period and in a manner perhaps most likely to engage the child's interest and commitment to the mastery of a highly evolved field of knowledge. In other words, a "coincidence" occurs, more remarkable even than the awesome talents which make it possible. This subtle, delicate coordination of elements of human potential and cultural tradition is to me even more dazzling than the abilities characteristically attributed to these children. (p. 151)

The various strands of coincidence discernible in the lives of famous (and infamous) prodigies can be seen in the specific case studies that

Feldman has conducted over the past several years. For example, one of the chess prodigies studied by Feldman is an eight-year-old New Yorker who ranks in the top twenty players in the country under the age of thirteen. This youngster, currently being trained by a chess master, plays chess with total concentration, spending up to eight hours at a chessboard with only a brief break for lunch. This gift is amply supported by outside aid. His father spends much of his free time arranging schedules, transporting, waiting for, and otherwise encouraging his young chess-player son: he does this less out of ruthless ambition than from a desire to help his son carry out what is obviously of central importance in his own life.

Another youngster studied by Feldman is a nine-year-old composer and violinist who lives only two hours away from Boston. Described by his teacher as the most promising student he has ever known, the child has been composing since six, sometimes writing works he could not himself perform. Chauffeured regularly by his mother, he goes to seven different kinds of lessons given by at least five teachers at three locations around Boston. Like the chess player, he is totally absorbed in his work and never loses his aplomb; indeed, he loves to perform and to receive congratulations, though he is rarely surprised or overwhelmed by it.

We occasionally hear of the "omnibus" prodigy—the individual, like the young Goethe or John Stuart Mill, who is reputed to excel "across the board." But such individuals, who sprint simultaneously along multiple tracks of excellence, must be exceedingly rare. For example, in the six youngsters whom Feldman has studied intensively, and in the dozen or so others that he and I have heard about, there is little evidence for such "transfer of prodigiousness." These youngsters, who include gifted artists, writers, and a young scientifically oriented child, are certainly bright and often very appealing personalities. But when Feldman gave three of them batteries of tests, including measures of operational intelligence, moral reasoning, social perspective-taking, and map drawing, they performed like their bright age-mates, not like individuals who were "off the scale." Nor do the few case studies that have been published support the notion that a prodigy is a prodigy in everything. Brightness (as in Terman's subjects) may cut across domains, but prodigiousness does not.

If all goes well for the prodigy as *Wunderkind,* will he naturally attain the heights of productivity in a chosen domain? Certainly a display of early signs of prodigiousness and a culture that recognizes the importance of that talent are essential components in ultimate achievements. But of equal importance, it seems, are the particular facts of the individual's own life. At a certain point in development, an individual must become self-reflective: he needs to address his own activities, evaluating them in terms of his own goals as well as the values of the culture in which he lives. With prodigies, such reflectiveness often occasions a so-called "mid-life crisis" in adolescence. The youth begins to ask, "Why am I doing this? Is it for me or for other people? Is it all worthwhile?" Those who cannot fashion a satisfactory answer often cease their creative efforts.

There is a risk entailed in *not* having such a crisis, in avoiding self-analysis: the individual may continue to be fluent and glib, but he may never deepen his talents. Numerous cases can be cited of youthful prodigies who did not "pan out" in the long run. It was quipped of the prodigious composer Camille Saint-Saëns, "He had everything, but he lacked inexperience." In fact, the opportunity to have diverse experiences and to reflect upon them clearly is crucial in areas like philosophy or literature, and may be important in such fields as the sciences, music, and perhaps even chess. Possibly the most profound achievements involve the whole person, an individual who has sought to come to grips with himself: only through unsparing self-examination is such deepening likely to come about.

Certain personal traits contribute to the requisite developmental history. An individual who would be great needs to be daring, able to take risks, willing to confront the unknown. But even that is not enough. If his contributions are to be sustained, the individual must also display staying power: he must have the fiber to transcend an early triumph (or disaster) and continue to deepen. The presence of sensitive models and teachers, the existence of an audience to appreciate his inventions, and a healthy injection of luck—all these are at a premium.

Even if this model serves as a viable framework for the development of talent, one can still ask whether it can help to illuminate individual cases. We can test our model by returning to the four-year-olds introduced at the beginning of this essay.

First, our young autistic child. This hapless youngster serves as an example of an individual with a fantastic native gift in the domain of musical perception and recall. This gift is the sole reason the child is able to learn and sing back entire pieces upon a single hearing. However, this gift unfolds largely apart from a cultural context. It is simply a "well-prepared computer" unfolding at great speed—possibly because of genetic inheritance and possibly also because of great powers of concentration and the absence of competing stimuli. As long as the child remains autistic, he will be unable to relate this gift to the interests and concerns of the culture, and, even more important, he will be unable to benefit from the psychological deepening which ordinarily occurs during youth. In fact, unless this orientation is radically altered, he is destined to produce (or reproduce) works which, while skilled technically, cannot be considered genuinely artistic. They will lack that sense of originality, that essential tension, that emotional range which we associate with the most valued performances. Genetic endowment is not enough.

Consider, in contrast, the young Suzuki student. Such youngsters do not necessarily have unusual music talent as part of their birthright, though it may well be that musical families are more likely to gravitate toward a Suzuki school. These children benefit, however, from living in a culture where tremendous attention is paid to the development of musical skill and, more generally, to the attainment of artistic sensitivity.

Suzuki students travel amazingly far on the basis of shrewd teaching and the contributions of a culture that cares deeply. They remind us of the role a culture can assume when it chooses to pour considerable resources into a field of endeavor. However, without a generous dollop of native talent, and without the kind of ever-deepening personal history to which I referred above, it is unlikely that the Suzuki children will eventually become notable adult musicians. It is interesting that Shinichi Suzuki regards his program as a means of training character and discipline, not as a means of producing hundreds of virtuoso violinists. And perhaps not surprisingly, most of his students cease playing at or before adolescence.

Finally, our third child, a future Mozart. In his case, we can examine the historical record for guidance. As a prodigy, Mozart represented the rare "coincidence" of all the aforementioned factors: an individual of unquestionable individual talent; a field that allowed prodigious accomplishment; life in a cultural and family setting that (in his formative years) was highly supportive of his talent; a developmental history that, in its combination of vicissitudes, triumphs, and tragedies, led to remarkable deepening—a maturing testified to by the power of *Don Giovanni*, the later concerti and symphonies, and the final *Requiem*. In this unique instance, natural gifts, cultural support, and personal developmental history combined, as perhaps never before and never since, to yield unsurpassed accomplishment.

Even armed with this model, it may still be impossible to predict *which* gifted young children will eventually achieve mastery, even as it may be impossible to tell, given an adult master, exactly what his youthful work was like. There is simply too much variance. Even as experiences in a person's life can change the appearance, if not the actual structure, of one's face, so, too, the twists and turns of one's own history can prove critical in determining the relationship between youthful giftedness and adult mastery.

Nonetheless, based on our hypothetical examples, it is possible to offer a relatively simple formula for success. First, take an individual who, initially with little support from the environment, exhibits a strong proclivity toward a particular medium of expression. Place that child in a family and a culture that cares about this particular medium and that provides the child with plenty of opportunity to explore and to master the medium. Add the requisite experiences in the rigors and vicissitudes of life—pleasures, pains, conflicts, opportunities for self-reflection and self-examination. Finally, recreate the atmosphere of classical Athens, Renaissance Florence, or turn-of-the-century Vienna. If such a recipe could be followed, it might actually produce a bevy of innovative individuals. But until this model is subjected to considerably more testing, it had best be restricted to texts in psychology rather than be offered in tracts on child rearing.

PART III

ON EDUCATION
AND MEDIA:
THE TRANSMISSION
OF KNOWLEDGE

INTRODUCTION

DEVELOPMENTAL PSYCHOLOGISTS subscribe to a convenient fiction. Just as Rousseau was fond of talking of a "state of nature" untrammeled by any effects of the corporate state, members of the corps to which I belong enjoy discussing "pure" or "natural" development: the unfolding of an individual's cognitive and affective capacities with only minimal interventions by others, such as family members, peers, or the more impersonal institutions of the external society.

But this is a fiction, and perhaps a not altogether appropriate one. Just as Rousseau could not really rear his fictional Émile without any interventions by others (many commentators view Émile's Rousseauan tutor as a master manipulator of development), so, too, the notion of an individual developing to any significant extent in the absence of a cultural milieu is untenable. From the very first days of life we live in a meaningful environment, surrounded by symbol-using creatures who are conveying messages to us, who are constantly interpreting our behaviors, and who soon show us which interpretations "matter" in our environment. Before long, more formal kinds of educational intervention are taking place in school, through other social institutions, and at the feet of various media of communication. Take away culture and the result is autism or death.

As behavioral scientists, we have no choice but to unite insights from the biological and psychological realms (where growth may be thought of as a largely individual preordained matter) and findings from anthropology, sociology, and education (where the formative nature of our milieu is taken for granted). In the essays in this section we turn our attention directly to various forms of education in order to discern the effects they exert upon the developing child who has thus far occupied our attention, as well as the effects upon the learner who continues to exist in all of us. In essay 18, which contains some musings on the proper course of artistic education, we encounter the interface between naturally occurring developmental processes and more focused interventions on the part of educators and educational institutions. I argue for a proper rhythm in the educational processes, with external interventions relatively ineffective (and inappropriate) in the first years of symbolic exploration, but increasingly opportune (and necessary) during the middle years of childhood. Still in the area of art education, I go on to describe in essay 19 one approach which greatly impressed me when I happened to encounter it at an exhibition in Minneapolis. This discussion also serves as a tribute to one of the great art educators of our time, Rudolf Arnheim.

The remaining essays in this section deal more directly with new forms of educational technology, forms that are effecting a revolution in the ways in which all of us process information, learn, and teach. During a time when we cannot escape inundation by the electronic media of communication, it is difficult to remember, but important to recall, that even the medium of written language is but a few millennia old, and that until a few centuries ago it was the possession of only a small élite. Now, however, schoolrooms that concentrate on the three R's are considered "old hat," and any school system worth its salt has its bevy of portapaks and microcomputers. There are even certain circles in which these are required items in the home if you want to keep up with the Joneses.

Once again, as at the Minneapolis exhibition, the potential pedagogical power of these new media was brought home to me most vividly by a seemingly small incident—my children's reaction when they received as gifts a few small computer-style toys. The vast learning that can emerge from direct contact with cleverly programmed machines is described in essay 20, "Toys with Minds of Their Own."

Beyond question, the most powerful medium—for good or ill—in our society today remains television. So much has been written about its effects, however, that it is with some reluctance that I have inserted my own "cognitive" and "developmentive" perspective into current discussions. Fortunately, my colleagues and I have had the opportunity over the past several years to conduct research on television's effects on children, and so we are at least able to marshal some data in support of the relatively modest conclusions we have so far reached.

In the first of the trio of essays on television, I introduce some methods we have devised for contrasting this medium with more traditional modes of communication and education. The second recounts a study in which we eavesdropped on children's initial encounters with television in an effort to tease out those effects that are peculiar to television from those that seem part of the "natural developmental processes," which have earlier occupied our attention. In essay 23 I offer some of my own speculations on a much-debated issue: Does television stimulate or stultify?

Though I would rank low in any listing of individuals who are enamored of the new technology, I have been receptive to its positive effects and have even engaged in a little applied experimentation concerning the effects of media on my own thought processes. A case in point is my switch from "composing at the typewriter" to "writing by dictation." I remain skeptical that any technological innovation will ever replace "sheer mental sweat" in the process of creation, but I am impressed by the extent to which media can serve as significant adjuncts in any cognitive undertaking. Properly used, they are indeed extensions of the mind.

18

UNFOLDING OR TEACHING:

ON THE OPTIMAL

TRAINING OF ARTISTIC SKILLS

TWO WIDELY diverging views can be found on the optimal means for developing artistic talent, for fostering creative artists, performers, and perceivers in the visual arts as well as other aesthetic domains. One view might be termed the "unfolding" or "natural" perspective. The child is viewed as a seed, which, though small and fragile, contains within its husk all the necessary "germs" for eventual artistic virtuosity. The role of the naturalist or gardener who tends the seed is primarily preventive: to shield the young shoots from malevolent influences— violent winds, fiendish crows—so that the seeds have the opportunity to unfold on their own into uniquely beautiful flowers.

By analogy, in the field of art education every normal child is seen as (at least potentially) a productive and imaginative practitioner of the arts. The art teacher must play the role of a Rousseauan tutor— shielding the innocent and fragile young child from pernicious forces in the society so that his inborn talents can flower. Other than providing a comfortable setting and minimally equipping the child with paints, clay, or blocks, the teacher does little that is active; his task is preventive rather than prescriptive.

Unfolding or Teaching

The opposite point of view, if somewhat less in favor today, is no less familiar to those who have toiled in the fields of the arts and education. This perspective, which can be termed the "training," "directive," or "skills" approach, holds that, at the very minimum, unfolding is not enough. Like a young seedling abandoned on the shady side of a hill, the child artist, left alone, will never achieve his potential. Special cultivation or perhaps even transplantation is necessary if the immature plant is to survive or thrive. By the same token, the young child, even one displaying considerable promise, will come to nought without firm guidance and active intervention on the part of more knowledgeable adults. Proficiency in the arts entails the attainment of many highly intricate skills, ones that can be acquired only under the direction of a gifted teacher or practicing artist.

It is an established ploy—in teaching, writing, and even thinking—to set up two such antipodes, or straw men, and then to declare sagely that both sides have a point and that the truth lies in a golden mean, located just about midway between equally untenable extremes. I will succumb to this spineless stance to the extent of affirming that both of these positions on art education have a solid cipher in their favor. Yet I hope to go beyond the obvious by insisting that a deeper understanding of both views—unfolding as well as training—may emerge from a developmental perspective and that, indeed, questions in art education in general benefit from such an examination.

Developmental studies are today much in vogue. Almost everyone quotes Jean Piaget or Jerome Bruner or Erik Erikson whether or not they agree with or even understand them. This is not the occasion for a minicourse on child development, but it may be opportune to offer a few asides regarding the developmental perspective. To be specific, one is not being "developmental" simply by looking at children or by noting the ways in which they change over time. To say that the average three-year-old is thirty-three inches in height and that the average twenty-year-old is sixty-six inches in height is to make statements about children and their growth but to abjure a developmental approach. One can have a developmental perspective only when one begins to focus on such questions as the rate of growth, the meaning of spurts in growth, the organization of physiological systems, and, most centrally, the possibility that physical growth in two periods of life—such as infancy and adolescence—may be mediated by different physiological mechanisms and affect different portions of the body. For it is the burden of developmental psychology to discern qualitatively different stages in physical, intellectual, and affective growth, the fundamental units and operations entailed in each stage, the factors contributing to the growth of each, and the interrelations among them.

It is no more possible to give a capsule summary of the "state of knowledge" in developmental psychology than to give a foolproof definition of the field but, again, a schematic description taken from the work of Piaget may help to orient our inquiry. As I have discussed in the first essay, Piaget sees intellectual development as consisting of four broad stages: a *sensorimotor* stage, occupying the first two years of life, during which the child gains a practical knowledge of the physical world about him—coming to understand, for example, that objects have a permanent existence within a framework of space and time; an *intuitive* or *symbolic* stage, covering the period from age two to six or seven, during which the child explores various kinds of symbols and images representing the world, but does not yet do so in a systematic or logical way; a *concrete-operational* stage, extending from about the age of seven to the age of twelve, wherein the subject becomes able to think logically about objects, to classify them consistently, and to appreciate their continuity despite alterations in their momentary appearance; and a *formal operations* stage, commencing in early adolescence, at which time the child becomes able to reason logically, using words and other symbols in order to create a world and make deductions about it without departing from the "abstract" or "theoretical" level.

Piaget's work is absolutely fundamental to any study of children and their minds. This is true even if one has not yet been converted to his developmental perspective, even if one does not share his convictions that each stage represents a qualitatively different way of thinking about the world, indeed of thinking altogether, or that each stage follows logically after its predecessor, in turn becoming the necessary ingredient for progress to subsequent stages. To conduct research in the area of developmental psychology without knowing about Piaget is about as sensible as pursuing biological studies without taking note of recent developments in genetics and molecular biology or of pursuing physics while ignoring Einstein's conceptual breakthroughs.

Having thus praised Piaget, let me add that I think his view can be seriously misleading to those involved in art education. Piaget's model of mature adult thought, as implied above, involves scientific thinking in the manner of the physicist or chemist. Piaget explicitly states—and his candor is refreshing in this eclectic era—that he is not interested in creativity as it is usually defined, or in the arts. It is quite possible, however, that if "involvement in the arts" is seen as a final stage of development, one might arrive at a rather different set of elements and stages, which, while not directly contradicting Piaget's works, possess a strikingly different flavor.

My own work has been devoted largely to the building of an informal model of artistic development. Portions of the model are based upon empirical research conducted by many investigators, including those of us associated with Harvard Project Zero; large portions of the model are based on my own observations, impressions, and intuitions as a parent, teacher, and reader. No doubt the model will be tinkered with and revised in the years to come, and that is to the good. But I feel that the model casts some light on the central question raised at the outset, and for that reason I propose to sketch it briefly.

During the opening years of life, as Piaget has shown, the child is indeed involved in the development of basic sensory and motor capacities and in the parallel enterprise of constructing knowledge about the physical and social world. These activities are evidently a prerequisite for artistic activity—for instance, in awakening the child to various means of communication—but are not in any powerful sense involved with the arts. That is because, in my view, the arts are integrally and uniquely involved with symbol systems—with the manipulation and understanding of various sounds, lines, colors, shapes, objects, forms, patterns—all of which have the potential to refer, to exemplify, or to express some aspect of the world.

To come to grips with the world of symbols, a world in large part designed by the culture, is the principal challenge of the years following infancy. The most familiar example is, of course, language: in the course of two or three years the child catapults from a phase during which he can utter or understand a mere word or two to one in which he can effortlessly issue sentences of almost any length, at the same time understanding a dizzying variety of structures and messages. But equally stunning progress occurs on all other symbolic fronts. Children with a musical flair can sing long and complicated pieces of music, assimilate the basic components of a musical style, and, in some cases, even compose works of interest. And by the time they enter school most children have also advanced from the merest capacity to scribble and form simple geometric patterns to the ability to make complex and aesthetically satisfying paintings.

I view the period from age two to seven, then, as a time during which the child's capacity to use, manipulate, transform, and comprehend various symbols matures at a ferocious pace. These processes can be seen in at least two ways: in watching the same child over a period of many months, as he advances from simple forms and patterns to complex configurations with many integrated portions; and, within a briefer interval, as he explores the potentials and possibilities of particular graphic patterns, often making inferences not apparent initially or combining the pattern with another scheme on which he has also been working. This kind of rapid "microgenetic development" is, in its own way, as amazing as the more leisurely "ontogenetic development," or evolution over a matter of months or years.

What is most striking, however, about the events of this period is that they seem to be similar in most children and that specific instruction has relatively little effect on what the child does. Let me be clear about what is meant here. There are indeed differences in children. Some favor one medium over another. Children also differ in the kinds of patterns they come to fix on, in the various set ideas or themes that recur in their works, and even in the extent to which these themes are beneficial or counterproductive.

Yet over and above these differences in style and preferences, the principal stages affecting young children across cultures, and across media, are persuasively similar. And, as far as we know, this parallel artistic development occurs despite the fact that educational procedures in various cultures may differ enormously. My best guess is that during this symbolic period the child is propelled by a dynamism that is largely his own. Like the seed with its own plan for development, the child is following the inner logic dictated by his own sensorimotor development and the nature of the particular symbols with which he is working. While children will naturally (and properly) draw what they see about them and tell stories about beguiling objects in their environments, external interference and efforts at explicit instruction rarely prove valuable or productive.

By the age of seven or eight, and sometimes earlier, the child has achieved an initial grasp on the major symbolic media of his culture. In our society, for example, a child of this age understands what makes a story (and what does not), and he can produce a literary work that, at least in its broad lines, conforms to the general cultural model. He has a sense of what occurs within a piece of music and, in many cases, can combine fragments in order to produce a new piece on the basis of a familiar style. Finally, his works in the visual or plastic arts also exhibit a sense of composition, balance, and construction, which indicates an awareness of the constituents of executed works of art, and he has long since learned to "read" the various representations contained in pictorial productions.

With what I hope will be regarded as benign exaggeration, I have suggested that the young child of this age is an incipient artist. By this I mean that he now possesses the raw materials to become involved in the artistic process: a "first draft" notion of how symbols work in a raft of symbolic media, some knowledge of how to construe a work, some capacity to construct one on his own. Indeed, he can enact the roles of performer, artist, and member of an audience. Only when it comes to the task of being a critic—who, like Piaget's formal operator, must be able to reason on the level of words or logical propositions— is the young school child significantly deficient.

It would be absurd, of course, to view the child of seven or eight as a mature artist. He requires, at the very least, additional knowledge about the medium, more understanding of the culture in which he lives, increased flexibility in the way he regards artistic objects, and greater psychological insight into human nature, as well as superior technical skill to permit him to realize desired effects in particular media. Indeed, to become acquainted with all the potentials of the medium, the multifarious ways in which it has been and can be employed, is perhaps the central task of artistic development and the one that most clearly differentiates this form of development from other realms, including those detailed by Piaget. It is my feeling, however, that these tasks involve quantitative rather than qualitative change. That is, while the acquiring of technique, of cultural understanding, of knowledge of feelings and thought may well require a lifetime, probably a very full and complete one, no new level of cognitive operation is required. The seven- or eight-year-old has the mental equipment to become an artist, and he need not pass through qualitatively different stages in order to participate fully in the artistic process. Here, then, I part company with Piaget. While he highlights the advent of concrete and formal operational thought, rightly perceiving these forms as central to the achievement of the scientist, he does not focus on other forms of thought, and so he does not confront the possibility that concrete and formal operations are not directly relevant to the artist's task, or the contention that versatility with a medium represents an extremely sophisticated cognitive achievement.

This formulation is very controversial, and many scholars would not endorse my conclusions. Two worthwhile points may nonetheless emerge from this controversy. First, there is renewed recognition that artistry is not just "less developed" science but rather involves different processes of thought with their own evolution; artistic cognition may not involve qualitative changes after early childhood, but it continues to deepen and evolve for many years. Second, this perspective helps to explain why individuals in other cultures, including the so-called primitive societies, who do not exhibit types of thought crucial to Western science, nonetheless produce artistic works and exhibit an aesthetic awareness commensurate with, if not superior to, our own. We need to acknowledge forms and intensities of thought other than those upheld by Piaget; the particular genius of "medium knowledge" and "symbol use" has to be recognized.

We find, then, that the seven-year-old has gained enough of an intuitive familiarity with symbol systems to be able to work with them adequately. However, he knows little and can accomplish little that is subtle and complex. At the same time, he is superbly equipped to learn. Throughout the world, schooling commences at about this time, and during the years from approximately age seven to thirteen the major lessons of the society are transmitted to offspring. The child of this age group seems superbly equipped to learn just about everything—not merely reading, writing, and arithmetic, not merely farming, fishing, and hunting, not merely reasoning, religion, and rhetoric. As V. S. Pritchett has pointed out in *The Cab at the Door* (p. 102), "That eager period between ten and fourteen is the one in which one can learn anything. Even in the time when most children had no schooling at all, they could be experts in a trade. The children who went up chimneys, worked in cotton mills, packed coster barrows, may have been sick, exhausted, ill-fed but they were at a temporary height of their intelligence and power." If one has any doubts about the particular learning facility of this period, he should travel with a preadolescent to an exotic land and note who picks up the language, and without a trace of an accent.

Many of our data about children's artistic capacities describe this period of life. Since much of this research has been described elsewhere in this volume, I shall not dwell on it here. We have found, basically, that children around the age of six or seven suffer from a number of woeful aesthetic misconceptions or impairments, which, fortunately, prove to be quite reparable. Youngsters of this age do not, for example, exhibit sensitivity to painting style: they view paintings chiefly in terms of subject matter. A few weeks of training, however, in which children look at paintings and are directed to notice stylistic features produce a dramatic increase in their sensitivity to artistic styles. Indeed, so fertile are the minds of these subjects that their sensitivity to style is enhanced even if they are merely drilled in grouping together animals of the same phylogenetic group.

We also find that children of this age display little tendency to produce metaphoric figures of speech in tasks where they are requested to produce such figures. Indeed, their responses exhibit a literal, concrete, trite, or realistic trend. Again, however, a majority of these youngsters can be trained within just a few weeks both to recognize and to produce metaphoric language.

Finally, I should mention an informal study by Judy Burton, who has worked intensively over a period of weeks with sixth and seventh graders. She finds that such preadolescents initially possess little sense of how to produce a third dimension in their drawing. However, after some experimentation with various two- and three-dimensional materials such as paper, wire, or lines, and after some guided practice in producing the subject matter of greatest interest to them—the human figure—the youngsters undergo a quantum leap in their artistic productions. In a matter of weeks they become sensitive to the details of the human figure and to the potential for producing depth relations, in a way previously inaccessible to them. Children of this age generally exhibit a tremendous ability to acquire within a short time new skills in the arts; they enjoy doing so; they are not overly distraught by terminology, by errors, or by empty verbalisms. They are ready to plunge in, to forge ahead, to gain mastery.

And it is in this respect that they differ so demonstrably from other children just a few years older. It is not that adolescents are in some absolute sense less intelligent or even necessarily less motivated. But for a reason that we do not yet completely understand, enthusiasm about acquiring skills in the arts and the ready capacity to immerse oneself fully in an expressive medium seem lacking in most adolescents, at least in our culture.

Piaget may have uncovered one reason for this. During adolescence the child is developing his critical reasoning skills to a new level. For this very reason he may adopt a much more critical opinion of his own work, comparing it unfavorably with what highly skilled individuals are accomplishing. If he finds his own capacities inadequate in comparison, he is no longer motivated to continue producing, and he remains at most a perceiver of the arts. Here, then, we encounter an important lesson for art education. If we are to prevent this decline of interest (and possible decline in skill), our pedagogical efforts during the preadolescent period become extremely important. Sufficient progress in teaching or training should, therefore, be realized so that when the child finally gains in critical acumen, his works will not seem so inadequate that he quits in despair.

At least two measures would seem helpful. First, skills should be developed to a sufficiently high level so that the child's work will, objectively, possess merit; he will then feel less need to reject what he has done. Second, and of equal importance, the child should be encouraged, gently but definitely, to take a somewhat more critical stance toward his work during preadolescence. He can be presented with problems, exposed to various solutions, and given practice in evaluating and improving them. Through such measures he gains familiarity with the practice of criticism; he employs it himself; he benefits from it. By the time he enters adolescence, criticism is already a familiar tool that he can now apply by himself as well as accept graciously. In the cultivation of this critical capacity, I think, lies our best hope of maintaining a garden of young painters instead of a barren row of survivors during the interval from childhood to adulthood.

Perhaps in a sense Piaget has been vindicated. In the end I have returned to his scheme to explain one of the most striking and troublesome events in artistic development: the frequent decline of artistry during adolescence. But it should be noticed that what, for Piaget, is a clearly beneficent event—the advent of formal logical operations— proves severely problematic for the child. Indeed, some of our studies have even indicated a high point in artistic creativity *before* adolescence, with the reasoning capacities of this later period proving more of a hindrance than a boon.

There is, then, a central enigma pervading the development of the child. While in the sciences development is completely linear and progressive, at least through adolescence, in the arts the picture is rather different. If anything, there is a kind of golden period during the first years of life in which every child can be regarded, in a meaningful sense, as a young artist. And while many children continue to participate in the arts in middle childhood, it is often with much less of a sense of inner direction, with much more of a searching for a model, and with a considerable amount of mindless repetition and pointless stylization, especially when no inspiring teacher is present. The development of scientific capacity is, generally speaking, a straight line upward; the lifeline of artistic development is punctuated by ups and downs.

Yet if the emerging picture of artistic development is less simple than one would have liked, our developmental analysis does provide one potentially useful prescription. As already suggested, the early years of life constitute a time of natural development of artistic competence. And during this period the approach of unfolding, of giving full rein to natural development, seems indicated. During middle childhood, however, a more active type of intervention is called for. Rigid drill is not necessary; what is wanted are recipes that give the child tools for achieving the effects he wants, that open up rather than foreclose possibilities. He should have some questions to ask and some ways for trying to answer them and an incipient acquaintance with standards and with criticism. This calls for the more active type of intervention involved in the teaching approach. It occurs, I think, at a time when the child is especially open and undefensive and is receptive to aid, suggestion, and inspirational models. As the noted art educator Viktor Lowenfeld once remarked,

If we can stimulate the child's unaware production to such an extent that it reaches in his unaware style a creative maturity which will be able to stand the critical awareness which once will set in, we have kept the child from making a sudden change and have protected him from disappointment or shock with regard to his changing imaginative activity. (p. 233)

I submit that both approaches we have contemplated are appropriate. The one that accentuates unfolding displays its particular virtue during the first years of life, from the period of two to seven. With the development changes accompanying the years of schooling, a more active and interventionist stance seems advisable, especially in a milieu virtually bereft of societal support for artistic (as opposed to scientific) endeavors. By the time of adolescence, it is in all probability too late to begin a rigorously structured educational program, and if natural development has not exerted its effect by then, it never will. Instead, one hopes that by adolescence the child will have attained sufficient skills and a sense of critical awareness, as well as ample ideas and feelings he wishes to express; then he can continue on his own to gain sustenance from whichever artistic medium he selects.

19

ILLUMINATING COMPARISONS:

LOOKING AT FAKES

AND FORGERIES

DURING THE SUMMER of 1973 the Minneapolis Institute of Arts mounted an exhibit of several hundred works of art drawn from diverse persons and schools. It included works representative of several aesthetic media, ranging from paintings and drawings to book covers and pottery. The show was billed as an "educational exhibit." This struck me as a curious designation from one point of view, since a noneducational museum exhibit is difficult to envisage. And yet, as the exhibit lent itself superlatively to pedagogical purposes, perhaps the description is justified. I had the opportunity to attend the exhibit on a number of occasions; it proved a singularly entertaining and edifying aesthetic experience. In this essay I will seek to uncover the reasons for my positive reaction and consider whether some wider principles might be culled from this experience. Using the exhibit as a point of departure, I will examine the technique of the "illuminating comparison" as a means of heightening aesthetic awareness in individuals of diverse ages and backgrounds.

Fully half of the works on display in Minneapolis would normally have been a source of keen embarrassment to the curators and trustees of a museum, for the director and the curatorial staff had assembled a collection of "Fakes, Forgeries, and other Deceptions." Deceits of every variety were conveniently juxtaposed alongside the originals they were purporting to represent. By this happy arrangement the viewer was granted the invaluable opportunity to compare and contrast originals and forgeries.

Unquestionably, such a collection constituted a veritable feast for the connoisseur. Not only did he have the opportunity to examine works seldom on display, but he could also bring to bear varied tools of technical analysis, ranging from knowledge of the methods and materials available in different historical periods to details of the ways in which specific artists signed, dated, and otherwise incorporated distinctive marks onto canvases. Indeed, a wide array of scholars and critics visited the Minneapolis show, delivered suitable lectures, praised its catalogues, and urged the preservation of the displays in one form or another.

Too often exhibits are mounted just for the *cognoscenti*. The hypothetical average viewer may well feel alienated or abandoned by such professional tours de force. Lacking the necessary background and training in analytic procedures, the untrained observer cannot fully appreciate the rationale for the show, the significance of particular selections (and omissions), the technical language of the catalogue, and the intent and impact of this or that curatorial aside. At best, the typical gallery-goer may gain some pleasure from one or another work, or from the elegance with which the show was assembled.

The special power of the Minneapolis assemblage lay in its vast potential for aiding the unsophisticated but motivated viewer to gain insights hitherto available exclusively to the connoisseur. The expert is equipped to honor Rembrandt, for he understands the master's technical innovations, heightened expressive powers, special use of color, and unsurpassed capacity to compose a scene and capture an emotion. What the average viewer had only glimpsed in a traditional show could now become manifest; as if magically supplied with the critic's lens, he too became capable of contrasting Rembrandt with his lesser contemporaries and, more especially, with those poseurs of later periods who unsuccessfully attempted to pass for the Dutch master. And particularly when given the opportunity to examine several fakes, forgeries, and deceptions, the untrained viewer could gain a feeling for the range and depth of Rembrandt's powers; the chance to survey a variety of would-be masters, each failing (in instructive ways) to achieve a desired effect, was invaluable.

Derogating the fake may be unnecessarily argumentative. To be sure, when it comes to a genius of Rembrandtian proportions, almost any comparison is likely to be at the expense of the deceptive work. But prior to, and perhaps more important than, the ultimate evaluation in terms of good and bad, better and worse, is the vital capacity to *discern*, to *appreciate differences*. What renders the work effective or ineffective to the viewer is the manner in which the numerous choices and challenges confronting the artists were resolved. Viewing the finished products, we confront records of the artists' choices— the differences in the final canvases—and from these derive our final evaluation.

All judgment, all evaluation, necessarily presupposes and depends upon comparison. In most exhibitions and displays, the comparisons are implicit: the viewer must compare what he sees with what another artist, given similar goals and means, but having different abilities, plans or techniques, might have done. The connoisseur is prepared for these implicit comparisons, for he has seen the absent works so many times that they have been deeply engraved on his mind's eye, but the average viewer is only rarely so equipped. At the "Fakes" show all viewers had the opportunity to be connoisseurs, for the raw materials were provided from which informed comparisons could be made and reasoned judgments achieved.

Indeed, the opportunity was more than merely present; the invitation to compare was compelling. Faced with two apparent Botticellis and with the knowledge that only one was the "real thing," a virtually irresistible temptation arises to examine both closely, to peer back and forth, to focus on respective attempts to realize details, capture expressions, achieve certain hues, and, after detecting the differences, to make an informed guess about which is the "real Botticelli." Cleverly exploiting the pervasive human proclivity to enter into such a game, the museum placed in every municipal bus a poster bearing two Mona Lisas with the enticing caption: "Will the real Mona Lisa please stand up?" The stagers of the exhibit had exploited the human tendency to search for similarities and differences among objects or displays, to represent to oneself the meanings of such resemblances and disparities, and to evaluate works on the basis of such a survey.

In a way, adoption of the phrase "illuminating comparisons" may yield a deceptively simplified view of this process; in fact, achievement of such comparisons is a lengthy, painstaking process, fraught with the possibility of uninstructive contrasts and misleading conclusions.

By no means will any set of objects or artworks lend themselves to comparisons, let alone to relevant and enlightening ones. Rather, like the physician who draws on his memory in making a diagnosis of a rare disease, a curator or instructor must search through a mental (or physical) catalogue of many hundreds of objects in order to select the pair or trio that drives home to even the most uninitiated individual the salient points of a lesson or a comparison.

Had the Minneapolis exhibition contained an endless series of originals juxtaposed to fakes, it would have been interesting and at least moderately entertaining, but not to my mind especially memorable. Again, however, the unseen hand that mounted the exhibit was guided by a basic tenet of human psychology: that there are many ways to stimulate a comparison, and that our minds are well served by a multiplicity of exploratory routes. Thus a wide array of comparisons was featured. Nearly every set of works posed a new challenge; no solution generalized automatically to the succeeding alcove; and yet there were enough possibilities for success and sufficient emerging patterns for the viewers so that, rather than despairing, they were instead stimulated to proceed on their course through the gallery.

Let me record a few of the pedagogical techniques that effectively stimulated comparisons. To begin with, one might speak of a *distance* principle: some works were directly juxtaposed to facilitate comparison; others were mounted at some remove so that one had to stroll back and forth to effect a comparison. This device brought home the lesson that the expert does not always have the original available to him; it stimulated the viewer to remember or to reconstruct the original, so that he might achieve the present comparison and be better equipped for future ones. In addition to geographical distance, disparities in quality were included. Sometimes the difference between the original and fake was quite evident, so that even the least trained eye could detect it; at other times it was so subtle that supplementary aids were needed. The museum provided a magnifying glass in one such instance, and it was constantly employed by visitors.

Further cognitive exercise was insured by the inclusion of a wide variety of comparisons. The sets included, for instance, an original and a fake, an original and two or three fakes, lithographs produced in different periods, an original and a copy by a member of the artist's own school, innocently produced copies that had been provided with false signatures, copies supervised by the artist himself, and a whole group of fakes collected by one individual. These assemblages revealed that the expert is continually confronted with new problems and questions, that there is no unequivocal line between fakes, forgeries, and harmless exercises. The viewer was challenged to take on the task of the expert and to learn from each of these confrontations. Every set conveyed new messages or presented old messages in slightly new ways.

Furthermore, to warn the viewer against facile conclusions, some presentations were deliberately misleading: originals without signatures; originals of poor quality; a whole set of fakes without a reassuring original. Again these unexpected twists provided special insights into the expert's dilemmas and conferred a light touch to the exhibit as well. Finally, the show featured some unfrocked forgeries, in which the forged work was partially removed, revealing part of the previous worthless painting on top of which the forger had labored. An apparent El Greco which had been partially defaced served as a dramatic and jarring reminder of the manner in which forgers work.

A third distinctive feature of the exhibit was the way in which it emphasized diverse historical and stylistic features. Included were several works by a single forger (for example, van Meegeren) as well as attempts by different artists to imitate one particular artist (several fake Rembrandts). The viewer could gain a feeling for the style of the forger (who often revealed his own period when sufficient examples of his work were gathered in one place) and also an appreciation for the subtlety of the original artist's style (by seeing the manifold ways in which it is possible to disfigure a Rembrandt).

Forgeries date back to ancient times, and fakes have been elicited by diverse circumstances at different epochs in history. The special problems raised by contemporary forgeries were clarified by the exhibit: we have no distance from our own era; sophisticated methods of mechanical reproduction are available; certain works (such as conceptual or pop art) seem particularly easy to duplicate, at least to our own eyes. Nonetheless, clear differences could be seen between the original and a copy of Claes Oldenburg's "Baked Potato" (1966).

Finally, the exhibit conveyed a sense of the task an expert faces when he encounters a suspected deception. Insights were provided into the different cues available to the expert: analysis of signature, size of work, age of canvas, x-ray methods, tiny details of shading, awareness of anachronistic details or colors, construction of the frame, knowledge that an artist favored certain themes and spurned others, failure to capture a certain facial expression. These methods differ greatly in their objectivity, their reliance on technology, their dependence on acquaintance with other works by the artist, but all are helpful. The exhibit also revealed that some attributions are disputed; and it illustrated how a convergence of reasons, none of which is individually decisive, can nonetheless lead to authoritative conclusions. The viewer was thus enabled to draw on multiple criteria in making his own judgments.

Though tremendously impressed with, and delighted by, the stunning exhibit, I was conscious of a number of problems that it raised. Although described as educational, it is unclear that the exhibit educated anyone. I believe that it did, and so did the staff at the museum, but there is no proof. It does not suffice merely to assume that displays intended to stimulate comparisons have had that effect: they may have had unintended consequences or no consequences at all. To evaluate the educational success of an exhibit, no elaborate machinery or high-powered statistical techniques would be necessary: a common-sense approach and perhaps consultation with a psychologist should yield suitable and unobtrusive measures of audience learning.

Another difficulty centered around the level of audience sophistication assumed by the displayers. Though in my view most visitors enjoyed and profited from the exhibit, a significant number commented that it was too difficult. Some viewers failed to see the differences alluded to in captions; others expressed disillusionment about the whole connoisseurial enterprise: "Well, if the experts make all these mistakes, how can I ever hope to tell?" "Who knows, perhaps half the pictures we admire are fakes." "The experts don't know any more than we do." These latter comments are particularly disconcerting. They suggest that for certain viewers the comparisons may have failed in their intended effects. True, their awe of art may have been healthily reduced, but at the bitter price of a general cynicism.

The expert's role vis-à-vis the audience is a challenging one. It does not suffice to say, "I have chosen this work: therefore you must like it." After all, the expert does not casually decide which classical vase to display: he knows and he cares about mythology, Greek methods of sculpture, the materials available to artists of two millennia ago, the clothing, religion, philosophy, mores, likes, and prejudices of individuals of that era. It is not enough simply to declare this knowledge to the viewer; such technical detail cannot be absorbed by the unprepared mind. Rather, an exhibit should be so staged that the viewer is led, subtly and entertainingly, yet authoritatively and convincingly, into the reaches of the expert's own knowledge. Only then can the nonexpert appreciate why *this* artwork is worth exmaining today. The Minneapolis exhibit was most successful when it made the world of the expert come alive for the viewer, less successful when it simply paraded knowledge or assumed understanding.

Finally, some comments are also in order about the supplementary information sources—the labels and program guides—that adorned the exhibit. There is no question that some labeling is essential in an exhibit of this type—how else can one tell if his guesses are correct or what features to look at if he is incorrect? Without good labels, the exhibit would not work. The labels should be placed in a nonprominent spot: indeed, it might be optimal if the viewer were not allowed to scan the label until he had spent some time examining the canvas. It is too easy to conclude that you have seen what you are supposed to see after you have been told what it is and where to look for it.

In general, I encountered two difficulties with the labels in the "Fakes" show, difficulties by no means restricted to the present exhibit. First of all, there was a fair amount of technical material—recondite references to the styles of painting, characters from mythology, methods of production and detection, which were doubtless devoid of meaning for many viewers. Such references could intimidate them. Second, there was too much empty display of erudition.

An effective label is one that points to a difference that can then be seen by the viewer: "In the original the shading runs directly into the clouds; in the fake there is a gap of two millimeters"; "In the original the numeral five has been printed backwards." An ineffective label is one that is too vague or that requires specialized knowledge. Here are some labels that I found unhelpful:

The piece is mechanical and dull, displaying nothing of the fine concern for life and death which characterizes Aztec religion.
The difference between the pieces is in essence, not in substance.
While superficially Renaissance in style, the triptych is really purest nineteenth century.
The artist expresses awe whereas the copy is merely coy.
The forgery captures none of the subtle qualities of the original.
Out of character in terms of the artist's true style.
It fails to capture the artist's deeply felt religious feeling.

It might have been helpful to categorize the kinds of differences cited; at least then label-writer and viewer alike would acknowledge the differences between an objective technical reason (age of frame), an objective nontechnical reason (the shading does not reach to the clouds), an interpretation that can be readily verified ("The Madonna in the original is looking directly into the eyes of the child"), an interpretation that does not lend itself to such verification ("The forger fails to capture the religious spirit of the original"). I do not mean to imply that the latter reason is irrelevant, only that in the present context it could have so many possible meanings that it does nothing to sharpen the viewer's appreciation.

Discussion of labels and their applicability to works of art raises the vexing question of the relationship between visual displays and linguistic instruction. The question is especially crucial in the present context, given the goal, on the one hand, of improving the viewer's perceptual skills, and the risk, on the other hand, of his failing to draw valid inferences from the comparison before him. And yet the question is extremely controversial. One school of thought is deeply suspicious of any linguistic comments about "ineffable" works of art, while another equally vociferous group considers verbal instruction the optimal means for enhancing aesthetic sensitivity.

In this dispute, the views of Rudolf Arnheim are especially instructive. As one who has devoted a lifetime to the understanding of art, and who writes eloquently about what he has seen, he is keenly sensitive to the advantages and the drawbacks of linguistic and nonlinguistic modes of communication. Arnheim has offered a needed corrective to the uncritical overuse, and frequent misapplication, of linguistic instruction in our educational system. Without questioning the essential communicative role of language and its appropriateness for transmitting certain subject matters, he challenges the widespread belief that language provides the optimal means for presenting the full range of information and capturing the entire gamut of thought processes. Arnheim demonstrates that thought processes rely heavily on the effective functioning of our sensory modalities and on the role of nonlinguistic symbol systems.

By theoretical conceptualization, as well as by example, Arnheim has helped to specify the appropriate role of ordinary language in explicating the arts. Often, as at certain points in the Minneapolis exhibit, the correct point will be grasped without recourse to verbal documentation; at such times linguistic elaboration is neither necessary nor desirable. At other times, however, a pictorial display may be subjected to numerous interpretations, and the intended pedagogical principle, the illuminating comparison, is likely to be missed. At such times verbal labels can provide useful supplements, directing the viewer toward points worthy of his consideration, helping to explicate the significance of elements that have been but dimly discerned. The shortest distance to effective communication is not always a direct or literal line, however. Metaphors, personifications, and other figures of speech may well succeed in conveying a crucial point in an especially succinct and effective manner. Particularly in the arts, the connotative and allusive qualities of language constitute a rich resource for the sensitive teacher or writer. Certainly we must not delete words from artistic instruction; we must only deploy them with the precision and care with which a brush is wielded or a violin bowed.

A case could be made that all learning necessitates contrasts and comparisons. Where there is no change, no discrepancy, no gap, no perceived distinctions, we cannot learn. The Minneapolis exhibit overshadowed most other cultural and educational experiments because, by means of a simple yet elegant technique, the viewer was enticed into comparisons; owing to the aptness of the comparisons, significant new aesthetic insights could be gained. A simple example or an illuminating comparison of two works can form the beginning of a deeper understanding of a principle. But the future application of this principle requires that its underlying features be detected and formulated with some precision.

The inquiry prompted by my visit to Minneapolis suggests certain conclusions about the role of comparisons in artistic knowledge. First, the teacher or exhibitor must be clear in his own mind about what educational point is to be made and have some confidence that the point is worth making. Next, he should select a variety of examples that illustrate the point in a number of different and accessible fashions. He should consider the use of various linguistic and nonlinguistic supplements for conveying the point; and if such supplements are used, he must take care that they direct attention to the relevant details, rather than serve to obfuscate the point or to signal the brilliance of the writer. And, finally, he should engage in some modest experimentation in order to determine whether the point at issue has indeed been grasped by the intended audience. In addition to a set of guidelines like this, however, some models or examples of effective aesthetic education are also desirable. To those in search of such models, I can point with enthusiasm to the works of Rudolf Arnheim, in which are exemplified many of the principles touched on in this essay.

20

TOYS WITH MINDS

OF THEIR OWN

SOME TIME AGO, my children were given two attractive toys. One, a book-shaped console called Speak & Spell, consisted of an alphabetic keyboard with several buttons on it and a mechanical device that simulated human speech. The instrument pronounces a word, lets you try to spell it, and then informs you whether or not you are correct. The second toy was the Play'N'Playback Organ (P&P), which resembles a brightly colored xylophone bordered by a panel of pressable levers P&P lets you create a little melody and then plays it back.

At first I thought these games were just some gimmicky new toys and that the children would quickly tire of them. But that did not happen. My two older youngsters, then aged seven and nine, spent many hours with Speak & Spell and became absolutely livid whenever the batteries gave out. Their younger brother, then two, was equally mesmerized by the P&P organ. What is more, nearly every adult who came to the house, no matter how sophisticated, became fascinated with the toys; one "grownup" was even reluctant to relinquish Speak & Spell to an impatient child. Clearly, there was something special about the toys.

I soon learned that Speak & Spell and P&P were just two representatives of a new breed of computer toys now on the market. Called "computer toys" because they contain tiny computing devices that permit storage of a wide repertoire of messages, they are far more challenging than the teaching machines invented in the 1950s—devices based largely on a Skinnerian approach to learning. In my opinion, the designers of the new machines have bet on different, and more appropriate, models of how the mind works. I believe the "learning machines," as I call them, come closer to imitating the style of human intelligence than the teaching machines of the past and may well represent the educational wave of the future.

One can find computer toys for nearly every taste and intellectual level. In addition to a host of games, ranging from Electronic Quarterback to Electronic Soccer, there are any number of brain-stretchers and explicit teaching instruments, some of them quite elementary in format. In Quiz Wiz, for example, you simply select your answer to each of 1,001 multiple-choice questions on music, history, television, sports, and books. For example: Q: Which instrument is not in the woodwind family? A: piccolo, glockenspiel, flute, or oboe; Q: Which blues singer was a favorite of President Franklin Roosevelt? A: Leadbelly, Josh White, Lemon Jefferson, or Bob Milton; Q: In the story of the Three Bears, which things does Goldilocks not try? A: food, beds, clothes, or chairs. (If you answered glockenspiel, Leadbelly, and clothes, you outwitted the Wiz.)

In Chess Challenger, on the other hand, you have the opportunity to play chess against a computer programmed to respond at no less than seven different levels of competence, which range in mettle from *patzer* to master.

One of my favorites is Merlin, whose small and deceptively unimposing keyboard with ten numbered buttons allows you to engage in six different pastimes, in any order and as often as you like. In Merlin's version of blackjack, buttons one to ten represent ace-to-ten in a deck of cards; Merlin and whoever is matched against him both try to acquire the higher hand without exceeding a score of thirteen. The goal of Merlin's Magic Square game is to form a sequence of eight lines on a grid of lights, using buttons one to four and six to nine. The purpose of Mindbinder is to discover, through deduction, the mystery number stored in Merlin's computer brain; feedback indicates whether the proper digits and the correct order have been guessed. On Merlin's Music Machine, one can create any tune of up to forty-eight notes; after a brief pause, he plays it back. In Echo the machine plays a random set of notes and lights; then the challenge is to recreate them in exactly the same sequence. Finally, in Tic-Tac-Toe, the player tries to get three marks in a row before Merlin does.

Toys with Minds of Their Own

Some computer toys resemble one or another of the basic ideas in Merlin. The P&P organ is, of course, a more elaborate version of Merlin's Music Machine. Another new entry, Simon, a cousin of Echo, generates in rapid succession a random series of tones and lights; one is challenged to recreate such a series at four levels of difficulty.

Another of my favorites is 2XL, the robot with a personality. Simply by injecting a cassette into the robot's body, you can communicate with him/her/it about a variety of subjects, learning about them and having fun at the same time. For example, in the cassette devoted to Wonders of the World, 2XL poses twenty-five questions; each is answered by pressing one of four buttons (accurate, not accurate, true, false). Sometimes the phenomena in question are really true: "There are fish that climb trees," or, "It was once illegal to take a bath." At other times the wonders are foolish: "Most pretzels in the United States come from pretzel trees in California."

The 2XL does more than simply indicate whether you are right or wrong. It banters in the parlance of the ten-year-old, replying, typically: "Jeepers creepers, you are right, where did you get that brain?"; "If you were a flower you'd be a budding genius"; "You have answered false, as I would have done, but you are wrong." And it furnishes additional information about the topic: "The mud skipper uses front fins to pull itself up trees to catch insects for food"; "Taking a bath was once illegal in some states in America, and in Philadelphia you could only do it once a week." All in all, one has the eerie feeling that there is a real person lurking in the cassette tape—possibly a failed comedian from the Catskills or a precocious eight-year-old emerging from the pages of J. D. Salinger.

But let us return to the pair of toys that captivated my youngsters. Speak & Spell does more than simply test knowledge of 200 words at four levels of difficulty. You can also play an electronic version of the old game of Hangman. Your job is to discover the word stored in Speak & Spell by guessing its letters one at a time. The machine announces each error—seven letters and you are "out." The P&P organ is also multifaceted. By pushing eight single buttons, you can play eight different tunes. Moreover, you can vary the rhythm of your own composition by including rests. Like an improvising pianist, you can play on the keyboard for as long as you want.

These toys are relatively simple and, in view of their electronic complexity, surprisingly inexpensive. They foreshadow even more sophisticated and specialized future versions. There is no need to restrict them to the spelling of words: any kind of question—historical, scientific, or athletic—could be posed and answered. They could be programmed with a plethora of numerical challenges—games of skill as well as games of chance. While the P&P organ now has only eight familiar tunes in its memory, many more compositions and variations could be programmed into future models. And there is no reason why an invented tune cannot be altered in key, tempo, meter, or even given fugal treatment, complete with inversions, retrogrades, doubling of voices, and the like. The possibilities are virtually limitless. The more interest we consumers display in the machines, the smaller, cheaper, and more versatile they are likely to be.

Why are the toys so engaging? As I pondered that question, I inevitably recalled the teaching machines of the 1950s, which, at least on a superficial level, seemed like forerunners of the computer toys. With a typical teaching machine of that time, the child is presented with a question. He writes or types in a response, which the machine declares right or wrong. When correct, the child is rewarded in some way— for example, by being told he is right, by being allowed to go directly to the next question, or (in the case of small children) by a bell going off. Programs can be "branching": they can include a number of alternative routes that are geared to the abilities and interests of different pupils. The size of steps between items, as well as the amount of rehearsal permitted, can also be varied. Surprising success has been claimed for these devices: they have proved an efficient means of teaching a circumscribed body of information to a broad range of students. (Commercially, however, they have been less successful. The machines were unwieldy and expensive, and they were bitterly opposed by many teachers. Several companies took a beating in attempts to market them.)

Some differences between the two devices suggest the reasons for their contrasting fates. Computer toys are small, eminently portable (and, in some cases, pluggable), and brightly packaged and designed. With voices that sound like the computers in *Star Trek* or *2001*, they have a space-age sheen; their keyboards resemble an instrument panel more than a manual typewriter.

Beyond the surface, the computational mechanisms have a number of attractive features. They are much speedier, indeed almost instantaneous, in their responses. They contain many items that are immediately at one's fingertips, and new modules can easily be substituted in them; in Speak & Spell, cassettes can be inserted with whole sets of new words. And the possession of a human-sounding voice is by no means a trivial feature. The synthetic speech of Speak & Spell—

produced mechanically from digital memory without any kind of tape or record—reminds one of a well-meaning and empathetic school-teacher. One converses with a reliable, if somewhat stilted and stodgy, teacher, not a stupid—or omniscient—machine.

There is a still more fundamental difference between the teaching machines of yesterday and the learning machines of today. Growing out of respectable psychological research with pigeons, rats, and other laboratory animals, the teaching machine represented a view of the individual as an essentially passive organism into which information should be pumped. True, the teaching machine constituted an advance over the stereotypical classroom teacher, for it could be tailored to individual students. But basically the machine was equipped before-hand with all requisite information, which was then to be transferred to the student through a form of behavioral conditioning that stressed rewards. It proved most effective in presenting a sharply limited body of factual knowledge—such as the anatomy of the auditory system, or the names and dates of an historical era. But there was little room for imagination, for leaps (or even questions) on the part of the student, for unexpected moves or outcomes, for active engagement of intellect. The teaching machine reeked of routine.

Some electronic toys, such as Quiz Wiz, are merely updated versions of the traditional teaching machine. But at its best, the learning machine reflects quite a different view of the mind—one that resonates with contemporary cognitive psychology. Consider chess-playing programs, for example. In this fully interactive setup, the player can use his wits as inventively as possible and count on the machine to respond at an adult level. Moreover, one's style of play can be varied, and its effect upon the machine-opponent can be assessed. On a more modest level, a similar competition marks the Hangman game of Speak & Spell: once again, the players' wits are pitted against the machine's, and although they can ask for cues, the outcome can by no means be anticipated.

Inventive use of intellect is even more likely once the toys transcend conventional game situations. With P&P, even a toddler has the poten-tial for composing elaborate musical works. Although in the past such artistic creation presupposed time-consuming mastery of an instrument and of musical notation, the compositional process is now virtually instantaneous. All the "artist" has to do is press some buttons, play back the results, and, if he wants to, make changes in the composition.

In my view, the computer toys display humanlike intelligence in two ways. First, they resemble the ideal teacher model—recreating the fabled educational relationship with an eager student on one end of a log and the gifted teacher on the other. The computer models behaviors that students can emulate; it also serves as a prod, a corrective, a sly opponent against which they can exercise their wits. But the computer also accomplishes a second, equally vital, human intellectual function. It supplements the intellect of the learner. Individuals differ vastly from one another in such capacities as pattern perception, linguistic memory, or the ability to transform a formula. These differences often count mightily against otherwise motivated students. Like a hand calculator, computer toys can carry out assorted secondary features, thereby freeing the individual to focus on those achievements that truly demand his attention (and that no computer can yet initiate). Thus, the P&P organ stores a musical fragment; Simon helps to train nonverbal memory; Speak & Spell allows one to master arrangements of letters.

There may be an even more profound difference between the philosophies that have given rise to the two kinds of devices. The fundamental goal of the teaching machine is to secure from the learner a specific product—the "right" answer. The learner succeeds when he has mastered all the facts; the method used is not apparent to others and, in any case, is immaterial. The learning machine, on the other hand, need be only minimally concerned with mastery of facts. The goal of such interactive devices—some of which even allow users to do some programming on their own—is to stimulate the processes of learning, to give the user the experience of "thinking well." It is not important that they win the chess game or the round of Hangman. What is important is that they acquire strategies for manipulating letters, or tones, or chess pieces—strategies that will enable them to think better in the future, long after they have forgotten the particular moves of a specific game.

Evidence is accumulating that interaction with gadgets of the computer age has as its primary effect a stimulation of the learning process itself. Many parents and teachers report that children armed with new computer devices rapidly exhaust the "assigned" games and go on to devise exercises and challenges of their own. Competitions with video games and also with Rubik Cubes and other hand-held puzzles of the computer age often center around games of the children's (or the individual child's) own devising. The popularity of the book series "Choose Your Own Adventure" lies in the fact that, rather than reading a preordained mystery thriller, the child has the opportunity to contrive as many different plot sequences as he likes.

Perhaps most dramatic are the results reported when children learn a simple computer-programming language like Seymour Papert's LOGO. According to Karen Sheingold, head of the media laboratory at Bank Street College in New York City, children often set as a goal the programming of a particular game like tic-tac-toe or Space Invaders. Yet, paradoxically, once the program has been satisfactorily constructed, the children do not simply sit around and play the game. Instead, they try to create a more elegant program to achieve the same end or, more likely still, devise an even greater programming challenge for themselves. Clearly the processes of learning and of learning to learn have come to the fore.

Whether by luck or design, the inventors of learning machines have rejected a Skinnerian approach and have instead adopted a much more realistic and apt view of human cognition: how individuals learn, from whom they like to learn, what kinds of learning aids are suitable. I can envisage a time when these toys may allow each student in a classroom to locate his mental métier, to advance at his own speed and in his own way, aided by the very best "minds." Naturally, children will vary greatly in the extent to which they wish to play with the toys and in whether or not they exhibit a flair for the various computational activities; after all, it is much more difficult to fool a computer teacher than a live one. But this situation could free classroom teachers to focus on tasks for which they may well be better, and certainly more uniquely, suited: encouraging social and emotional development, guiding children in activities for which they may have relatively little knack, and providing special activities for the precocious or the handicapped.

In the last analysis, the learning machines may accomplish some of the very goals that B. F. Skinner (and, before him, the educational psychologist Sidney Pressey) entertained for the original teaching machines. After all, Skinner also wanted to use the most recent technology to motivate students of different levels, to allow self-paced interaction with a well-informed device, and to make possible an ever-expanding exploration of a field of knowledge. It is paradoxical that this analyst of human behavior, whose model of teaching and learning has undergone increasingly severe criticism, has nonetheless inspired—if by an unanticipated path—the devising of apparatuses that may have a truly revolutionary educational impact.

21

ARE TELEVISION'S EFFECTS

DUE TO TELEVISION?

NEARLY ALL of the ills of our sorely afflicted society have at one time or another been blamed on television. The drop in College Entrance Examination Board scores, the decline in literacy, the lack of political involvement on the part of many citizens, the upsurge in violent crimes, the mediocre artistic tastes of large segments of our culture—these and countless other lamentable trends have all been attributed to this pervasive medium. A deluge of articles, books, and even television programs have chronicled the evil effects of television. Marie Winn has deplored *The Plug-In Drug,* and Gerry Mander has issued *Four Arguments for the Elimination of Television.*

To be sure, one occasionally hears whispers about possible dividends from television: an earlier mastery of certain basic skills (courtesy of "Sesame Street"), greater access to information by neglected pockets within the society, an increase in the rate or efficacy of visual thinking, and, possibly, the speedier erection of Marshall McLuhan's "global village." Yet for the most part, when television is spoken of, the medium that has been viewed by more individuals for longer periods of time than any other in human history receives a dismal press.

When such a consensus is voiced, it requires some boldness (or foolhardiness) to call it into question. Yet in my view we know astonishingly little about the actual effects of television. For the most part, we do not know what things are caused by television. And even when we can establish probable cause, it is difficult to confirm that the medium of television *per se* is at fault. Put another way, it might be that any pursuit, or at least any medium with which one were engaged for twenty to thirty hours a week, would yield similar results—in which case the various trends cited above are hardly due to television itself. Our "vast wasteland" of ignorance about television's effects stems from the fact that researchers claiming to study television have failed to tease out those effects due directly to television from those that might have resulted from any mode of presentation. And so, to anticipate my conclusions, only if we systematically compare television to other media of communication will we be able to determine which sins— and which virtues—can legitimately be laid at the base of the ubiquitous console.

Television and Human Behavior, a recently published exhaustive compendium of more than 2,500 studies, provides an important case in point. This thoughtful book compiled by George Comstock and his colleagues inundates us with information about television in this country—the number of sets, the number of hours they are watched by members of every age and demographic group, and the preferences and dislikes of the gigantic viewing audience. Appropriately, the largest section of the book is devoted to the aspect of television that has generated the most controversy—the effects of the medium on children. In fact, it takes more than a hundred pages simply to survey the several hundred studies in this area.

I read through these pages with mounting disappointment. The millions of research dollars spent on this issue seem to have yielded only two major findings, each of which might easily have been anticipated by the experimenter's proverbial grandmother. As the authors constantly remind us, "it has now been established" that children will imitate behaviors they see on television, whether these actions be aggressive, violent, or benignly "prosocial." Moreover, "it has also been established" that the younger the child, the more likely it is that he will believe in the contents of commercials, urging parents to purchase what has been advertised and confusing commercial fare with other television content.

Some recent research efforts have adopted a more cognitive approach to children and television: they have implicitly viewed the child as a fledgling explorer trying to make sense of the mysterious lands visible on the handful of channels beamed to every household. And these studies have furnished the reassuring headline that, much as children pass through stages in the other realms of existence probed by psychologists, so children pass through "stages of television comprehension." But again, these pioneering studies have not revealed much that would surprise an observant parent or a shrewd grandparent.

Why do we know so little? Why have the thousands of studies failed to tell us more about television *per se* and about the minds of children who view it? A number of answers spring to mind. First of all, just as a new medium usually begins by presenting the contents previously transmitted through older media (for example, movies initially conveyed celluloid theater, and television at first amounted to visual radio), so, too, initial lines of research on television have largely adopted methods and questions that had once been applied to other media or to "unmediated" behavior. Only when a generation reared on television undertook research in this area did studies become attuned to the special or "defining" properties of television. Another limiting dimension has been the "mission" orientation of most television research. Because society has been (justifiably) vexed about violence and about commercials, it has twisted researchers' arms to grapple with these issues.

But probably the chief stumbling block to imaginative and generative television research has been the fact that everyone (and his grandmother) has a television set. Thus the crucial experimental control—comparing individuals with televisions to those without—cannot be done. The few eccentrics who do not have television are too different from their viewing counterparts to serve as a meaningful control group. Those scattered societies not yet blessed (or traumatized) with television are also sufficiently different to render comparisons of little value. When the gifted social psychologist, Stanley Milgram, was asked to study the effects of television on violence, he had a very logical idea which was, alas, soon dashed. Milgram's first impulse was to divide the country in half, remove all violence on television west of the Mississippi, enact laws so that no one could move from one part of the country to the other, and then observe what happened over a period of years. "It turned out not to be practical," he wryly admitted to an interviewer, "so I had to work with what I had" (p. 73).

I have recently encountered a few strands of research that address more directly the distinct features of television. In trying to determine which aspects of television compel children's attention, researchers Aletha Huston-Stein and John Wright of the University of Kansas have focused on the medium's "formal features"—the quick cutaways, sound effects, and frenetic activity, in which commercial television revels. They have documented that the younger the child, the more likely he is to attend to these features of television, independent of the kind of content being presented. In contrast, older children will watch a program for extended periods of time even when such formal features are not heavily exploited. Huston-Stein and Wright make the interesting suggestion that violence or aggression are unnecessary for capturing the attention of preschool children. So long as a show is fast-paced, contains action, and is laced with interesting visual and sound effects (as is, for example, much of "Sesame Street"), the youngsters will remain hooked.

Another innovative researcher, Gavriel Salomon of the Hebrew University in Jerusalem, has also focused on those features that prove unique to television. He has paid special attention to such features as the zoom—the shot that begins with a panoramic overview and then rapidly "zooms" in upon a tell-tale detail. According to Salomon, children with difficulty attending to relevant detail can be greatly aided by a television segment replete with zooms: the medium can "supplant" a skill that the child needs but that, for one or another reason, he has not yet developed on his own. Salomon has not only documented an effect linked specifically to television but has also pointed the path to a positive pedagogical payoff.

Yet because they employ only television, even these isolated oases in the wasteland of research do not permit a determination of the effects of televison *per se*. One line of research that *does*, however, was initiated by Laurene Meringoff, my colleague at Harvard Project Zero, and is now being continued in conjunction with several other colleagues. Exploiting the fact that television transmits certain contents, such as narratives, that have traditionally been conveyed by other media, these researchers have compared with as much precision as possible the differential effects wrought by such story content when it is presented on television, as opposed to when it is presented in book form. And they have uncovered some very intriguing findings.

Let me describe their procedures. To begin with, members of the research team select stories of high quality and interest. Using materials developed at Weston Woods, a studio which produces stories in various media for children, they prepare book and television versions that are virtually identical save in the medium of transmission.

As an example, the research team has worked extensively with *The*

Three Robbers by Tomi Ungerer. In this tale three hitherto ferocious bandits abandon their violent ways after stopping a stagecoach that was carrying the charming orphan Tiffany. Turning their backs on a life of crime, the trio of robbers goes on to help abandoned girls and boys throughout the land. In a typical study, one group of subjects hears the story read by an experimenter and sees the accompanying pictures—the "book version." Another group of subjects views a film of equivalent length, based on the book, on a television monitor; in this "television version," the specially recorded sound track uses the voice of the book narrator and the animated film presents the same illustrations that appear in the printed text. Thus, while respecting the essential properties of each medium (movement within the image in the case of television, discrete static imagery in the case of a picture book), the two versions are about as similar as can be imagined. (Of course, reading a book oneself is different from having it read aloud to one at a preordained rate, but the researchers were interested in attempting to simulate the latter experience.)

A quartet of studies carried out thus far by the Project Zero team revealed a consistent and instructive picture. To begin with, adults who watched the television program remembered about as much of the story on their own and were able to select as many items from multiple choice as did the matched adults who had the picture book read to them. But when subjects were asked to make inferences that went beyond the text, modest effects of medium were found. For example, subjects were asked to evaluate how a character felt or how difficult it was for the robbers to carry out an action. In these cases, adults who saw the story on television were more likely to make inferences based on the visual portions of the story (such as the expression on a character's face), while those exposed to the book were more likely to rely on the plot they heard (although both groups were exposed to identical sound tracks and saw a similar set of visual images, one static and one dynamic).

With children the differences across media proved far more dramatic. Compared to the video youngsters, the book children remembered much more of the story on their own and were also better able to recall information when they had been cued. When it came to recalling precise wordings and figures of speech, differences proved especially dramatic: the book children were surprisingly skilled at repeating just what they heard (phrases such as "visit her wicked aunt"), while the television children, when they remembered linguistically presented information at all, were prone to paraphrase.

238

Are Television's Effects Due to Television?

To my mind, the most intriguing differences with children emerged when inferences were called for. Both groups of children tended to reach the same conclusions—for instance, an equal number of television and book children concluded that the robbers' axe was easy to wield, or that Tiffany felt happy. But the lines of reasoning used to buttress the inferences were different. Television children relied overwhelmingly on what they had seen—how difficult an action looked, how someone appeared to feel. They rarely went beyond the video information, either to attend to what was said or to draw on their own experience. In contrast, book children were far more likely to draw on their own personal experiences or to apply their own real-world knowledge ("It's hard for me to hold an axe—it's way too heavy"). Estimates of time and space were also more constrained for the television children. That is, when asked how long an action took or how far from one another two sites were located, television children made more modest estimates, suggesting a reliance on the superficial flow of information rather than a consideration of what was plausible.

In all, television emerged as much more of a self-contained experience for children, and within this bounded realm the visual component emerged as paramount. The book experience, in contrast, allowed for greater access to the story's language and suggested greater expanses of time and space; it also encouraged connections to other realms of life—thus buttressing some of the very claims bibliophiles have made in the past.

One possible outcome of such research is to comfort critics of television—those troubled souls whose Cassandran cries I initially branded as premature. And it seems to be true that the younger the child, the greater the gap between comprehension of television and comprehension of books. Yet, in my own view, the significance of this research does not rest primarily in its favoring one medium over another. For one thing, the largely verbal measures used thus far could well be charged with being "pro-book." It could be that other more visual measures might have favored television, as has in fact proved to be the case in subsequent studies. Or it could be that the kinds of skills actually engendered by television (for example, being able to create or recreate in one's mind a vivid visual sequence) cannot yet be tapped by our experimental methodology. Rather, the importance of the research may lie in its demonstration of qualitative differences in the effects of these media: exposure to television apparently highlights a set of contents and engenders a line of inference quite different from that stimulated by experience with books. Thus the individual who views television intensively and extensively may well develop different kinds of imaginative powers or, as Marshall McLuhan might have claimed, a different "ratio among imaginations" from that of an individual weaned on another medium, such as books.

We are left with an even more tantalizing thought. Ever since the time of Immanuel Kant, it has been assumed by most philosophers that individuals perceive experience in terms of certain basic categories—time, space, and causality. Indeed, one has no choice but to conceive of life in such terms—they are "givens." While psychologists do not necessarily accept these categories as part of the human birthright, they assume that eventually all normal individuals will come to possess similar versions of these basic categories of knowing.

If, however, one adopts an alternative perspective, if one affirms that some of our knowledge of time, space, and causality comes from the media of communication that happen to proliferate in one's culture, then this research has an additional implication. Put simply, it makes little sense to talk of the child's sense of time or space as a single undifferentiated entity. Rather, the ways in which we conceptualize our experience may reflect the kinds of media with which we have been engaged. And so the temporal and spatial outlook—and, a fortiori, the imagination of the television freak may have a different flavor from that of the bookworm. While such a finding from television research is perhaps not as immediately sensational as those involving violence or commercials, it can have potentially far-reaching educational implications. For instance, the ways in which one teaches history (with its time frames) or geometry (with its spatial components) might differ depending on the media with which children happen to have been raised *and* the media in which lessons are conveyed. And the findings can also help to reveal something about our own era. Based on comparisons between two pervasive cultural media—books and television—research results can pinpoint differences between individuals of our era and those of earlier times, and also suggest which of those differences might be due to television alone.

22

CRACKING THE CODES OF TELEVISION: THE CHILD AS ANTHROPOLOGIST

WITH LEONA JAGLOM

THE ANTHROPOLOGIST occupies a unique position in our society. While most of us have little opportunity to visit exotic lands, such ventures constitute the anthropologist's central mission. It is a daunting one. Relying primarily on common sense and general knowledge of human nature, he has to describe and eventually to construct, almost singlehandedly, models of various aspects of an entire society—its language, its kinship structure, its values, and its beliefs. He must continue to test and revise his formulations as necessary, until he feels relatively secure in his characterizations. Even with the help of articulate informants, he is unlikely to grasp the culture in all its particulars. Indeed, if his description is even approximately right, his ethnography will be considered a success.

Though our daily routine may seem far removed from such an existence, most of us have been anthropologists early in our lives. For in being placed in front of a television set and being asked, in effect, to make sense of the innumerable fleeting images it presents, the young child of two, four, or eight years of age is a kind of anthropologist.

Indeed in many ways the job confronted by our young anthropologist as he steadily eyes a Sony portable set is even more challenging. He has spent but a few years on the planet. He must make sense of diverse and seemingly incommensurate forms of reality, including the technical apparatus placed in front of him, the various slices of reality it serves up, the complicated panoply of commercials, features, news, documentaries, entertainment, specials, and test patterns which constitute daily video fare. One might say that he has to decode or unravel a number of worlds—the world of television as a whole, the world presented on each channel, the world represented by each kind of program, each particular program, and each episode and scene.

To complicate matters further, the child must learn the visual language used by television (for example, closeups, instant replays, montages). And he must decode rules that determine the operation of commercial and public television, the relationship among the various channels, the motivations leading to the production of commercials and shows, the status of live shows, recorded shows, original productions, and reruns. These tasks might intimidate even an accomplished Oxonian ethnographer.

But amazingly, the average child, working largely on his own, succeeds in making sense of these worlds in remarkably short order. By the age of five, most of these understandings and discriminations have already been accomplished. In fact, so speedy and untutored is this process that it recalls the preternatural facility shown by children everywhere in mastering language and other symbol systems of their society.

All the same, the child's conquest of television is neither total nor totally even. Just as sophisticated aspects of language may elude the young school child, certain aspects of television, both technical and programming, remain opaque even to much older and more accomplished youngsters. And confusion attends such conventions as canned laughter, such distinctions as documentaries versus fictionalized history, such realities as the purpose of commercials. It is here that skilled informants—such as parents, teachers, or peers possessing higher levels of sophistication—may prove essential. An especially delicate matter involves the proper situating of television within the child's ongoing life stream, giving it a place that is neither too exalted nor too inconsequential. Like the anthropologist, the child must steer between excessive ethnocentrism and "going native."

At Harvard's Project Zero my colleagues and I have been studying the first years of television viewing. We have been observing a small group of first-born, primarily middle-class youngsters between the ages of two and five as they watch television. Donning the roles of anthropologists ourselves, we have observed the children as they ingest in turn a steady diet of "Sesame Street," "Mister Rogers," the assorted daily mix of cartoons, commercials, soap operas, situation comedies, and the occasional specials that punctuate the television season. Watching children watching television, we have documented the tremendously rapid mastery of basic video competence and detected as well some lingering problems in "reading" the worlds transmitted on television.

At the outset every child must achieve two fundamental understandings about television. First of all, the child must come to understand the nature and limitations of the *physical medium* of the television set. To the extent that a one- or two-year-old child attends to television (and most of them at least sample the wares of video), these youngsters accept the material presented on television as a natural part of everyday life and regard the television set as a member of the family. There is essentially no appreciation of television as a distanced medium, one whose content represents rather than constitutes the daily flux of experience. Thus, at twenty-five months one of our subjects, whom we call Johnny, sees a broken egg on television and runs to fetch a paper towel to clean up the egg. Donny, just two months older, is afraid that the Abominable Snowman on television will want to invade his room. Sally, at the same age, spanks a television personage and then kisses her. And at age three my son Jerry became terribly fearful when, while sitting next to me, he spied me appearing on a television talk show as well. Not until the child is four or five does he understand that what is presented on television exists in a world apart from his immediate life space.

A second and equally fundamental challenge facing the child during his first years of viewing is an appreciation of the *narrative nature* of much of television. For the one or two-year-old, television presents an army of isolated images that bear no connection to one another. Any image could appear at any time: no necessary order seems to govern beginnings of programs, commercials, or station announcements. By the age of three or four, the child begins to sense that television presents narratives that may be interrupted from time to time by commercials. However, even when the narrative purpose of television has been grasped, the understanding of individual narratives may remain extremely meager.

In an effort to trace the beginning of narrative competence, we studied several youngsters as they observed the "Sesame Street" bit, "The

Boy Who Cried Monster" (patterned after "The Boy Who Cried Wolf"). Over a period of three years, the children watched this bit dozens of times with undiminished interest, tinged during the latter years with fright at the sight of the scary cookie monster. Comprehension of the bit surely increased over this period. Children came to realize that the vignette did not depict merely a voracious monster who deprived a boy of cookies: by the age of four or five there was incipient awareness that the villagers played a role in the story and that the boy had antagonized them with false alarms. Yet we found that even the four- or five-year-old child had only a partial understanding of this still simple and familiar fairy tale—failing, for example, to grasp that this particular monster was actually a friendly and grateful devourer of cookies.

Any sophisticated relationship to television rests on these fundamental understandings: the world presented on television exists independently of the actions and thoughts of the television viewer; the bits presented on television programs are ordinarily related in a sequential order. Despite the various misinterpretations just described, most children do appreciate these concepts by the conclusion of the preschool period. It is worth noting that such understandings of how to "read" symbolic products emerge more readily in the case of books than of television. As physical entities, books seem less "true to life" than television and so are less likely to be confused with daily reality. Moreover, both the slower pace of books and the ways in which their contents are customarily shared between parent and child, encourage mastery. Still, whatever confusions may obtain with respect to the apparatus of television and its fundamentally narrative quality have largely been dispelled by the time children reach five years of age.

Three remaining puzzles perplex the youthful television viewer. The first is the need to relate what is presented on television to what is available in the rest of one's daily experiences. The child must arrive at the following conclusion: the world of television is not exactly the same as his everyday world, but at the same time it is not totally alien from that world either. As we have come to phrase it, the child must be able to appropriately construct that *membrane* which stands at the interface between the worlds of television and the world of daily life.

Recall that the child at the age of one and a half accepts television as an unquestioned part of his daily experience. By the age of about two, while acknowledging that materials encountered on television

244

may not be identical to ones from his own world, he remains mesmerized by similarity. Thus, at twenty-eight months Sally sees a frog on television and immediately runs to get her frog puppet and plays with it. Vocal comments at this time also simply underline the similarities between materials or events presented on television and counterparts from the child's own existence: "I go McDonalds," "Get Lego," "Let's fly plane."

Having been hitherto dominated by identities and similarities, the three-year-old child effects a transition to the noting of differences between the televised and real world. Sally at forty months sees a stuffed bear and comments sagely, "Polar bears have this many feet? I never saw that on 'Sesame Street.' " This detection of differences may eventually assume such ferocity that the child comes to deny any relationship between what is presented on television and what is encountered in the real world. Thus Donny at fifty-seven months questions whether sneakers seen on television could be like sneakers in his own house; Johnny at fifty-nine months denies that he could be on television even though he has recently seen himself in that medium; and Sally, nearly five, claims that real people could not be dressed as Wonder Woman because "they're not real when they're on television."

In the course of the first few years of television viewing, then, the child moves from a time when there is no membrane to a phase when the membrane between these two worlds is virtually impermeable—a sort of Berlin Wall separating television from daily life. By the age of five, however, the membrane has achieved a more appropriate, semipermeable status. The child regularly points out both the similarities *and* the differences between television and the real world. Seeing Kermit the Frog on television, Sally declares, "I have a puppet like Kermit too, but mine doesn't talk."

The emerging acknowledgment of semipermeability reflects increasing awareness of the symbolic or representational nature of television fare. For example, seeing a fire on a news program, Charlie, age four and a half, realizes with genuine surprise (and cognitive pleasure) that it is the same fire which had been discussed at his school earlier that day. Newly aware that television may sometimes (but only sometimes) represent a specific aspect of his own daily experience, the child becomes gradually more open-minded about the connections between the domains.

As part of our investigation of the relationship between television and real life, we wondered which domain serves as a primary point of reference for the child. Hence we searched for references to daily experience while the child was watching television, and for references to television during the child's non-viewing hours. Somewhat to our surprise (and to our considerable relief), we found that the world of mundane experiences typically functions as a backdrop against which television is viewed. Children often remark that something on television resembles experiences in the real world: they much less frequently characterize daily experience in terms of the extent to which it resembles television. At least in our small population, there was little indication that television serves as a "real basis" against which to evaluate daily experience.

A second major puzzle facing the young television viewer is the relation among the multitude of programs presented on a typical day. The solving of this task involves recognizing various shows as well as diverse kinds of programs and charting their relationship to one another. Entailed as well is an appreciation of the schedule that governs programs and the role of "central characters" in the definition of a program. We were interested in the kinds of program distinctions children could initially make, and in the factors that motivate these and further delineations.

In general, the child's discriminations among television fare echo the distinctions he is effecting between the televised and real world. In the beginning the membranes obtaining among kinds of shows are totally permeable. Any character or any segment can appear, willy-nilly, at any time or in any context. Indeed, the young child attributes to himself magical powers: if he wants a bit to appear, it simply shall. To the extent that shows have any definition at all, they are built primarily around their lead characters.

By the age of two and a half or so, the child does make certain very broad distinctions among television programs. For better or worse, the first reliable category to emerge is the commercial. At a time when the child has no understanding of the purpose of commercials, he is already able to identify and label those short segments as different from the rest of television fare. We believe that the brevity, clarity, and highly vivid character of commercials contribute to their recognizability. In contrast, though our children watch the television show "Sesame Street" much more frequently than they watch any commercials, they do not recognize it as a show. Possibly the "magazine format" of "Sesame Street" renders it much less identifiable as a specific program or program type.

Cracking the Codes of Television

By the age of three or three and a half the child can recognize and identify cartoons: he also comes to appreciate that the various magazine segments juxtaposed together all fall under the single rubric of "Sesame Street." Children prove to be instructively sensitive to a relatively rare feature of a television diet—the preview for a forthcoming special. We speculate that previews—a kind of commercial—are especially recognizable because of the great interest that these specials hold for children, and also because they serve as hypotheses of future events which are confirmed when the program itself eventually appears on television.

Certain telltale cues may signal specific programs or program types, but they do not in themselves allow for complete mastery of program distinctions. Thus, unless children also appreciate the temporal organization of television—when shows begin and end, how flexibly specific characters and bits may appear across time slots, the nature and timing of commercials and station breaks—they will remain confused. In fact, such organizational aspects pose profound problems at the beginning; at age two or two and a half children have little recognition of what should appear at a given time, confuse commercials with programs and beginnings with ends, and stubbornly insist that characters will return even after a show has been completed. By the age of three or four, children do recognize the most familiar beginnings and endings, have a sense of schedules for their favorite television programs, and acknowledge that when a character fades with the end of the show "he won't be back again 'til tomorrow."

Children's understanding of television fare takes a decisive leap forward in the period between age four and five. At last children have a firm sense of the beginnings and endings of shows, the times at which the shows and characters appear, and the mutually exclusive relationship between regular shows, advertisements, and specials. Certain other program distinctions continue to pose problems. Even though (or perhaps because) from the age of two children dislike "the news," they still have difficulty reliably identifying segments taken from news programs. They also fail to honor the well-worn programmer's distinction between "children's programs" and "programs for grownups." In fact, they make a charming confusion: children's programs are simply programs watched by children, whether they are opera, soap opera, news, sports, or a segment of the "Beverly Hillbillies."

This confusion highlights a revealing aspect of children's television viewing. While adults readily classify programs in terms of the intent of the producer and the designated target audience, children have great

247

difficulty appreciating these abstract modes of classification. They think instead in terms of particular shows or even particular episodes and resist grouping these together as instances of situation comedies, dramas, documentaries, and the like. To the extent that they ever offer overriding generalizations, they will classify on the bases of the affects they experience: "funny shows," shows that are "frightening," and "boring programs."

We again encounter the "membrane effect" as the child ponders the role of the central character in a program. Initially, as we have seen, children assume that characters can appear at any place and at any time. Later on, during the middle preschool years, children come to associate characters exclusively with particular programs: they refuse to acknowledge that a character associated with one program can appear on another. And so if Mr. Rogers happens to appear on a talk show, that talk show becomes "Mr. Rogers"; or if Flip Wilson appears on "Hollywood Squares," it is then the "Flip Wilson Program." Eventually the membrane softens. The child of seven or eight does concede that an individual character is somewhat mobile in the land of television: even though he has a primary home, he may be allowed to visit other houses on the block.

The final and perhaps most formidable puzzle confronting the young television viewer is the status of, and relation among, the multiple levels of reality and fantasy within the variegated fare presented. In artistic media, levels of reality and fantasy are typically mixed: television is perhaps the medium that serves the most notorious and dizzying ensemble of levels of reality. While continuing to remain confused about this mélange of "reality with tiers," children nonetheless do make significant progress during the early years of their lives in effecting some preliminary sorting.

Initially the child is likely to consider everything presented on television—live films, cartoons, photographs, fantasy, or news—as equivalently real. Reality is the background against which fantasy or non-reality stands out. The first distinguishing markers surround abnormal or superhuman figures like monsters, wizards, and freaks. Children sense their divergent reality status. But frequently the child's own wishes get in the way, as he declares that he wants to be (and could be) like the Hulk, or Superman, a prince or a king. And even when the child purports to recognize the lines between reality and fantasy, this understanding may cloak amusing ignorance. Consider the child who said, "I know Big Bird isn't real, that's just a costume. There's just a plain bird inside."

If the potency of the character provides one important clue to irreality, the medium of presentation is another. The closer to photographic reality, the more likely a character will be considered "real." And conversely, cartoon figures, figures executing impossible actions, or figures presented in strange iconographies are much less likely to be judged as real.

But to transcend this very preliminary and primitive sorting, the child must master two long-term agendas. First of all he must become alert to the various uses and tricks to which the medium can be put, to the effects that directors and editors can conjure up. Only then can the child peer through surface indications of what is real and what is not and make a cool assessment of the realistic status of a segment.

The second requirement is to go beyond the simple duality—possible-impossible, real-fantastic—and to render an assessment of plausibility. Among the innumerable scenes and situations presented on television, certain bear a much closer relation than others to events in the world of regular experience. Yet the capacity to invoke plausibility presupposes the ability to weigh numerous factors simultaneously and to render a probabilistic judgment—calculations far beyond the ken of the young child. And so children must fall back repeatedly on simple formulae and single markers, which often yield erroneous assessments.

To override these initial canons of classification proves challenging. Only during the school years do children become alert to the fact that one individual may look real but behave in fantastic ways (Gilligan, for example), while another may be animated yet undergo psychologically authentic experiences (Charlie Brown, for example). And only at that time does a child become even dimly aware that certain kinds of programs (such as historical fiction or documentaries) may entail a peculiar blend of veridicality and editorial judgment.

How then does our young television viewer stack up as an anthropologist? On nearly any criterion, he performs extraordinarily well. Some aspects of television—for example, its narrative nature—are solved early on. More challenging aspects—the schedule of television, principal distinctions among programs—are essentially understood by the time the child enters school. Given the child's meager experience and the relative lack of help from informants, his achievement is spectacular.

Nonetheless, as exemplified by children's continuing difficulties in sorting out various levels of reality, certain aspects of television viewing remain problematic. Separating the facts from the editorials in a news broadcast, the amount of staging in a game show, or the extent to which various celebrities on a talk show are "being themselves," prove extremely difficult matters.

Another problem of enduring difficulty is to determine the accuracy with which the world is portrayed on television. While our young children consider the real world as the basis against which to assess television, the steadily accruing experience that children have with the various stereotypes fostered by television may ultimately tip the balance. Children may know so much more about law courts, operating rooms, or racial groups from their viewing experience than from their daily lives that they will inevitably attribute a high reality status to these video stereotypes and come to evaluate their occasional actual experiences against this idealized reality. As Jerzy Kosinski remarks in *Being There*, "In this country, when we dream of reality, television wakes us" (p. 89).

More complex narrative materials on television pose continuing challenges. While even the young child frequently gets the basic point of the plot, there is mounting evidence that important aspects of television programming continue to pose difficulties for children and even adults. In addition to the work in our own laboratory, we can invoke the recent report of Gavriel Salomon that American school children cannot answer even simple facts about television programs viewed on the previous day, and the findings of Purdue's Jacob Jacoby that a very high proportion of television viewers misunderstand at least part of what they see on short thirty-second segments of programming or public-service commercials.

Some of these aspects of television would prove difficult for any individual. Assessing the plausibility of a deliberately ambiguous film like "The Autobiography of Miss Jane Pittman" or the televised series "An American Family" would challenge even a philosopher. Even if these deliberately provocative examples are bracketed, it seems clear to me that children can be helped in dealing with questions of ambiguity, authenticity, and stereotypy. This is where parents, older siblings, friends, and educators can make a contribution; indeed, the people working in television can themselves perform a public service. If the brains that are customarily put to work in fashioning effective commercials were instead (or in addition) marshaled to clarify the nature of challenging materials presented on television, progress could be made in sealing various knowledge gaps confronted by the school-age child and by many adults as well. Dorothy and Jerome Singer of Yale University have made promising efforts in this direction through the devising of segments that take viewers "behind the scenes" of television.

Television can be mastered. Indeed, human beings seem extraordinarily well equipped to make initial sense of this complex medium. But even as language has its arcane and complex aspects, involving abstract argument, rhetoric, or figurative expression, so too can television present excessively challenging material and may, if somewhat inadvertently, foster obfuscation rather than clarity. Equipped with a good handbook, a skilled informant, and his own intelligence, the competent anthropologist eventually learns even the most difficult native tongue. Given analogous help, children can equally master the full range of television fare and will certainly enjoy it better. They may even succeed in becoming superior producers of television material. Quite possibly those whose "native tongue" is television will eventually become its greatest poets.

23

TELEVISION'S EFFECTS ON

CHILDREN: DOES IT

STIMULATE OR STULTIFY?

DURING the past twenty-five years two starkly contrasting myths have grown up, almost side by side. The first portrays the child as an active agent, an individual perpetually solving problems and inventing meanings. The second myth, equally prevalent, portrays the child as a passive victim of certain forces in his society, chief among them being television. According to this myth, television wreaks its destruction upon the hapless youngster, destroying any budding powers lurking within. It is difficult to see how both these legends could endure. If the child is truly a constructive being, he should exploit materials on television and thereby develop his mental and imaginative capacities. If, however, the child has been immobilized by television, his mind should stultify and his imagination wither away.

Though the final score card from scientific research has not yet been filled in, it is possible to begin to assess these myths. In my view, there is considerable support for the view of the young child as an active transformer of video fare and little, if any, convincing support for viewing the child as a passive "victim" of television. Television may actually exert positive effects on the child's imaginative powers.

Television's Effects on Children

Let us turn first to the image of the child that is emerging from psychological research. Investigators have provided considerable documentation to show that, from the very first moments of life, the young child is a vigilant attender to his environment and a keen solver of problems presented by the world around him. By dint of his constructive powers, the child becomes able to recognize persons, objects, and events and to master language, drawing, and other symbol systems of the culture. At the age of five, six, or seven he is already a very competent participant in his world.

Far from thwarting this active stance, television becomes a principal arena in which it is manifest. Even as a child is making sense of other media in his world, from the age of two to five he is also aggressively making sense of the diverse worlds presented on television.

Consider this accomplishment, as already sketched in the preceding essay. Within a few short years the child learns about the physical operation of television. He comes to appreciate that he cannot have any effect on the images presented on television but that often they will resemble the events and persons that fill his daily life. He learns about the routine of television—which shows appear at specified hours, which feature particular personalities or characters, which furnish news, comedy, or adventure. He ferrets out commercials, previews, test patterns, and the multitude of other bits that populate the television screen. By the age of three he can already monitor television, attending to those bits that interest him, "tuning out" when the message becomes too verbal or abstract.

Most remarkably, this rapid learning about television takes place with little, if any, formal tutelage from the outside world. At a time when the child cannot yet read or write, he already has, like a superior sleuth, achieved an amazing amount of comprehension of a very complex medium of communication.

By and large, then, studies of children watching television support the general view of the child as a clever and active problem-solver. But what about the more subtle facets of the child's development? In particular, what about the growth of the child's creative and imaginative powers? Can television make a contribution here as well?

Admittedly, it is very difficult to study children's imaginations. Scientists do not agree on how best to study imagination or creativity; nor do they even agree on exactly what these entities are. Also, so much of imagination occurs invisibly inside that other box—the head—whose private recesses scientists cannot yet probe. But one can look at the products of children's imaginations—their stories, their songs, their dances, their drawings, and the like. And this repository of the child's imaginative powers can provide some evidence about the effects wrought by television and other media.

My own observations, as well as those by other researchers, document that television can fuel the child's imagination. In years past children's imaginations were stimulated by the events and characters they encountered in fireside 'ales; or, in somewhat more recent times, by the pictures and stories they encountered in book form. Now, however, these sources have largely been supplanted by those characters and events that youngsters encounter on television. Mickey Mouse and other Disney characters have yielded to the "Muppets" and "Sesame Street." The kings and witches of the Brothers Grimm have been replaced by the superheroes who populate the television on Saturday morning. The child's imagination scoops up these figures from the television screen and then, in its mysterious ways, fashions the drawings and stories of his own fantasy world.

The drawings made by my son Jerry during his preschool years underscore an important point: in no sense did the child passively imitate the figures presented on the screen. Rather, as illustrated in essay 12 on children's drawings, Jerry portrayed them in his own style, with his own points of emphasis. He constructed new events and situations that reflected not only those situations conventionally depicted on television but also the concerns, anxieties, and desires that he was facing in his own life.

Like a vehicle equipped with proper fuel and allowed a suitable track, every preschool child provided with the media of expression—pens, markers, clay, puppets, and the like—will draw upon the images presented on television in fashioning creative products. Somewhat later in childhood, however, such activity becomes less common. And so one is less likely to find the child of ten or the adolescent drawing pictures or writing stories based upon characters encountered on television.

Revealingly, however, the children most gifted in the arts, those who continue to draw or compose in an imaginative way, rely heavily upon the characters encountered in the popular media, including those on television. In fact, as Brent and Marjorie Wilson of Pennsylvania State University have shown, superheroes often are the chief supplier of images and narrative material in the products of talented "middle-aged" youngsters.

Far from stifling the child's imagination, then, television can often aid its flowering. Yet a skeptic might still contend that there is nothing special about the contribution of television. On such an account, *any* source of imagery would have the same liberating effect. Indeed, to the extent that television presents uninteresting images, it might prove a relatively ineffective fuel for creative powers.

Scientists have culled little evidence to answer the skeptics' case. Nowadays, nearly every child has a television set, and, short of depriving youngsters of the beloved box, it is very difficult to determine what the imagination would be like in the absence of television. Moreover, we lack sufficient information about children before 1950 to allow a judicious comparison of imagination before and after the advent of "I Love Lucy."

Nonetheless, it should prove possible to find out more about the powers and liabilities of television as a stimulator of imagination. One way to do this is to present essentially "the same story" or "the same scene" to children across a variety of media of presentation. By looking at the children's products in the wake of such an exposure, one can make tentative statements about the contributions of the medium of television *per se* to the child's imaginative output.

It is just such a line of study that my colleagues Laurene Meringoff and Martha Vibbert have been pursuing. They allow children to encounter "the same story" in such diverse media as radio, picture books, and film. Then, at various points during and after the presentation, they ask children to draw pictures. At the very least, these pictures tell us about the effects of these media on the child's creative powers: at best they allow us to peek inside the child's imagination, discover his "mental images" and ultimately gain an impression of how these have been stimulated by presentations on rival media.

Though still at an early stage, these studies have already provided some suggestive results. It is not at all the case that one medium promotes imagination while the other undercuts it. Rather, each medium can fuel the imagination but is likely to do so in characteristically different ways.

A radio presentation, for example, while encouraging recall of ornate language, will yield drawings that are prosaic and standardized. Images are "stock" and finished. On the other hand, a video or film presentation, even one conveying the same auditory information, encourages a fixation on the visual image and a relative neglect of ornate language. The child is attracted to vivid and dynamic visual images which he can reproduce or transform; often the "video" child will draw a feature in a less stereotyped and more unusual fashion, and the canvas as a whole is less likely to host a standard "composition." In addition, television's penchant for depicting dramatic action stimulates drawings that feature dynamic movement and a rich assortment of facial expressions.

Such evidence declares television innocent of the charge that it destroys or radically reduces the child's imagination. The impact of television on imaginative powers might be even more evident if the child were given the opportunity to serve as a television director. Perhaps the chief creative skill inculcated by television is the ability to plan and "script" dramatic scenes. However, since most children do not yet have at their disposal videopacks or other film-making equipment, it is not possible to determine whether an extensive exposure to television actually stimulates such directorial powers. About the only hint we have that this might be so is found in the frequent playground games in which children re-enact exciting episodes from favorite television programs.

In my own view, the charge that television destroys or reduces imaginative powers is largely unfounded. In fact, rather than undermining the child's active creative and problem-solving tendencies, television during the early years of childhood can be a major stimulator of imaginative capacities.

Nonetheless, there may be some substance to the frequent criticisms we hear of television's effect on children. The view of television as a stunting influence gains in persuasiveness once the child has passed the years of early childhood and is well into school. At this time, artistic and other forms of symbolic activity often take a back seat in the child's development. The child becomes instead increasingly oriented to verbal and logical discourse, and increasingly caught up in the abstract arguments of science or history classes. Children's cognitive powers are often marshaled in new ways in dealing with such material. Rather than making drawings or acting out dramatic events, youngsters are more likely to compose essays on these topics, to discuss and argue about them with their friends, and to begin to ponder more abstract concepts, like democracy or demography, electricity or evolution.

Perhaps television as a medium has the potential to help children explore such concepts. In fact, some of the best material on educational television may well have this positive effect. However, it certainly seems to me that at present television does a much better job of stimulating that sensory imagination so important in the life of the young child than in undergirding the more abstract, conceptual lines of thought which become critical just a few years later.

24

DICTATED BY NECESSITY,

OR EVERYMAN HIS OWN

BOSWELL

MOST PEOPLE engaged in a creative enterprise, such as writing or composing music or painting, spend a fair amount of time musing on ways to increase their productivity. Either alone or with colleagues, they may ponder a variety of prods to "getting started," better ways to plan priorities, more efficient methods of revising and correcting errors, or the use of mechanical, "prosthetic" tools for enhancing their output.

By no means immune from this vanity, I recently began to dictate my manuscripts into a tape recorder rather than compose them on a typewriter. The transition has created at least the illusion of a tremendous increase in the speed of production and, possibly, an improvement in the quality of my work. Even with a tape recorder, I will not equal the output of Samuel Johnson, who in one two-and-a-half-year period produced half a million words of reportage on the debates in the British Parliament. Still, I have begun to sing the glories of dictation and have even begun to consider using some other prosthetic devices, such as computer word-processing systems.

These aids seem to make life easier in the way that a supermarket eliminates the strain of visiting a dozen specialty markets. But do they really sharpen thinking and writing skills? To begin looking for an answer, we might consider how the cognitive processes involved in dictating may differ from those of writing, either by hand or on a typewriter. Since to my knowledge there is little research around on the subject, I have no choice but to begin with some subjective impressions.

While use of prosthetics is exciting to some people, it is threatening to others. Many writers need the mental set that accompanies banging away on an old clunker of a typewriter. Others are absolutely wedded to the pencil, if not to a row of sharpened pencils. (For that matter, Proust could work only in a cork-lined room. Schiller had to sniff rotten apple cores before the verbal juices would begin to flow.)

In college I underwent considerable anxiety in weighing whether or not to switch from writing by hand to typewriting. However, the speed and efficiency I gained from typing was such that no one— least of all my professors—regretted the retirement of my script.

The move to dictation was dictated by necessity. On returning from a long trip, I discovered I had so much work that it seemed I could never catch up. I went out and bought a tape recorder. I knew that I could compose short notes orally, because I had dictated some to an assistant when pressed for time. First I began dictating long letters. In short order I found that I could also compose entire articles and essays while talking into the machine.

Before I start to dictate, I prepare for writing just as I did before. I do the required reading, digest the material, and think about it. I then jot down an outline of a page or so, listing in order the major points I want to make. Then, instead of composing a legible draft on the typewriter, I begin talking into the machine as if I were lecturing to a small group of students.

As a primarily auditory person, when I speak I appear to be following the dictates of an inner voice—that is, I do not see any words in front of me, but I hear what I am about to say and find myself virtually transcribing the sounds of the words with my tongue. Often I proceed as quickly as if I were talking to a class, though at other times I slow down, or even swear to myself.

From my conversations with others, I have learned there may be different cognitive styles involved in dictation. For example, those who are more visually oriented appear to see a sentence in their minds— sometimes visualizing a whole paragraph as they construct it. (In my own auditory imagination, I can hear some of what came before and some of what is to come, but little more.) The relationship between dictated copy and final copy also seems to vary from one person to another. Some people, myself included, are excessively wordy and have to prune the dictated copy; others are oversuccinct, composing in outline form and later filling in details and supplying the connecting links.

I have found that dictating is not only faster than typing or handwriting but also permits closer synchrony between thoughts and word production and enables me to avoid annoying interruptions, like correcting typos or putting new paper into the carriage. Lack of back pain is another dividend.

There are a few unanticipated problems, however. I have difficulty in estimating the length of the material I have produced, in remembering the wording I have used, and in judging just where paragraphs should begin and end. The material that comes out is sometimes wordier, more repetitive, more colloquial than I normally like. I also regret not being able to peek back at what I have written, to make sure I have laid a firm foundation for what follows. But slowly each of these hindrances has been disappearing, and I would not be surprised if my first drafts of a dictated piece were soon indistinguishable from their typed predecessors.

Once I have finished dictating and my secretary has prepared a legible typed manuscript, I then edit in the usual pen or pencil method. However, I could use another prosthetic aid in the editing. After dictation the entire piece could be keyboarded into a computer word-processing terminal. With some of the fancy new programs available, I could shift whole sections of the text from one place to another, move words, phrases, or sentences within paragraphs, perhaps even make use of word definitions, lists of synonyms or antonyms, and "trees" describing relations which obtain among a network of words.

To understand the advantages—and limitations—of dictating, it is helpful to compare the processes of writing with those of speaking. Initially, of course, we all speak and none of us writes. The development of writing skills is a lengthy and not yet well-understood process that begins in the drawings of childhood and has, in its initial stages, little if any connection with speech. It takes years for a child to master the technical aspects of penmanship and spelling and to know enough about sentence, paragraph, and essay construction to produce passages that compare in interest and complexity with what he can readily utter.

Though some of the best writing sounds as if the author were simply speaking to the reader, the two processes are radically different. In speaking, a person can rely on gesture, tone of voice, and the response of an audience to guide the style and substance of what he is saying. In writing, all information must be carried by the written word, and one runs the risk of being misunderstood—or of not being understood at all.

Nevertheless, speaking and writing obviously have a lot in common. Both depend upon sufficient mastery of the *forms* of a particular linguistic entity (be it the letter, report, or poem) so that each realization of that form observes its basic rules. Thus in delivering a campaign speech, politicians know the general form and the points they wish to make with sufficient intimacy to present on each occasion an acceptable, if modified, version of "the basic speech." By the same token, the writer of a daily newspaper column—James Reston or Ann Landers, for example—has mastered several forms that such columns usually take and can plug the specific content into the pattern easily and quickly.

This particular technique has been carried to exquisite heights. We learn from Walter Bate's biography that Samuel Johnson could write three columns of 600 words each in one hour, faster than most people can dictate the same amount of material today. When it came to the writing of books, Johnson was even more amazing. Approaching a superhuman pace, he drafted his entire *Life of Savage*—a book of 186 pages—in about thirty-six hours. In fact, he wrote the first forty-eight printed pages at one sitting, though, as he said, "I sat up all night."

Johnson knew his subject matter so intimately that his views were fully crystallized by the time he turned to actually producing a work. His memory was so well honed that he could maintain gigantic units of material in his mind. Finally, he had so thoroughly mastered the literary structures and formulas of the day that he could write at breakneck speed. But even he used prosthetics—notably James Boswell, through whom he transmitted some of his prose and much of his wit.

Without doubt, dictation can increase output. It can perhaps also improve the quality of that output in at least two ways. First, dictating forces one to outline the whole argument or piece in advance—a skill that can significantly increase the coherence of the final product. Second, it permits thinking to unfold in a natural and unimpeded way, at the speed of speech and with fewer interruptions. Another advantage in dictating is that we are more likely to capture fleeting thoughts and sequences of thought than if we had been writing by hand or on a typewriter—thus avoiding the uncomfortable feeling that some brilliant idea was irretrievably lost while we were slipping a new sheet of paper into the typewriter.

In my view, prosthetics can help some people improve the quality of their writing. However, truly creative people must rely primarily on internal processes. That is, to be able to think in an original way about a topic, a person must have the material so organized in his mind that he can readily juxtapose and combine it in a variety of unexpected ways, proceed in a number of directions with the same information, and shuttle with ease from one set of issues to another.

All these capacities presuppose that the individual can organize information in a number of complex and flexible ways. And that may be why many creative people monitor their thought processes constantly and search for more efficient ways to record their more striking conceptions. The resulting work is highly individual, idiosyncratic, and impervious to formula.

I take issue with books that purport to teach people to think better—laterally, generatively, creatively. It is not that they do not provide some modest clues to how an individual might jack up his performance by 10, 20, or even 50 percent. It is, rather, that they often hold out the false hope that one can be transformed from what Johnson called "a harmless drudge" into an individual of superior thinking powers. Whatever their uses in today's productivity-oriented world, neither tricks nor prosthetics can erase the gap between drudgery and mastery.

PART IV

THE BREAKDOWN

OF THE MIND

INTRODUCTION

ON THE SURFACE few worlds seem more different from one another than that of the normal young child and that of the brain-damaged adult. In the first instance, the child is in the course of development, with his skills gradually unfolding and with an unknown but, it is hoped, bright future ahead. The young child is in many ways at the height of his creative powers. He is also in an unequaled position to benefit from special interventions and support systems, even as he proves to be most resilient in the case of physical injuries as well as other setbacks and obstacles. We can only agree with poets and sages that the hope for the race lies in its children.

For the person who has suffered brain damage as an adult, the outlook seems bleak. Formerly at the height of his powers, he has now been struck down by a malady from which very few recover completely and which usually entails severe setbacks. Far from exploring new interests or visiting remote sites, the brain-damaged patient is often bedridden and seems unable to enjoy even familiar pursuits. Forced to spend time in the often depressing rooms of a hospital or a rehabilitation center, he may well be estranged from family, friends, and the vocation and interests that earlier occupied him. The road to recovery is long and difficult, and even with the most diligent and caring assistance he may well not make it.

Such, at any rate, were my attitudes as I first began to work with brain-damaged individuals a decade ago. As I relate in my autobiographical notes in essay 30, I found myself working with this population quite by accident and had little knowledge of it beyond superficial appearances. As I came to know many brain-damaged individuals, however, and to work with some of them intensively, my stereotyped initial views were gradually overcome and I became able to think of them as persons in their own right, with their own personalities, thoughts, and aspirations.

From a scientific point of view, the world of the brain-damaged individual is initially fascinating and potentially enlightening. Many aspects of human thought and personality can be approached and clarified through an understanding of what happens to the individual who has suffered damage to the brain. In particular, many aspects of creativity, artistry, and symbol use which have been reflected upon throughout these pages are freshly illuminated by studies with this population. The experiences of brain-damaged individuals turn out to be far more varied than I had thought. While some have suffered so grievously that they are no longer at all the same persons as before and show little improvement over time, many other individuals have considerable insight into their condition and draw upon these insights to ease the road to recovery. Many brain-damaged patients are able to retain good relations with those individuals they knew before and can even forge new and meaningful relations with other patients and with personnel at their health-care facility. Perhaps most important, life does not finish with brain disease: even impaired and elderly individuals have an inspiring capacity to make the most of their spared abilities, to set reasonable goals for themselves, and to display satisfaction and happiness when they achieve them, while redoubling their efforts when they are not successful.

Unfortunately, the lessons for rehabilitation which emerge from a better understanding of brain disease are not always apparent or straightforward. The art of rehabilitation is by no means coterminous with the science of neuropsychology. And yet there is to my mind no question that progress has been made in the treatment of the brain-damaged and other disadvantaged populations and that some of it came as a result of scientific advances. Further, I am convinced that the greatest hope for future breakthroughs lies in a constant and mutual collaboration between scientific researchers and experts in rehabilitation. Not infrequently, insights obtained from individuals in other fields can prove of help in this effort: in fact, some of the principles obtained in educational work with children have proved applicable to brain-damaged individuals.

In my view, then, the scientific study of brain disease can yield insights of the first magnitude for the understanding of normal human cognition, even as it holds out limited but genuine promise for more successful rehabilitation of the victims of brain disease. There are two perils that must be avoided. One is the tendency to make excessive claims about the findings of neuropsychology, or about their implications for present treatment. The second is the temptation to tamper with the work of scientists in this area, whether out of unimpeachable or suspect motivations. These aspects of scientific practice become increasingly evident in an area such as brain disease, which is filled with vexing problems and strong feelings, and so it will occupy us in the essays that follow.

The lead piece is a general introduction to the study of brain damage. It chronicles some of the scientific lessons that can be learned from this line of study and indicates as well some promising modes of rehabilitation. The second, essay 26, is a cautionary note that designates some of the pitfalls of accepting the excessive claims made in neuropsychology—in this particular case, the notorious exaggerations about the functions of the two halves of the brain.

The area of cognition that has been most informed by neuropsychological studies is language, and so it is fitting that two essays in the central part of this section deal with linguistic disorders resulting from injury to the left (or dominant) hemisphere. The first of these essays describes aphasia—the loss of language following damage to the brain. The second focuses on what is for me the single most enigmatic instance of cognitive dysfunction—selective loss of the ability to read in the face of the preservation of other visual and linguistic functions. In a final essay on language, I turn to recent work on patients' abilities to appreciate sophisticated forms of language, such as stories and jokes. In this connection, the focus shifts from patients with left-hemisphere disease to those with an equally devastating but far less well-understood condition that emanates from injury to the right (or nondominant) hemisphere. Some clinical impressions about the behavior of Justice William O. Douglas after he suffered a debilitating stroke to the right hemisphere raise the delicate issue of how a society should react when one of its leaders has sustained cognitive impairment.

My own studies of brain damage arose in the course of an effort to understand better the nature of human artistry. An essay reports what I have learned about art and the brain through studies of both gifted artists and normal nonartistic individuals who have had the misfortune to suffer brain disease.

I conclude this section with a tribute to one of the outstanding scientists of our time, the Russian psychologist and neurologist Alexander Luria, an individual who pioneered in exploring the relationship between the study of normal children and the investigation of brain-damaged adults. Luria's scientific legacy is a magnificent achievement. It has stood as a model for me as I have sought to collate findings from the seemingly diverse populations of normal and exceptional children on the one hand, and brain-damaged adults on the other. But the story of Luria has a depressing side as well. This good man had the misfortune to practice science in a land where political considerations typically overran the pursuit of knowledge. The way Luria gradually came to lose touch with his own thoughts and beliefs stands as a poignant reminder of the dangers to free inquiry which extreme political forces—of the left or the right—are prone to pose.

25

BRAIN DAMAGE: A WINDOW

ON THE MIND

OVER the past decades our understanding of brain chemistry, of neural circuitry, and of sensory and motor processes has so increased as to render obsolete the medical textbooks of an earlier generation. But how much have these lines of neurological investigation—usually conducted with "lower" animals and dependent upon microscopic preparations—revealed about the functioning of the human mind? Can we draw from studies at the cellular level insights about these intellectual, emotional, and social capacities of pivotal importance within human society? In truth, it must be said: the gap between most work in the brain sciences and the elucidation of our own "higher functions" remains enormous.

Over the past century, however, there has accumulated an unexpected but highly revealing set of insights that illuminates precisely those functions central in human intellectual activity. From the careful study of normal individuals whose brains have been injured, we receive penetrating insights into the nature of such cerebral activities as reading, writing, speaking, drawing, doing mathematics, and making music. We can uncover the links—and the distances—between such activities. And we can gain fertile clues about those enigmas that have long intrigued both philosophers and laymen. What is the nature of memory? Can one think without language? Are all art forms cut from a single cloth?

269

An uncomfortably large number of circumstances can injure the adult brain, but by far the most common and, as it happens, the most revealing is the cerebral vascular accident, or stroke. Each year in this country alone approximately 300,000 individuals suffer strokes; they occur when blood vessels leading to their brains are occluded by deposits of fat, when a clot lodges in an artery, or when an artery bursts. These events threaten the loss of the two elements upon which the brain is crucially dependent: oxygen and glucose. Deprived of these precious substances for more than a few minutes and having no reservoirs upon which to draw, brain tissue is damaged or destroyed. And, once destroyed, it cannot be regenerated. Instead, one may expect an unpalatable set of failures in those functions controlled by the brain cells: loss of motor and sensory capacities, failure of "high cognitive functions," and perhaps coma and death.

In the most fortunate cases, injury to the brain caused by a stroke may be so slight that it remains undetected; on other occasions death or total disability occurs. But a sizable number of strokes each year prove to be of intermediate severity—insufficient to kill, yet virulent enough to affect permanently the individual's mental functioning. By what they can (and cannot) do, these unfortunate victims yield invaluable information to the neurologists, psychologists, and other scientists involved in the study of the brain.

Were the destruction wrought by a stroke, tumor, or head trauma completely general so that all mental abilities were reduced by an equivalent proportion, little knowledge could be gained about the nature and organization of intellectual skills. (The victim would simply be a "dulled" normal individual; any insights gained from studying him might as readily be procured from the investigation of other normal individuals.) In fact, however, brain damage is highly selective. The victim may lose some abilities completely, while others remain wholly or virtually unaffected. An individual with a lesion in his left hemisphere may be completely unable to speak, while remaining able to draw or hum with skill. An individual with a lesion in his right hemisphere may be unable to dress himself properly and may lose his way in the hospital, while he can read and speak just as before.

As a result of these somewhat surprising circumstances, the brain-damaged patient constitutes a unique experiment in nature. What could never be done experimentally occurs daily as a result of inexorable fate.

As a neuropsychological researcher at the Aphasia Research Center

of the Boston Veterans Administration Medical Center, I have come
to know several hundred victims of brain damage. Most of our patients
are aphasic: their language abilities have been disrupted as a result of
damage to the brain, such injury implicating their left cerebral cortex
in nearly all cases. About one third of our patients suffer from other
kinds of brain injury in other sites, which, while sparing their language
functions, vitiate other abilities. And so I have had the instructive
opportunity of comparing the functioning of two kinds of patients—
those whose language is impaired but who have retained other abilities
and those who, while losing other capacities, retain the abilities to
express themselves verbally and to understand spoken language. In
what follows, then, I shall sketch some of the insights that other researchers and I have obtained from studying various brain injuries that
may befall the normal adult.

One of the first lessons gleaned from work with brain-damaged patients is that common-sense notions of the relationships among abilities
may be invalid. Take, for example, the set of symptoms encountered
in a bizarre but not infrequent condition called *pure alexia without
agraphia.* Patients afflicted with this disorder are unable to read text
(they are alexic) yet remain able to write (they are not agraphic).
One's immediate thought is that they must be in some sense blind;
but in fact the patients can copy or trace out the very letters and
words that they fail to read. To complicate the matter even further,
the same patients are often able to read numbers. They may even
read "DIX" as "509," while proving incapable of reading it as "diks."
They are able to name objects but are frequently unable to name samples of colors shown to them.

On its own, this syndrome confounds a raft of intuitions about how
the mind works. Reading can be separated from writing; verbal symbols
differ from numerical symbols; objects are named in a way different
from the way colors are. No one completely understands pure alexia,
but the major facts of the syndrome described above have been repeatedly described and are widely accepted. Some researchers hold that
the individual's visual powers and his verbal-language capacities are
reasonably intact but that the connections between them have been
disrupted. As a result, purely visual configurations—like letters or colors—cannot be named (or read). But those visual configurations that
arouse sensory or tactile associations (like objects or numbers) can
be satisfactorily processed. Evidently such findings not only undermine
common sense; they also challenge the researcher to devise a model

of mind that can account for this bizarre blend of abilities and disabilities. And they provide intriguing clues about why some normal individuals can master arithmetic before they can read or why others can more easily remember the names of rare objects than rare colors.

Pure alexia demonstrates that symbols which might have been thought similar (numbers and words) are processed in different ways by the brain. In a condition that accompanies injury to the parietal and occipital lobes of the left hemisphere, patients can understand single words and declarative sentences but fail to decode utterances that employ prepositional phrases like "on top of" or "next to," possessive constructions ("my brother's wife"), or the passive voice ("the lion was killed by the tiger"). Other syndromes demonstrate precisely the reverse situation; skills usually thought independent of one another in fact turn out to be closely related. Further investigations with these patients reveal difficulties in carrying out mathematical operations and in analyzing a spatial array. These disabilities co-occur with sufficient regularity to suggest that the same underlying "mental operations" may be drawn upon in understanding certain linguistic structures, in performing arithmetic, and in comprehending a spatial layout. And so, in this instance, the modeler of mental processes is challenged to unite skills that, on intuitive grounds, may appear quite unrelated. By the same token, the schoolteacher receives an impetus to use linguistic examples to aid mathematical understanding or to draw upon mathematical exercises in explicating the principles of grammar.

In most cases the deficits exhibited by brain-damaged patients are only too apparent—to the victim as well as to those who know him. Sometimes, however, a victim may be completely unaware of his deficits, and they may even escape the casual observer as well. An instructive example of this is Korsakoff's disease, a syndrome that results from damage to the mid-brain and is often the pathetic climax of many years of alcoholism.

The Korsakoff patient exhibits no evident physical disabilities. He may perform at an average or above average level on an intelligence test. He can solve a variety of problems posed to him; he can converse in an intelligent manner for hours. And yet, once his deficit has been revealed, it becomes painfully obvious. For a victim of Korsakoff's disease cannot remember anything that is told to him or anything that has happened to him since the onset of his disease.

Few medical demonstrations are as powerful (and memorable) as that of Korsakoff's disease: one tells an apparently normal patient one's name, engages him in distracting conversation for a few moments, and then hears the patient not only claim ignorance of one's name but also deny that it has ever been told to him. Yet, if all memory were of a single piece, the mechanisms underlying this process would not be illuminated by Korsakoff's disease.

In fact, however, the Korsakoff patient *is* able to learn things providing only that one does not accept his testimony concerning what he knows. For instance, one can teach such a patient to play a new piece on the piano; the next day he will deny ever having learned the piece, but, once given the opening bars, he (or his fingers) will play the piece perfectly. One can teach a Korsakoff patient a complex new motor skill—say, solving a maze or copying an intricate pattern; once again, despite his sincere protestations of ignorance, the patient (or his hands) will reveal mastery of this new skill. And, most surprisingly of all, one can even teach such a patient a new line of verse, a nonsense slogan, or a series of answers to questions, though, instructively, this verbal information cannot be "accessed" unless the right semantic trigger is pulled by the questioner.

Such findings document at least two forms of memory. Given sufficient drill, the brain of the Korsakoff patient can learn new patterns—motor, musical, even verbal—and can spew these patterns back under appropriate circumstances. But the Korsakoff patient has largely lost the ability to learn something new—particularly if it is verbal. And he is completely incapable of knowing what he has learned or of drawing upon such new skills in the voluntary way available to normal individuals.

The Korsakoff patient, finally, illuminates some of the quirks of our own mnemonic capacities: we can now better understand why we may be able to repeat a game, a motor activity, or a prayer that apparently had been forgotten; why a line of verse may be more effortlessly retrieved when its meaning is ignored and its syllabic sequence is allowed to unfold without interruption; why a forgotten town becomes instantly familiar once we return to its environs; or why we can sometimes parrot back a recently heard phrase whose meaning has totally eluded us.

Study of the brain-damaged individual can not only illuminate the ordinary processes of ordinary individuals; it can also help to unravel highly developed skills possessed by talented individuals. Among the individuals who have proved extremely difficult to study under ordinary conditions are artists; such creative persons are few, display little sympathy toward empirical investigators, and possess skills of such fluency that they defy dissection and analysis. Here again the accidents of brain damage offer a unique investigative opportunity.

Only on rare occasions has an artistically knowledgeable neurologist encountered an accomplished artist whose brain has been damaged. But from such rare happenings considerable insight has been gained into the operation of the artistic mind. As I note in greater detail in essay 30, "Artistry After Brain Damage," painters can, typically, continue to create significant works after their language powers have been seriously disturbed; indeed, more than one researcher has claimed that visual artistry actually improves as a result of aphasia. But, interestingly enough, painters with right-hemisphere disease—whose language has remained unaffected—often exhibit bizarre patterns in their paintings: they may neglect the left side of the canvas, they may distort the external form of objects, or they may portray emotionally bizarre or even repulsive subject matter. Apparently painting and linguistic capacities can exist independently of one another.

On the other hand, the relationship between linguistic and musical skills seems more complex. Some aphasic musicians prove able to compose or perform; some (among them the composer Maurice Ravel) lose the ability to create musically even though their critical powers seem to be intact; still other musicians have been completely disabled by aphasia.

The striking individual differences found among brain-damaged musicians suggest that musical capacities may be organized in idiosyncratic ways across individuals. Perhaps most individuals learn in rather similar ways to speak and to draw, but the organization of music in the brain may differ dramatically depending on whether one has learned an instrument, what instrument one favors, whether one plays by ear, the extent to which one sings, and so on. No wonder that the preparation of musical exercises suitable for all students poses enormous challenges to even the most gifted and enterprising musical teacher!

Of the diverse conundrums that populate the area of human neuropsychology, none is more persistent and more endlessly fascinating than the relationship between language and thought. Opinions on this issue vary enormously. Some investigators (for example, those influenced by the American linguist Benjamin Lee Whorf) view all thought processes as shaped by language and consider aphasia the death of cognition. Other researchers (for instance, those influenced by the Swiss psychologist Jean Piaget) see language and thought as separate streams; they believe that thought can proceed in a virtually unimpaired manner despite a pronounced aphasia.

Dozens of studies inspired by this vexing question reveal quite clearly the inadequacy of both extreme positions. Unquestionably, certain cognitive and intellectual abilities depend quite heavily on linguistic intactness: the ability to reason about abstract issues, the capacity to solve scientific problems, and, in most cases, skill at mathematics. (Just try to think about a comparison between socialism and communism without resorting to words.) However, an equally impressive list details reasoning powers that may be well preserved despite a severe aphasia: the ability to solve spatial problems, sensitivity to fine differences in patterns or configurations, and alertness to the emotional contours of a situation. (Just try to describe a spiral staircase using only words.) And, though this area has not been much studied, it seems probable that an individual's sense of himself is not noticeably affected by linguistic impairment—even as "the self" can be decimated while linguistic powers remain completely unaffected.

With every passing year new neuropsychological laboratories are opened; virtually every issue of the leading journal documents fascinating new cases or pivotal experimental discoveries. Our knowledge of the skills detailed above, as well as many others not alluded to here, is certain to increase and to change. And yet it is already possible, on the basis of well-documented findings, to posit reasonably convincing models of human mental processes, particularly in the area of language. Moreover, it should be possible within the next decade to begin integrating what is known about relatively discrete cognitive functions—such as reading, memory, or visual recognition—with insights concerning such subtle and elusive areas as the individual's emotional life, his preferences and fears, his relations with other people, and, most intriguing of all, his consciousness of his own experiences and of the world about him.

Understanding the brain-damaged individual and extrapolating to the normal person is a worthwhile scientific endeavor in its own right. I do not at all wish to detract from it. However, work with the victims of brain damage provides both an opportunity and a challenge to aid these often hapless individuals. It is therefore encouraging to report that in the area of aphasia the increased understanding obtained from neuropsychological investigation has suggested some promising avenues of rehabilitation.

Once it had been established that skills in musical and visual tasks could be at least partially dissociated from linguistic skills, the possibility arose that such spared capacities might be marshaled to aid individuals in communicating with other persons. At our own research unit, novel forms of aphasia therapy have been devised for use with patients who have not benefited from traditional language therapy. The most successful of these new therapies, one devised by Nancy Helm, Martin Albert, and Robert Sparks, involves the use of singing (or melodic intonation) in order to aid the patient who is unable to express himself orally. A still-experimental therapy, developed in association with Edgar Zurif and several other investigators, involves the ordering of visual symbols drawn on index cards. Patients learn to associate these symbols with objects and actions in the world and then communicate their wishes and thoughts by manipulating the cards. Still other therapies, designed with the aphasic patient's strengths and limitations in mind, draw on sign language and on manipulation of an artificial speech synthesizer. It is still too early to pass final judgment on the efficacy of these therapies, but they at least offer hope that those areas of the brain that have been spared may to some extent be placed in the service of apparently destroyed functions.

Because the patient ordinarily studied by neuropsychologists was once normal, those parts of his brain that are still functioning are presumed to reflect the way in which mental capacities are typically organized in the intact individual. In this respect he differs from the young child whose brain is much less differentiated into specific zones and, at the same time, is much more flexible. The adult with even a small lesion may suffer permanent disruption of major skills; the toddler can lose as much as half of his brain (via the removal of a hemisphere) and yet remain able to operate reasonably effectively in intellectual matters, presumably because spared areas "take over" functions.

Despite these telling differences in brain organization and potential, knowledge about children's learning abilities and disabilities can be obtained from a study of the brain-damaged adult. In my view, the kinds of brain injury that befall adults often seem to reveal conditions found, perhaps in somewhat less clear-cut form, in school children with learning disabilities. For instance, individuals with acquired alexias (or reading disorders) often resemble children with dyslexia (otherwise-competent children exhibiting special difficulties in reading). Similarly, adult patients with selective disorders in calculation often resemble children who experience special difficulties in learning arithmetic. (Selective sparing may also prove illuminating: patients who can decode written symbols or who can repeat language without understanding resemble certain autistic or retarded youngsters.)

These clinical findings suggest that some children may be born with neurological abnormalities that yield the behavioral pattern found in certain normal adults whose brains have been injured. The rehabilitative clue here arises from the fact that the brain-damaged adult could once perform the now-disrupted function. Should one succeed in devising a way to "reactivate" this skill, using a channel that is as yet unimpaired, one might accomplish two goals. Even while aiding the adult in recovering an ability of importance, one has developed methods that may facilitate the acquisition of these same skills by the learning-disabled child. For one has developed an alternative-training regime that, while unnecessary for the completely normal child, may prove highly serviceable for the child with a slightly atypical brain.

Returning to our original example of pure alexia without agraphia, one finds further applications of this procedure. Studies have documented that, if given three-dimensional letters to touch, alexic patients can read with greater skill. And, most intriguingly, studies of alexic patients in the Orient have revealed that they may be able to read ideographic characters while they fail to read phonetic characters. Just these insights have been drawn upon in the education of American children with selective disabilities in reading. Thus Paul Rozin and his colleagues at the University of Pennsylvania have developed an ideographic system effective with inner-city dyslexic children. And psychologist Jay Isgur, working with learning-disabled youngsters in Pensacola, Florida, has reported marked success in a program that builds upon the use of three-dimensional "objectlike" letters.

Whether such rehabilitative measures prove to be potent prosthetics or of only marginal assistance remains to be determined. Once destroyed, brain tissue is forever beyond repair, and the loss of this precious substance almost invariably involves serious cost. Yet given that some brain damage is inevitable, and that transplants of neural protoplasm will not soon be with us, efforts to assist the injured child or adult must certainly be encouraged. And, indeed, such efforts constitute one of the most rewarding portions of research on brain damage. Even as insights into our own minds, and into mental processes generally, have been coming forth rapidly, it has proved possible to apply what has been learned to those individuals who, willingly if inadvertently, have contributed to our understanding.

26

WHAT WE KNOW

(AND DO NOT KNOW)

ABOUT THE TWO HALVES

OF THE BRAIN

IT IS BECOMING a familiar sight. Staring directly at the reader— frequently from a magazine cover—is an artist's rendition of the two halves of the human brain. Surprinted athwart the left cerebral hemisphere (probably in stark blacks or grays) are such words as "logical," "analytical," and "Western rationality." More luridly etched across the right hemisphere (in rich orange or royal purple) are "intuitive," "artistic," or "Eastern consciousness."

Regrettably, the picture says more about a current popular-science vogue than it does about the brain. Claims about the division of labor between its two halves are becoming increasingly remote from what is known or even suspected. Indeed, the current packaging of human-brain research threatens to reveal more about academic huckstering than about neurological function. It is time, at least provisionally, to set the record straight.

Such an evaluation should begin with the recognition that heightened interest in the brain is warranted today, as in the scientist's desire to grasp the "brass-ring" secret of the brain's organization. As we uncover the biological origins of life and unravel the structure of the physical order, the nature of the human brain remains perhaps the chief and most profound enigma confronting the scientific community. Furthermore, the particular problem posed by the coexistence of *two* cerebral hemispheres is especially alluring, since initial appearances so long misled investigators.

Superficially similar in appearance and functioning, the hemispheres of the brain have gradually revealed their individual identities. Not only does each half control the movement of limbs and sensations on one side of the body, but the left and right hemispheres seem to play distinct roles in thinking, perception, feeling, and memory. Moreover, left-handedness—and who has not pondered the reasons for that condition?—seems integrally tied to an atypical relationship between the two halves of the brain.

In view of these and other considerations, curiosity and speculation about laterality in the brain are certainly proper. But leapfrogging the facts is not. When the journals of pop psychology are joined in that enterprise by the most respected general magazines and newspapers, the moment for a more sober assessment is at hand.

It has been known since classical times that the human brain is composed of two massive, physically equivalent halves. More recently, we have learned that each half controls movement in the opposite half of the body. Only in the latter part of the nineteenth century did physicians first conjecture that higher cognitive functions might be organized asymmetrically in the left and right cortices (or outer mantles) of the two hemispheres. Careful study of patients who had lost language functions after their brains had been damaged revealed that this condition, known as aphasia, predictably follows injury to the left cerebral cortex, but occurs rarely after equivalent damage to the right hemisphere. Gradually, higher reasoning powers also came to be attributed to the left hemisphere. By 1950 it began to appear that the left was the hemisphere to have. But in the past few decades complementary evidence has suggested that the right hemisphere also has its special genius.

As we shall see, the precise nature of that specialization (or "dominance") remains a subject of heated dispute. Evidence has also emerged that not all human brains are organized the same way: for example, many left-handers—and even some right-handers—turn out to have significant linguistic capacities in the right hemisphere.

Knowledge about brain and hemisphere function has come from three principal sources. The first—and in all probability the most revealing—has been the study of once-normal individuals whose brains have been injured by a stroke, a missile wound, an accident, or a tumor. When such patients lose the ability to perform a task, the inference is made that the injured region played an important role in the execution of that function, as when a patient with significant injury to the left hemisphere becomes aphasic. Conversely, if a brain-injured patient retains the ability to perform a task, the crucial capacities are thought to reside somewhere in the remaining intact portions of the brain.

Interpreting these forms of injury, however, can be somewhat problematic. Although the injury resulting from a stroke can be assigned to a well-demarcated region of the brain, stroke patients often have deteriorating blood vessels, hardening of the arteries, and heightened susceptibility to other strokes. All these debilitating factors tend to dilute the value of observations based on stroke victims. Weapons and accidents are apt to produce "messy" and unlocalized wounds. And tumors—masses that change in size and create high pressures within the skull—may exert effects at a considerable remove from their original site, perhaps even at the opposite end of the brain. Surgical intervention can also produce unintentionally messy consequences, and in any case is undertaken almost exclusively in patients whose brains are already diseased.

Although the consistent relationship between a given state of brain damage and impaired functions has yielded valuable information, the findings must still be regarded as tentative. Even though a function is impaired by damage to a specific site, it cannot be proved that the function is *housed* there: the functioning of a radio can be terminated when the plug is pulled, but we would delude ourselves if we concluded that the operation of the radio is "explained" in any meaningful way by the fact that it must be plugged in. In brain damage we always see what the surviving parts of the brain can accomplish, not what the injured portion used to do.

A second source of insight, studies with normal individuals, relies on various ingenious "indirect" methods to yield information about which half of the brain plays a dominant role in processing various kinds of stimuli.

In "dichotic listening," for example, stimuli are presented simultaneously to both ears. It is assumed that each ear has its stronger connection to the opposite hemisphere: if the individual hears or remembers a certain kind of information more accurately when it is presented to one ear than when it is presented to the other, the opposite hemisphere is considered "dominant" for that kind of information. Such techniques have revealed that the left hemisphere (or right ear) is better at processing verbal stimuli (say, words or a set of consonants), and the right hemisphere is analogously, though less strongly, dominant for musical stimuli and certain other nonlinguistic sounds.

Another road to the normal human brain exploits the anatomy of the visual system. Because of the pathways favored by the nervous system, information presented briefly (for perhaps a tenth of a second) in the left field of view proceeds with greater dispatch to the right half of the brain, while information presented briefly in the right field of view similarly favors the left half of the brain. Myriad studies using the tachistoscope, an instrument that flashes visual information to the desired visual field, document the left hemisphere's preference for linguistic stimuli, such as words and letters. Again, the right hemisphere seems to prefer various kinds of nonlinguistic stimuli, ranging from sets of dots to unfamiliar ("nameless") human faces.

Both dichotic listening and tachistoscopes present stimuli in unfamiliar ways, and inferences drawn from them about normal processing are quite possibly erroneous. The "hemisphere effects" are, to be sure, relatively reliable, but not absolutely so. The left hemisphere favors verbal materials and handles them more efficiently, but this tendency varies markedly from subject to subject and is influenced by the conditions under which the stimulus is presented and the time of testing. In any case, the correlations are far from overwhelming. Because each ear and each visual field is actually connected to both hemispheres, further caution in interpretation is needed.

Most critically, nearly every study is open to multiple interpretations and confounded by numerous variables. For instance, studies of reading ability in the two fields have yielded conflicting findings. The length, time of exposure, and meaningfulness of the words have affected the results, as have the language used, the reading habits of the subjects, the horizontal or vertical alignment of stimuli, the kind of response demanded, and a host of other nasty little variables.

Some exciting new procedures have been developed to test laterality in normal persons. One that is surprisingly simple follows eye movement after a question is posed. A movement to the right is thought to signal heightened activation of the left hemisphere, as might be expected if the subject were asked to solve an anagram, and thus to

281

use language skills. Eye movement to the left, then, would indicate that the right hemisphere has been activated, as might be expected with a problem requiring visual and spatial analysis.

Euphoria first greeted this method: the reliability of the procedure and the specificity of findings were extolled. It is disappointing and sobering to report that an army of new researchers have encountered difficulty in seeking to replicate the effects that were originally reported. With this technique, as with others, new insights into brain laterality are obtained only by some researchers, and only some of the time.

A brain researcher somewhere must once have dreamed that the mystery of brain organization could be penetrated if one hemisphere could somehow be observed in complete isolation from its companion. This fantasy was suddenly realized when a new surgical technique was developed to control violent epileptic seizures. The technique—our third avenue to the organization of the brain—requires complete separation of the two hemispheres; when the commissures (heavy bands of nerve fibers joining the hemispheres) have been completely severed, it becomes possible, at last, to see what each hemisphere can do "on its own."

Many of the most dramatic findings and claims have been based on careful study of the few dozen patients on whom this operation has been performed. A patient, speaking with his left hemisphere, reports that he has seen object A, and at the same time, guided by his right hemisphere, points to object B. Another patient hits his spouse with one hand and protects her with the other. Yet another effortlessly solves a simple jigsaw puzzle with his left hand but fails the same task a moment later with his right. Such findings, as reported by Nobel laureate Roger Sperry and his colleagues at the California Institute of Technology, drew a dramatic portrait of each hemisphere's genius.

But how valid are these findings? There is no disputing the facts, but much controversy surrounds their interpretation. First of all, findings differ markedly across patients, rendering any generalizations difficult. Some patients can perform impressively with both hemispheres; others function adequately with only one; and others are only capable of inferior performance with both. Indeed, as new patients are added to the series, claims have repeatedly been revised. And of course it is highly questionable whether findings obtained from such a grossly atypical group can justifiably be applied to the normal population. For this radical surgery is performed very rarely and only as a last resort on patients with longstanding, uncontrollable epilepsy. Early in life loss of neural tissue (for whatever reason) is followed by considerable compensation, as the spared portions of the brain step into the breach. By the same token, the disease treated by the brain-splitting operation has, in all probability, led to reorganization in an individual's brain. All in all, study of such patients may tell us only how the human brain under extreme duress can be reorganized; what it reveals about the brains of normal individuals is far from clear.

While study of brain laterality by each of the principal methods has yielded results with intriguing implications, technical difficulties have clearly been minimized in the popular press. It should nonetheless be possible to reach at least some tentative conclusions, ones more faithful to the experimental facts.

As I read the scientific literature, the left hemisphere has manifested a clear advantage in dealing with language, particularly with consonant sounds and rules of grammar. Processing of vowel sounds and access to the meaning of words seem to reside in both hemispheres. The left hemisphere also assumes a more dominant role than the right in classifying objects into standard, linguistically defined categories; it can ferret out from a heterogeneous set of objects all the large red cones or all the pieces of silverware.

The right hemisphere has no cognitive superiority equivalent in strength to the left hemisphere's dominion over language. Nonetheless, the right hemisphere does seem relatively more important in spatial tasks. We may tend to rely on it in finding our way around an unfamiliar site or in mentally manipulating the image of a two- or three-dimensional form. The right hemisphere also seems crucial in making fine sensory discriminations, which range from the recognition of faces to the detection of unfamiliar tactile patterns.

So much can be said with confidence—not as much as we might have hoped, but certainly nothing to apologize for. Pursuing their separate interests, neuroscientists have converged impressively in their views about the forte of each hemisphere. New findings emerge monthly, contradictory findings are being reconciled, and cognitive functioning of the brain is increasingly well understood. Indeed, precisely because scientists have been making steady and sometimes even spectacular progress and because their own quest has such intrinsic interest, overblown claims about brain laterality are especially vexing.

Where, then, have the popularizers gone overboard? Musical abilities, painting abilities, numerical abilities, and a host of other important cognitive functions have been studied but not conclusively localized. Sometimes conflicting assignments of these abilities seem to be supported by equally persuasive evidence. Sometimes individuals seem to differ one from another. And frequently it seems that both hemispheres contribute to the task but in different ways. For example, to draw an accurate representation of something, we seem to need the right hemisphere for the overall contour and the left hemisphere for identifying details and internal elements. My hunch is that this picture of differing, but complementary, contributions by the two hemispheres will hold as well for other realms of thought. And I also expect that we will discover more ways in which the two hemispheres can interact.

So far I have not mentioned artistry or logical capacity, let alone intuition, consciousness, or the Western mind. There is a reason for this silence: little scientific evidence bears on the notion that such general traits of personality are located on one or the other side of the brain. I seriously doubt that we could recognize such information if it *were* available to us. The truth is that scientists and philosophers, as well as the lay public, have little clue as to what "intuition" or "consciousness" may be. None of the competing conceptions of these treasured capacities enjoys widespread acceptance. As far as I know, those who make "brain claims" about such vital but dimly understood capacities have failed to reveal—let alone experimentally "operationalize"—their definitions.

To put it bluntly, academic hucksters have engaged in a scientific shell game. They have taken a hodgepodge of tasks and have simply claimed that these test intuition or consciousness, though they do not even attempt to give these terms an operational meaning. Then they have leaped to the conclusion that one ill-defined faculty resides in one hemisphere and some other contrasting trait in the opposite cortex.

I do not mean to suggest that it is impossible in principle to make meaningful statements about these capacities. One could devise tests for intuition (though no one has done so) and try to find where it is housed. My own guess is that there exists a set of intelligences (far more than two); that intuition and consciousness are not single faculties. Rather, separate forms of intuition and consciousness, as well as separate memories and reasoning powers, correspond to each of these several kinds of intelligence. In this view, intuitions and consciousnesses are localized in several different portions of the brain. Since this "theory of intuition and consciousness" is sheer speculation, I shall clearly label it as such.

What We Know About the Two Halves of the Brain

I do not impugn the motives—though I do question the judgment—of the brain's great dichotomizers. Many, for example, sincerely detect faults in our society, especially in its educational system, and are eager to use any method at their disposal to bring about desired changes. But the scientific enterprise is too precious to be sacrificed to any cause, however worthy it may appear. It is high time for investigators conversant with brain lateralization to announce that the unknowns in the field dwarf the little that is known, and the little more that is suspected. Once we concede the improbability of a brass ring's existing, we can, perhaps, get down to brass tacks.

27

THE LOSS OF LANGUAGE

SKILL IN LANGUAGE develops so quickly and operates so smoothly that we take our linguistic capacities largely for granted. Most three-year-olds can speak simple grammatical sentences and execute simple commands. Nearly every ten-year-old in our society can read and write at the primer level, and most adults can read a novel in an afternoon or write several letters in an evening.

Our linguistic potentials are even more impressive. Placed in a foreign culture, particularly as children, we readily learn the basic phrases of another language; and all of us, bilingual or not, are capable of mastering various language-related codes—the number system (Arabic or Roman), musical notation, Morse code, or the familiar trademarks for commercial products.

The loss of various language abilities in the otherwise normal adult is tragic, and the consequences are as devastating as those of blindness, deafness, or paralysis (which often accompanies it). Deprived of the power to communicate through language and languagelike channels, the individual is cut off from the world of meaning. Though loss of language is relatively rare among young persons, who are less susceptible to many of the causes of brain damage, it becomes increasingly common with age. About one quarter of a million individuals suffer linguistic impairment each year. The extent and duration of language disability vary greatly, but a significant proportion of the afflicted individuals are left with a permanent impairment. Those who suffer language loss as a consequence of damage to their brains are victims of the strange condition called aphasia.

Aphasic individuals are not always immediately recognizable. One patient whom I recently interviewed appeared to be normal when he entered the room: a nice-looking, well-groomed sixty-two-year-old retired bookkeeper. He answered my first questions appropriately and with a speed that suggested nothing was amiss. When asked his name, the gentleman responded, "Oh, my name, that's easy, it is Tuh, Tom Johnson and I . . ." It was only when I gave Mr. Johnson a chance to speak a bit more that the extent and nature of his aphasia became clear:

"What kind of work have you done, Mr. Johnson?" I asked.

"We, the kids, all of us, and I, we were working for a long time in the . . . you know . . . it's the kind of space, I mean place rear to the spedwan. . . ."

At this point I interjected, "Excuse me, but I wanted to know what work you have been doing."

"If you had said that, we had said that, poomer, near the fortunate, forpunate, tamppoo, all around the fourth of martz. Oh, I get all confused," he replied, looking somewhat puzzled that the stream of language did not appear to satisfy me.

Mr. Johnson was suffering from a relatively common language disorder called Wernicke's aphasia. Patients with this disorder have no trouble producing language—if anything, the words flow out too freely and it sometimes proves difficult to silence them. Nor do Wernicke's aphasics have any trouble producing the words that structure and modulate speech—"if," "and," "of," and the like. But when they try to come up with specific substantives—nouns, verbs, and adjectives that specify persons, objects, events, and properties—these patients exhibit great difficulty. As Mr. Johnson exhibited several times, aphasics frequently cannot issue the precise words they want to say, and they wander from the stated topic to another, the meaning of which remains obscure to the listener.

From my description of the interview, it may seem that Mr. Johnson understood what I was saying but was simply encountering trouble in responding appropriately. This supposition was quickly and dramatically dispelled when I took a key and a pencil from my pocket and asked him to point in turn to each one. These two simple words, known to any child, eluded him. When asked to point to other objects and to body parts, he also fared poorly, as he had when trying to name certain objects. He could not read words aloud correctly, nor could he understand most written commands, though he did read letters and numbers aloud. Any bystander would have inferred that Mr. Johnson's understanding was very limited (as indeed it was).

One fascinating island of preserved comprehension remained, however. Toward the close of the interview I said, almost out of the blue, "Oh, Mr. Johnson, would you please stand up and turn around twice?" Suddenly, as if his comprehension had been magically restored, Mr. Johnson stood up and proceeded to rotate in just the way I requested. He was also able to carry out several commands that involved his whole body (like "Lean forward" or "Stand at ease"). However, this preserved comprehension could not be elicited in any other manner.

Mr. Johnson, a Wernicke's aphasic, can be instructively contrasted with another patient whom I recently met. Mr. Cooper, a forty-seven-year-old former Army officer, was seated in a wheelchair, obviously paralyzed on the entire right side of his body. A slight droop on the right side of his face became more noticeable when he opened his mouth or smiled. When I asked what was wrong with him, Mr. Cooper immediately pointed to his arm, his leg, and his mouth. He appeared reluctant to speak at all. Only when I pressed him did he point again to his mouth and with obvious effort blurt out the sound "Peech."

I posed Mr. Cooper a number of questions that could be answered by "yes" or "no," and in each case he nodded appropriately. I then said that it was important that he try to speak. Noting his wedding ring, I asked, "How many children do you have?" Mr. Cooper looked blank for a time. Then he peered at his fingers and began to raise them, accompanying the motion with low and strained sounds: "one, two, tree, pour, no, pive . . . yes pive," he said triumphantly.

Next, I asked him to tell me about the kind of work he had been doing.

"Me . . . build—ing . . . chairs, no, no cab—in—nets." The words came out slowly, taking him forty seconds to finish.

"One more question," I said. "Can you tell me how you would go about building a cabinet?"

Mr. Cooper threw up his left hand in frustration, and after I gently insisted that he attempt a verbal explanation, he said, "One, saw . . . then, cutting wood . . . working. . . ." All of this was said with great effort and poor articulation, which left me (and Mr. Cooper) unprepared for a sudden oath, "Jesus Christ, oh boy." This was uttered effortlessly, as if another language mechanism—an island of preserved production—had temporarily been stimulated.

During the rest of our examination, Mr. Cooper performed well on tasks that required little language production. On request he pointed easily to objects around the room. He read simple commands silently

and carried them out clumsily but properly. He could name some familiar objects and read aloud some names of objects, though he failed
at reading aloud letters of the alphabet and small grammatical words
such as articles and prepositions. He could read aloud the word "bee,"
but not "be," though the latter occurs more frequently in spoken and
written language. He could carry a melody and sing lyrics to familiar
songs more readily than he could recite those same lyrics.

But Mr. Cooper had definite difficulties in understanding. Although
he could designate a series of two objects when their names were recited
in order, he sometimes failed at three, and he never succeeded at four—
the level of success achieved by most normal adults. He caught the
drift of nearly all questions in casual conversation, and could almost
always produce at least a minimally appropriate response, but he experienced significant problems with questions that involved careful attention to word order and inflection. I could stump him with sentences
like "Do you put on your shoes before you put on socks?" or "The
lion was killed by the tiger: Which animal is dead?" or "With the
pen touch the pencil." Just as Mr. Cooper's spontaneous speech was
limited largely to nouns and verbs and virtually devoid of words that
modulate meaning, so too he often failed on questions and commands
that required him to note the order of words and the meanings of
prefixes, suffixes, and other grammatical fixtures.

Mr. Johnson and Mr. Cooper illustrate two of the most common
forms of aphasia. In my years of work with aphasic patients, I have
seen dozens of patients whose symptoms closely resemble those of
one or the other man. Mr. Johnson is a victim of Wernicke's aphasia;
as a result of damage to the left temporal lobe of his brain, his auditory
comprehension has become severely impaired, but he remains able to
produce long, often obscure, strings of speech. Mr. Cooper has Broca's
aphasia, a condition caused by damage to the left frontal lobe. He
understands language, although not perfectly; his chief difficulty is
in producing words, specifically those that modify nouns and verbs.
The language of the Broca's aphasic is called agrammatic (or telegram-
matic), and such a patient's understanding suffers from some of the
same limits that affect his spontaneous speech.

These and other aphasic syndromes are the regular and nearly inevitable consequences of significant damage to the left hemisphere of the
brain in normal right-handed individuals. As a result of a stroke, head
injury, or brain tumor, cortical (or surface) tissue is destroyed in this
half of the brain. Such lesions impair linguistic functions and frequently

cause paralysis and loss of sensation in the opposite (right) side of the body. (The situation is somewhat different, and much more complex, in left-handers.)

The precise location and extent of the brain damage determines the nature of the linguistic disorder. There are forms of aphasia (called alexia) in which an individual's ability to read is most severely impaired; agraphia, in which disorders of writing are most pronounced; anomia, in which most language functions are preserved but there is magnified difficulty in naming objects; conduction aphasia, in which speech and understanding are relatively intact but the patient experiences enormous difficulty in repetition; and a bizarre complementary condition called mixed transcortical aphasia, in which both conversational speech and comprehension are almost entirely destroyed, yet the patient retains the capacity to repeat, and even to echo, long strings of meaningful or meaningless words (it makes little difference which). The striking predictability of these syndromes reflects the uniformity with which language abilities are organized in normal right-handed individuals.

Each of these conditions cries out for explanation. There are alexics who can read numbers, including Roman numerals, but not words or letters; transcortical aphasics who understand nothing but who will, in their repetitions, spontaneously correct grammatical errors; anomic aphasics who cannot produce a familiar word (such as nose) but will readily produce a highly improbable substitute (proboscis). To be sure, not all aphasics show such clear syndromes; the syndromes are most likely to occur in males of middle age or older who are fully right-handed and who have suffered a stroke. Yet nearly every aphasic patient exhibits some bizarre combination of symptoms, and many exemplify the textbook descriptions in the preceding paragraph.

A first meeting with aphasic patients is often dramatic; their symptoms are frequently fantastic and disturbing. A person's first impulse is to aid these victims of brain disease in any way possible. But the study of their condition has an importance that goes beyond helping victims of aphasia; it holds the promise of clarifying a host of philosophical and psychological issues about the nature of language and the mind.

Reports of aphasia can be found in many classical writings and even in the Bible. Yet the serious scientific study of aphasia began little over a century ago when in 1861 Pierre Paul Broca, a French anatomist, described two cases whose symptoms resembled Mr. Cooper's. Broca's cases were important not because of the way he described their behavior patterns but because he made an analytic leap. Noting that both of these cases had brain damage in the anterior portion of the left hemisphere, Broca proposed that this part of the brain played a special role in language. Besides immortalizing his name (Broca's aphasia, Broca's area), this discovery laid the groundwork for all aphasia research.

The reason for this breakthrough was simple but instructive. Until Broca's time, nearly all scientists assumed that the two halves of the brain, which on casual inspection look alike, carried out the same functions. It had often been observed that aphasia accompanied strokes and paralysis, but Broca was the first to argue publicly that language disorders are linked to the left portion of the brain. Though his announcement provoked controversy, supporting cases were quickly reported. Thirteen years later Carl Wernicke, a German neuropsychiatrist, described another set of symptoms, this time primarily affecting comprehension. He linked them to the left posterior (particularly temporal) lobe of the brain, thereby contributing his name to another brain area and another type of aphasia. Even more than Broca's discoveries, Wernicke's work stimulated scientists to construct models of language based on the behavior of brain-injured patients.

Broca and Wernicke gave impetus to a group of neurologists who have been called "localizers." Adherents of this approach carefully investigated the anatomy of the human brain, the structure of the cortical tissue, and the connections between the different parts of the nervous system. Building on this refined knowledge of human neuroanatomy, they sought to discover the functions that were governed by each part of the brain. Their first step was to locate the motor functions (or voluntary actions), which are associated with sites in the frontal lobe, and the sensory functions, associated with sites in the parietal, temporal, and occipital lobes relatively (see the accompanying drawing of a specimen left hemisphere). But the localizers went beyond these relatively elementary processes and tried to apportion even the highest intellectual and emotional functions to specific regions of the brain.

Findings about language function spurred them on. Researchers had discovered an indisputable "high" human function—one denied all other animals—occupying specific regions in the brain. The type of aphasia discovered by Broca and the startlingly different one described by Wernicke were but the first manifestations of this line of analysis. Within twenty years, a gaggle of aphasias had been described, each traced to a specific area in the brain, each exhibiting its own enigmatic symptoms.

Researchers transcended these correlations between brain and behav-

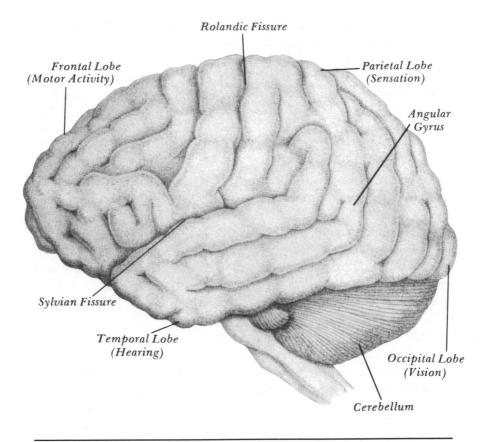

Rolandic Fissure

Frontal Lobe
(Motor Activity)

Parietal Lobe
(Sensation)

Angular
Gyrus

Sylvian Fissure

Temporal Lobe
(Hearing)

Occipital Lobe
(Vision)

Cerebellum

Figure 27.1. A specimen left hemisphere, with principal lobes demarcated.

ior to propose models of language function. In one popular version the language signal entered Wernicke's area, where it was comprehended; then a return message was fired forward to Broca's area, where it was fitted out with grammatical trimmings and ultimately spewed forth to the world. It naturally followed that a lesion confined to Broca's area allowed comprehension at the cost of grammatical speech, whereas destruction of Wernicke's area impaired comprehension but allowed a stream of grammatically rich, but often meaningless, speech.

The localizers probably went too far in their approach. In the early part of this century, a rival school reanalyzed Broca's original cases and announced that there was but one type of aphasia, the form stemming from lesions in and around Wernicke's area. Broca's aphasics, they said, were linguistically intact individuals who suffered only from problems in articulating their speech. Followers of this theory pointed out that not even textbook cases of Broca's aphasia showed all the observed symptoms and that some displayed additional symptoms. In their view, lesions anywhere in the left hemisphere could produce aphasia, and its severity reflected primarily the size of the lesion rather than its site. These partisans went on to argue that every aphasic exhibits difficulties in all language functions. Differences among the so-called syndromes, they said, are differences in degree (a little more reading difficulty in one case, a little more repetition difficulty in another) rather than in kind.

Today, after a century of research, there is little sympathy for the extreme versions of either of the conflicting theories. Owing in large measure to the efforts of Norman Geschwind, professor of neurology at the Harvard Medical School, the genuine contributions of the localizers are again appreciated. At the same time, a range of factors that modulate the classic syndromes—such as the nature of the brain disease, the age of the patient, or the situation of testing—are also recognized. The classic syndromes are seen as useful signposts for describing patients rather than as fixed descriptions of what a patient with a given lesion can and cannot do.

Progress has been stimulated by a number of factors. In the wake of this century's wars, researchers have seen many hundreds of patients with aphasia. The publication of numerous cases and countercases has clarified our knowledge of the incidence of full-blown examples of the classic syndromes and produced precise descriptions of the symptoms of aphasia.

But perhaps the biggest contribution has come from interactions among specialists from diverse disciplines, each of whom had approached aphasia from a different perspective. In my own view, the most important infusions have come from linguists, who have brought to the study of aphasia logical and well-conceived categories for the analysis of language, and from psychologists, whose accurate experimental techniques have supplemented the important but necessarily superficial methods of bedside examination evolved by attending physicians.

Issues raised by routine bedside testing often stimulate research by interdisciplinary teams. Consider, for instance, Mr. Cooper's apparent success at understanding spontaneous conversation. Such observations have led many neurologists to conclude that a patient with Broca's aphasia has no difficulties in comprehending language. Teams of linguists and psychologists noted, however, that when such patients were tested, they received multiple cues from the context in which a question was posed and from redundancies within the message. Accordingly, they devised questions that could be understood only if one were processing grammatical inflections and exploiting cues of word order. Deprived of the redundancy of ordinary conversational speech, individuals with Broca's aphasia showed far more impairments in comprehension.

Turning to issues raised by Mr. Johnson, experimenters have also clarified the nature of the comprehension defect in Wernicke's aphasia. Because these patients have difficulty understanding auditory messages and decoding single isolated words, some aphasiologists concluded that the primary impediment for the Wernicke's aphasic lay in his inability to decipher individual phonemes—the smallest discrete sounds of language, such as "p" and "b." Careful experimental studies have documented, however, that Wernicke's aphasics can readily discriminate between individual phonemes; they may surpass Broca's aphasics at this task. Their difficulty in understanding occurs at a higher level of semantic interpretation.

Not all the contributions have come from research scientists. Demonstrations by clinicians sometimes challenge—and even undermine—the workaday categories embraced by researchers. None of the categorical distinctions honored by psychologists or linguists can explain Mr. Johnson's curious ability to carry out commands that use the whole body. If, however, one takes into account certain anatomical considerations, this behavior becomes clarified. Unlike commands demanding the use of the face or individual limbs, which are carried out by the major pyramidal motor pathways running from the cortex to the spinal cord, these commands are executed by the alternative nonpyramidal tracts of the nervous system. A lesion in Wernicke's area usually spares these tracts. Here is a case where an anatomical point of view advances the explanation of aphasic behavior.

Constant interplay between bedside testing and experimental work proves crucial, since experimenters tend to devise careful but artificial test situations. When a patient fails on such a test, it becomes difficult to determine whether the patient lacks the ability in question or is simply confused by the instructions or by the task itself. Sometimes a patient fails on an experimenter's test only to demonstrate the skill in question when a natural situation arises in his life. A patient may fail to repeat an arbitrary set of phrases spoken by an experimenter and yet produce just these phrases in situations where they are warranted. Thus, in a curiously productive way, clinicians and experimenters keep one another honest.

It is impossible to understand the mind without considering its linguistic capacities. Yet both linguists and psychologists face a fundamental problem: the categories, distinctions, terminology, and levels of linguistic competence are based on the study of individuals in whom all linguistic capacities are operating efficiently. These individuals can produce the proper sounds, combine words according to the structure of a language, understand the meaning of the words they use, and use language appropriately in natural situations. Scholars have divided the study of language in the same way, analyzing it in terms of its phonological, syntactic, semantic, and pragmatic levels. No independent means exists for examining the validity of these categories, for determining whether another means of slicing the linguistic pie might not prove more comprehensive and accurate.

Here is where aphasia can make a unique contribution. Were it the case, as some researchers once implied, that all language skills break down simultaneously in aphasia, this pathological condition would hold little scientific interest. But aphasia proves remarkably selective in its damage. A patient may have an impaired ability to read while still being able to write, fail to comprehend and yet be able to speak, fail to understand and yet be able to repeat accurately. These and numerous other dissociations can demonstrate the validity of certain categories of analysis. For example, both Broca's aphasia and transcortical aphasia provide evidence for a separate level of syntactic analysis in the brain.

At other times the dissociations call into question some of the distinctions made by linguists. Aphasia gives little support for the linguist's distinction between competence and performance. Symptoms that violate our expectations can suggest new distinctions and categorizations that linguists have ignored, as in the case of the dichotomy in the brain's response to "whole-body" and other kinds of commands. Aphasia provides a testing laboratory for the distinctions made by those who study human languages—the primary window to the mind.

The study of aphasia may help to clarify several long-standing philosophical questions. Is language the ultimate symbol system on which all other modes of symbolization are parasitic? Or do other symbol systems exist that are relatively autonomous of language? Results from the study of aphasia indicate that language is but one of man's symbolic competences. Once a person's language ability is impaired, he ordinarily shows a lessened capacity to "read" other symbols. Yet this is not always the case. Many severely aphasic patients can carry out calculations, gesture meaningfully, or read musical notation.

Research on aphasia also pertains to another philosophical chestnut: the extent to which thought depends upon language. Aphasia exacts toll on performance in various concept-formation tasks, as do all forms of brain damage. Yet it is by no means uncommon to encounter a severely aphasic individual who can solve a difficult maze or puzzle, play a game of chess or bridge, or score above normal on the nonverbal section of the Wechsler Adult Intelligence Scale. Other aphasic individuals have continued to paint, compose, or conduct music at a professionally competent level.

Mental functioning in aphasia is relevant to an issue of great current interest: the functions of the left and right hemispheres of the brain. In nearly all right-handers, the left hemisphere of the brain is specialized for language; lesions there will result in significant impairment of language. Such an injury spares right-hemisphere functioning and the aphasic patient remains relatively skilled in those functions for which the right hemisphere is superior—visual-spatial orientation, musical understanding, recognition of faces, and emotional appropriateness.

In working with hundreds of aphasic patients, I have been impressed by the extent to which they seem to be well oriented, generally aware of what is going on around them, and appropriately attuned to emotional situations. And I have been struck, in contrast, by the frequently inappropriate and disoriented behavior of patients with right-hemisphere lesions—individuals whose language remains essentially intact but whose intuitive understanding of the world seems to have gone awry. In these areas, which have remained recalcitrant to formal testing, one may secure the best evidence that common sense does not depend on competence in language.

Anyone who has spent time with aphasic individuals will recognize the need to help these victims; their personal frustration is so glaring. In the wake of experiments by aphasiologists, speech pathologists have been able to begin rehabilitation with a greater understanding of the processes (and limitations) of language function, and with a heightened ability to exploit those mental powers ordinarily spared in aphasia. To be sure, no rehabilitation can fully compensate for destroyed brain tissue; the best healers are still time, youth, and—at least in matters of language—the degree of left-handedness in one's family.

The Loss of Language

Research on brain function has led to certain significant break-throughs in aphasia therapy. As noted in essay 25, speech pathologists at the Boston Veterans Administration Medical Center have devised a training program that significantly boosts language output. Their work is based on the clinical observation that Broca's aphasics can often sing well, and on experimental findings that musical and intonational patterns are mediated by structures in the right hemisphere. During the first phase of this rehabilitation program, called Melodic Intonation Therapy, patients sing simple phrases; in ensuing phases, they learn to delete the melody, leaving only the words. Mr. Cooper, who could sing lyrics to songs but had difficulty reciting them, would seem a likely candidate for this therapy. If he succeeds as well as other patients, in about three months he should be able to produce short but grammatical and appropriate sentences.

The study of aphasia is still in its infancy, but interest in this field has grown so rapidly that advances in understanding and rehabilitation are likely. Few areas of study feature as close a linkage between the medical and the scientific, the clinical and the experimental, the concerns of the theorist and the practitioner. And the mysteries to be solved are inextricably linked with the vast enigmas of language, brain, and mind. It is paradoxical—yet in a strange way heartening—that those who can say little may help us answer questions that have until now eluded even the most eloquent philosophers.

28

THE FORGOTTEN LESSON

OF MONSIEUR C

READING has been an important skill in Western society for many hundreds of years. Yet even at a time when universal literacy is at a premium, a significant number of people seem to have serious difficulties learning to read. Furthermore, a smaller number, perhaps 3 percent of the population, find themselves unable to read at all. Some are educationally deprived or have emotional blocks; others are mentally retarded or brain-damaged. But some nonreaders are of normal or high intelligence, have gone to the best schools, and appear free of personal problems, retardation, and brain damage. They seem blind to words as some people are blind to colors. They exhibit a syndrome that has been called developmental dyslexia.

There is considerable disagreement among those who study reading problems about what causes dyslexia and how it should be treated. Psychologists interested in personality development often invoke a motivational explanation, while those who study cognitive processes may attribute dyslexia to perceptual or learning disorders. I believe that a clue central to the mystery of dyslexia was uncovered in France nearly a century ago.

In October 1887 Monsieur C, a wealthy businessman in his late sixties, experienced several attacks of numbness in his right leg, some feebleness in his arms, and a little trouble speaking. When his symptoms disappeared, he returned to work and thought little more about it until he discovered he could not read a single word. He made an appointment to see his ophthalmologist and be fitted with an adequate pair of glasses.

Much to C's surprise, his opthalmologist did not prescribe a new pair of glasses but referred him to Joseph Déjerine, a neurologist at the Bicêtre Hospital in Paris. Both men agreed that C's reading difficulty could not be rectified by glasses, for his failure had nothing to do with visual acuity. They concluded that C had suffered a relatively rare yet fascinating type of stroke that made it impossible for him to see objects in one half of his visual field and destroyed his capacity to read but affected little else. For the next few years Déjerine followed C's case very closely. He discovered that while C could copy letters with ease, he could neither recognize nor name them. He also noticed that when C copied, he treated letters as designs, and carefully traced each stroke. He described the letter Z as a serpent, P as a buckle, and A as a trestle or stand. He did not understand them as graphic units to be recast in his own characteristic penmanship. C protested that he was losing his mind, for he knew that the signs were letters even though he could not identify them. The meanings of words were also lost to him although, again, he could copy perfectly. An intelligent man, knowledgeable about political and cultural affairs, C had been blinded to the symbolism of print and was, medically speaking, *alexic*.

He was still able to express himself fluently, recognize and name obscure technical and scientific instruments, remember the most minute details of past events, and understand everything said to him. Even more surprisingly, he could still write without difficulty, both expressing his thoughts spontaneously and transcribing what was dictated to him. Yet he failed when he tried to decipher his own penmanship, unless he could remember what he had written. In fact, he preferred to write with his eyes shut, for he got "tangled" if he monitored his own writing.

When someone etched a letter on his hand or guided his fingers through the air in the form of a word, he could instantly identify it. In short, all his language functions were preserved, except the ability to decode words and letters presented to his eyes.

Yet there were certain written materials that C could understand. He could not identify the letters *R* and *F*, but when a circle was drawn around them thus— (RF) —he instantly reported *République Française*; (RF) was like a traffic signal or a cattle brand, not a group of letters enclosed in a circle.

Monsieur C was too active and energetic to be felled by his misfortune and continued his favorite activities. Since he could no longer read musical notes or lyrics, he had his wife perform opera parts which he learned by ear and later sang. He continued to play cards, for he recognized the different numbers and suits, and he even followed his business and stock-market investments, for he was able to perform elaborate calculations. Indeed, until ten days before his death, C led a normal existence—at least as normal as imaginable for an individual who had been selectively blinded.

Early in 1892 C suffered a second, more serious stroke, which still spared his general intelligence but left him unable to write—he became *agraphic* as well as alexic. Within ten days he died, and Déjerine was permitted to come to his home and remove and examine his brain. Cases of alexia had been reported previously, but there had been no adequate anatomical evidence about its cause. Déjerine's examination left little doubt, however, about the origin of C's language difficulties.

Part of his visual area—the right occipital cortex—was intact; therefore he could see lines and objects. His language area—the left frontal and temporal cortices—was also intact; therefore he could speak, understand, and write. But because of the structure of the human nervous system, C was not able to transmit information from the undamaged part of his visual center in the right hemisphere to the areas in the left hemisphere where the concepts and names of lexical items are processed.

By the same token, C could see forms and copy them adequately, but, because of an interruption of crucial pathways in his brain, this visual information could not travel to the language area. C could write what was dictated to him and even recognize letters etched on his hand, for the necessary pathways within his language system and between his language and tactile systems had been preserved, but he could not recognize and name a printed letter or word.

Déjerine could not explain why C was still able to recognize and name persons, objects, playing cards, and even numbers when part of his visual center was "disconnected" from his language center. Nearly a century later we are not much closer to the answer.

The role of the brain in linguistic activity was first clarified in 1861 when Paul Broca, also a French physician, demonstrated a connection between injury to the left hemisphere of the human brain and an impairment of language ability. Broca found that similar damage to the right hemisphere generally produced no language impairment, and this striking asymmetry in the brain became a major riddle. Scores of case reports about particular disorders (alexia, agraphia, aphasia—impairment in language production or comprehension; agnosia—inability to recognize objects; apraxia—disturbances of voluntary movement) followed Broca's discovery, and scores of anatomical localizations for each of them were proposed, some contradicting others.

In 1917 a Scottish ophthalmologist named James Hinshelwood summarized the accumulated reports on alexia. He pointed out that reading disorders caused by brain damage were of two principal sorts. The first, epitomized by C's condition after his first stroke, might be called *pure alexia,* or word blindness. A person with this condition is entirely normal in his language functions except for a selective blindness to the printed word. He still understands letters and words as "graphic entities" but cannot relate their appearance to their sounds and meanings. The second variety, epitomized by C's condition after his second stroke, could be called *alexia with agraphia.* Here the person can still speak and understand perfectly, but cannot read, write, or spell. He no longer understands words or letters as graphic entities.

Some of Hinshelwood's cases were as amazing as that of Monsieur C. One person, skilled in languages, found himself totally unable to read the words of his native English. Yet he could read some French, more Latin, and perfect Greek. Another patient was unable to read or name a single letter but could effortlessly read such difficult words as *stethoscope, electricity,* and *infirmary.*

Hinshelwood's consuming interest, however, lay in another group of patients whom he described as "congenitally word-blind." These were children who could not learn to read. They had no trouble seeing lines and forms and experienced no difficulty talking, recognizing numbers, or executing other school tasks. They were like C in the last days of his life. Hinshelwood was perhaps the first to make this connection explicit in his insistence that, "without an adequate knowledge of [acquired word blindness] congenital word blindness cannot be properly understood." In his view, these children lacked certain connections between the visual and speech centers of their brains and therefore had the same difficulties as adults whose left hemispheres had been injured.

It would seem natural that the discovery of a relationship between acquired and congenital defects would have resulted in revised theoretical notions about the brain, as well as practical applications in training those with reading problems, whatever their origin. But the fields of psychology and neurology were moving in a different direction, and the entire approach that related specific cognitive defects to discrete brain lesions was soon in disrepute. The existence of the kinds of cases that Déjerine and Hinshelwood had reported was questioned or even denied. These early physicians, the argument went, did not know how to examine patients properly, nor did they have acceptable histological methods for studying brain tissue. What they thought were isolated disorders were actually more-widespread difficulties that affected language and perception generally and resulted from injury to larger portions of the brain. For perhaps thirty years the notions of alexia, alexia with agraphia, and the relation between congenital and acquired disorders of reading were either forgotten or discredited, particularly in the English-speaking world.

In the past poor readers and nonreaders were regarded as retarded or dull. Often they were banished from school and work, compelled to repeat grades until they learned to read, or simply allowed to lag behind their classmates in any subject that involved reading. After repeated documentation that many nonreaders were (in other areas) as bright as, or even brighter than, their reading peers, some authorities allowed that reading problems might be selective disabilities. Children with these disabilities were then labeled and treated in a variety of ways. Often it was assumed that they did not see as well as they should. Such children then spent a great deal of time with an eye doctor or with a teacher who drilled them on discriminating signs of similar size, shape, or orientation. Sometimes nonreaders were called minimally brain-damaged, and efforts were made to correct their difficulties through medical intervention. Psychologists frequently tied reading problems to emotional blocks or attacks of anxiety. They urged the children and their families to undergo counseling or therapy, expecting that dramatic progress on standardized reading tests would result.

While any of these approaches may help in selected cases, it is widely conceded that none have proved totally effective for children with developmental dyslexia. These children have reading difficulties because their brains mature more slowly or are deficient in the anatomical connections needed to learn reading in the usual ways. Their brains are not damaged from birth trauma or a fall, but they *are* different, just as the brains of people who are tone-deaf or "all thumbs" appear to be organized in a different manner.* In a nonreading culture no

* Evidence of abnormal brain organization in an adult with developmental dyslexia comes from a recent post-mortem report by Albert Galaburda and his collaborators at Harvard Medical School.

one would ever notice these deviations from the norm, but in our society the variation creates enormous problems. With the proper education, many dyslexics can reach superior levels of accomplishment as mathematicians, painters, or musicians. Some have made substantial contributions in their chosen fields, and one, Hans Christian Andersen, became a masterful writer even though he never mastered spelling.

In an effort to help children with reading difficulties, many competent investigators have devised novel instructional techniques. Educator Caleb Gattegno's "words in color" is one example of the numerous systems that have been tried. The basic idea of Gattegno's method is that if each letter is printed in a different hue, the child has two distinctive cues to help him connect sound and image. Another example is the psychologist O. K. Moore's "talking typewriter": a picture is flashed on a screen and identified by a voice; the child then tries to spell the word correctly through the use of a typewriter that remains locked until the correct keys are pressed.

These techniques have proved effective for perceptually impaired children who have difficulty distinguishing one written letter from another, and for unmotivated children for whom reading must be made more meaningful or colorful. But they are of little help to those who have trouble breaking a spoken word into its component phonemes and relating them to arbitrary visual configurations on a page.

Samuel T. Orton's work in the 1920s opened the door to more effective treatment of children with "congenital word blindness." While the works of Déjerine and Hinshelwood were in disrepute, this physician was examining children with congenital word blindness in Iowa City. He observed the systematic irregularities and errors in the reading and writing of dyslexic children and found that they had a strong tendency to read words from right to left, confusing words like *was* and *saw*. They also had particular difficulties with letters whose orientation contributed to their identification (*p, q, d,* and *b,* for example) and often "mirror wrote" (writing *b* for *d,* or *p* for *q*). Some read as efficiently upside-down as right-side-up, and others could write equally well (or poorly) with either hand.

Orton believed that these irregularities held the secret to the riddle of dyslexia. He conjectured that by the time most children start learning to read, cerebral lateralization has already occurred. The term means that one hemisphere of the brain, in most cases the left (which controls movement on the right side of the body and is normally responsible for language functions), has established dominance over the other, usually the right. The right hemisphere controls movement of the left side of the body and normally plays a negligible role in language function. The two sides of the brain then work in synchrony, with the dominant hemisphere leading the other. Orton suggested that in dyslexics the two hemispheres still may be "competing" for dominance, that there may be no clear division of labor. He believed that dominance was necessary for consistent left-to-right reading, and he proposed that incomplete dominance could result in a tendency to read right to left as well.

In fact, he thought any activity might proceed equally well in either direction when the two hemispheres are competing. Thus writing might also go right to left, and letters might be read and written without necessary attention to their contour or to the direction and angle of their strokes. He suspected that "confusing memory images" from the nondominant hemisphere made reading even more difficult, and that dominance would have to be established before a dyslexic child could learn to read and write normally.

Orton named this condition *strephosymbolia*—"twisted symbol." He offered no ready-made solution but felt that repetitive drill would eventually result in the association of correct letter forms with their appropriate sounds. He favored strengthening the child's undeveloped capacities, rather than exploiting those that were normal (as the look-say approach to reading instruction did). Some of his followers have developed treatments aimed at accelerating cerebral lateralization, such as training one hand, foot, or eye. This approach is intuitively appealing, but there is little evidence that it succeeds. Many children seem to "grow out" of dyslexia, suggesting that their problems are chiefly due to a developmental lag like that described by Orton. But we can only guess whether such children would have been better or worse off had dominance been speeded up through clinical intervention.

Orton's approach signaled a healthy return of interest in the relationship between reading and the organization of the brain. Though a causal relationship between incomplete lateralization and dyslexia has yet to be confirmed, a correlation between a developmental lag in the attainment of dominance and a cluster of language problems has been well documented. In recent years several researchers have searched for brain-wave patterns that might distinguish dyslexics from normals. Bernard Sklar, working at UCLA's Brain Research Institute, used a computer to analyze the electroencephalogram (EEG) data he collected on a group of normals and a group of dyslexics. Although the EEGs looked similar to the human eye, computer analysis showed that the two groups differed in three ways. The dyslexics showed less synchronization between the two hemispheres of their brains, more synchronization within each hemisphere, and generally more theta waves (three to seven cycles per second). Surprisingly, these differences were more marked when the children were resting with their eyes closed than when they were reading. Sklar believes the first two findings support the theory that dyslexia is related to incomplete cerebral dominance. He also notes that increased theta activity is characteristic of people in new and novel environments (like the astronauts in space), and speculates that perhaps part of the dyslexic's problem is that his world never seems quite familiar to him.

Other researchers, inspired by the work of Norman Geschwind at Harvard Medical School, have returned to patients with acquired reading disorders to study the range of their difficulties and explore possibilities for remedial training. One of the more perplexing findings is that the brain lesion that produces alexia also usually destroys the ability to name colors but leaves intact the ability to read numbers and name objects. Geschwind observed that both color- and letter-naming involve arbitrary links between purely visual configurations and names, and that neither letters nor colors exist in the world as separate entities. In contrast, objects do exist separately in the world. Any individual makes multiple sensory associations with objects, including tactile, auditory, kinesthetic, and often olfactory impressions. While numbers do not exist in the world as objects do, we learn them by using our fingers. This method involves strong tactile and kinesthetic associations. Any activity in the realm of numbers entails an active manipulative process of counting, ordering, transforming, and coordinating.

Geschwind suggested that the differences between the relatively static and unisensory domains of letters and colors, and the relatively active, multisensory domains of objects and numbers are naturally reflected in brain organization. To recognize and name a letter or color, a person must proceed from the purely visual configuration to a name, and even a fairly discrete lesion in the brain could destroy the connection between the two domains. On the other hand, a person confronted by an object or number will have a larger number of associations aroused. Even if the purely visual-language connections have been destroyed, he has enough associations between visual and other sensory modes that he can recognize and name the target by taking an alternate anatomical route. For instance, the message "2" but not the message "D" might go from the visual to the tactile area, and then to the region of the brain where naming takes place.

Striking support for this line of reasoning comes from scattered reports of individuals who once could read two kinds of languages—a phonetic language like English and an ideographic language like Chinese. Certain lesions that impair the ability to read the phonetic language spare the ability to read the ideographic language. Presumably that is because the ideographic system, which involves symbols similar to objects or pictures of objects, aroused a wider range of sensory and motor associations, and is therefore more resistant to brain damage than the purely visual-phonetic language.

Systematic studies of alexics have also confirmed the clinical intuition that they have less difficulty identifying objects and symbols which they have learned in an active way and which arouse many kinds of associations, than identifying objects and symbols which they know only from their visual configuration and with which they have had less active and "transforming" contacts. Numbers are easier for them to read than words, number-related signs offer less difficulty than punctuation marks, and objects like telephones, fingers, or clocks are easier to name than such equally familiar objects as the sun, the moon, or the ceiling.

Careful examinations of alexic and agraphic patients have also shown that they can read much more than has been supposed if materials are presented to them in special ways. My colleagues and I recently saw a patient at the Boston Veterans Administration Medical Center who could neither read words aloud nor respond to written commands. Yet when we showed him a group of words, all but one of which belonged to the same category, he could pick out the exception, and when we gave him a category name, he could easily point out the word that belonged to the category. He could also answer many qualitative questions about written words—for instance, whether a word was large or small, good or bad.

We concluded that his ability to sound out words had been destroyed but that his "semantic reading," his understanding of the shades of meaning surrounding words, had largely been preserved. We have seen several other patients with similar problems, and often the way they misread words while remaining within the appropriate "semantic field" was revealing. One patient read *tape* as *reel, tallow* as *candle, learn* as *book,* and *elbow* as *macaroni.*

These findings suggest that, at least among some alexics, a considerable amount of reading capacity remains. The key lies in presenting the target item in the right context or asking the appropriate question. This discovery has important implications for therapy.

306

The first step is to determine which verbal materials the patient was familiar with before his disability, which words and abbreviations he could previously identify. Then when we write messages to him, it is important to include words with high semantic content and permit him different means of recognition, such as matching. The most difficult words for these patients are the "little words" like *and, but, if,* and *in,* because they lack strong semantic associations. An optimal rehabilitation program should include reactivation of the comprehension of familiar nouns and verbs, use of known trademarks and abbreviations, and intensive drill and memorization of those important "little words."

In 1915 one Bishop Harmon suggested that dyslexic children could be taught to read English on the principle of Chinese—that is, each word having its own unique symbol. Paul Rozin and his associates at the University of Pennsylvania recently described just such a method, which they used effectively to teach severely dyslexic children in the inner city. They gave an English meaning to each of thirty different Chinese characters. Their ideograms can be read from left to right and combined to form a variety of English sentences. After only a few hours of training, eight second-grade children were able to communicate with them in a flexible, nonmemorized manner.

Rozin's view is similar to the one I have been describing. He believes that the dyslexic's principal problem is blending a sequence of letters into an English word, perhaps because of a neurological deficiency. He recommends that these children be taught a system of easily recognizable characters that represent words rather than individual sounds. Since this method eventually runs into the same problem as Chinese— too many characters—he feels that perhaps a system of syllables, with one visual configuration representing a composite sound unit (like *can* or *er*) might be used to make the transition to normal English. He is currently experimenting with this method.

Rozin is by no means the only investigator who has come up with a successful program. There are others equally convinced that reading should be taught to dyslexic children exclusively by the look-say method, drill in phonics, tactile involvement with letters, teaching machines, artificial scripts which de-emphasize the importance of slant and orientation, or various kinds of pictograms. A similar range of alternatives has been recommended for patients with acquired reading disorders. Adapting David Premack's methods, Michael Gazzaniga and Andrea Velletri-Glass of New York University have reported success in employing with aphasic patients the same set of colored plastic symbols used to teach a chimpanzee to communicate. And several of us at the Veterans Administration Medical Center have found that an aphasic patient can more effectively communicate using a novel ideographic system than using his native English.

The number of remedial techniques increases almost daily. This variety and innovation should enable us to give better help to those with reading disorders. The real breakthrough will come, however, when we discover what Déjerine searched for a century ago: the neurological mechanisms that are involved in recognizing visual forms and associating them with sounds and with meanings.

29

MISSING THE POINT:

LANGUAGE AND

THE RIGHT HEMISPHERE

ON DECEMBER 31, 1974, Associate Justice William O. Douglas, long one of the most impressive and vigorous members of the Supreme Court of the United States, suffered a stroke. At first it appeared that Douglas would recover quickly and resume his place on the Court. Overly optimistic news reports indicated that "the stroke has not affected the Justice's brain [sic]"; other accounts dwelled on the fact that the Justice was still able to talk and, because the stroke had affected the left side of his body, was still able to write with his preferred hand.

As months passed, however, it became increasingly clear that Justice Douglas was seriously impaired and would not be able to resume his full duties on the bench. Rumors circulated, documenting surprising behaviors uncharacteristic of a distinguished jurist. It became a question of when, rather than whether, Justice Douglas would resign.

With the publication of a number of articles and books, in particular *The Brethren* by Bob Woodward and Scott Armstrong, more facts have come to light about Douglas's last months on the Court and the period following his resignation in November 1975. For all public purposes,

Douglas acted as if he were fine, as if he could soon assume full work on the Court. He insisted on checking himself out of the hospital, where he was receiving rehabilitation and then refused to return. He responded to seriously phrased queries about his condition with off-handed quips: "Walking has very little to do with the work of the Court" (p. 381); "If George Blanda can play, why not me?" (p. 385). He insisted in a press release that his arm had been injured in a fall, thereby baldly denying the neurological origin of his paralysis. Occasionally he acted in a paranoid fashion, claiming, for example, that the Chief Justice's quarters were his and that he was the Chief Justice. During sessions of the Court he dozed, asked irrelevant questions, and sometimes rambled on.

Finally, after considerable pressure from many quarters over a long period of time, Douglas did resign. But in the sad dénouement to this saga, the Justice refused to accept the reality that he was no longer a member of the Court. He came back to his office, buzzed for his clerks, and in general tried to inject himself into the flow of business. He took aggressive steps to assign cases to himself, asked to participate in, draft, and even publish his own opinions separately; and he requested that a tenth seat be placed at the Justices' bench. As Chief Justice Burger put it, he was like an old firehouse dog—"too old to run along with the trucks, but his ears prick up just the same" (p. 399). Only after each of the Justice's brethren, including his close friend Brennan, signed a letter in which they explicitly asked him to desist from interfering with the business of the Court, did Justice Douglas retreat from the scene. He continued to ail for the last six years of his life and received great honors and tributes when he died on January 19, 1980.

Not surprisingly, there was little discussion in the American press about the causes of Justice Douglas's bizarre reactions and behaviors. In addition to the propriety of such silence, it is impossible to determine in any single case *why* an individual behaves in an unfathomable manner. It might have been that Douglas was becoming senile, that he was reflecting (or emphasizing) aspects of his personality—always difficult, proud, narcissistic—which had been in evidence earlier. In my own view, however, it is most likely that Justice Douglas's behavioral patterns were a direct consequence of his stroke—a massive infarct in the right cerebral hemisphere, which left him paralyzed and in great pain for several years until his death.

To suggest that bizarre thoughts, words, and actions are consequent to injury to the right, or nondominant, hemisphere would have seemed an extreme statement some decades ago. For many years standard teaching has been that the left hemisphere of the human cortex is dominant for all linguistic functions. The right hemisphere, known since the 1940s to be crucial for visual and spatial functions, was said to have nothing to do with language.

Today, however, a spate of articles and books document the increasing number of linguistic abilities now thought to be subserved, at least in part, by the right cerebral hemisphere in normal right-handed individuals. Indeed, in November 1980, in an event impossible to have envisioned two decades ago, an entire conference was devoted to the linguistic capacities of the right hemisphere. Researchers vied with one another in their efforts to document the capacities that now seem the province of the right hemisphere. And in the light of the most recent research, the right hemisphere emerges as vital, perhaps even more important than the left hemisphere, in dealing with narratives, metaphors, jokes, morals, and other complex or subtle aspects of language.

To be sure, there were legitimate reasons for the original portrait of the left hemisphere as the linguistic zone par excellence of the brain. Since 1861 researchers have known that injuries to the left hemisphere (but not to the right) cause a normal individual to become aphasic—impaired in linguistic functioning.

A century later, studies of split-brain patients—mostly epileptics whose right and left hemispheres had been disconnected (by severing connecting tissue called the *corpus callosum*) to control seizures—strongly suggested that only the left hemisphere was able to process linguistic material to a significant degree. Many experiments with normal subjects also pointed to the left hemisphere as the dominant agent in all manner of linguistic functioning.

Brain scientists with more sophisticated experimental techniques and access to patients whose injuries can be precisely delineated have gradually been able to get a fuller picture of right-hemisphere functioning. The right brain is now thought to be important or dominant for a variety of cognitive capacities, ranging from musical fluency to the ability to act in an emotionally appropriate manner.

The most impressive evidence for that has come from the latest studies of split-brain patients. Although the first studies by investigators such as Roger Sperry at the California Institute of Technology did not seem to disclose significant linguistic capacities, several patients have now demonstrated a considerable ability to understand language when it is delivered solely to the right hemisphere. According to Eran Zaidel of the University of California at Los Angeles, two patients displayed a vocabulary about as large as that of a high-school student and the grammatical competence of a five-year-old, which, as both linguists and parents know, is very high indeed.

Two patients seen by Michael Gazzaniga of Cornell University Medical College are not only able to understand with the right hemisphere but can also use it to speak. The evidence comes from studies in which the subjects are exposed to written material in their left visual field, which sends information to the right hemisphere. For instance, the name of an object (say, an apple) is flashed briefly on a screen so that the information is received only by the right hemisphere. Then the subjects are asked to repeat the word or, if they are unable to do that, to choose the correct object from a group of objects presented to them.

Earlier subjects had sometimes been able to point with their left hands to the correct object, but they could never express the name orally. In fact, when they attempted to describe what the right hemisphere had seen and the left hand had touched, they spoke nonsense; in effect, the left hemisphere, which had never seen the word, was fabricating. But as Gazzaniga's two patients have demonstrated, the right hemisphere *is* able to name objects seen in the left visual field. In addition, both Zaidel and Gazzaniga now believe that some communication goes on between the hemispheres of the brain even after they are severed, thereby suggesting a richness of linguistic interconnection that had not been suspected before. (Just how this takes place remains a mystery. One theory is that the two hemispheres are communicating via subcortical connections; another, that they have a nonlinguistic way of cuing each other.)

A great deal has been learned from work with split-brain patients about the functions of the two halves of the brain. However, it must not be forgotten that these are extremely unusual and rare patients, whose brains must be abnormal. After all, they would not have undergone such radical and risky surgery unless they had sustained epileptic attacks for many years; moreover, the operations are usually performed during the teenage years, at a time when the nervous system is still quite plastic and may be able to acquire (or reacquire) language. Thus abilities imputed to the right hemisphere of split-brain patients may not exist to a comparable extent in the brains of normal people.

Missing the Point: Language and the Right Hemisphere

Recently Wendy Wapner, Suzanne Hamby, Dee Michel, Hiram Brownell, and I have been studying stroke patients who have suffered major injuries to the right hemisphere. We have focused for the most part on their ability to handle complex linguistic materials, such as stories, jokes, metaphors, fables, and the like. The basic linguistic capacities of these patients are in quite proper working order, we have discovered. They speak at a normal rate, have a rich vocabulary, and use grammar in an appropriate way. In this sense at least, the "language machine" in the healthy left hemisphere performs adequately. Indeed, it is suggestive to think of the isolated left hemisphere as a literal-minded talking robot: when asked, "Would you mind passing the salt?" such a dunce would reply, "No, I wouldn't mind," rather than handing the salt to the requesting individual. Accordingly, when we assess the performance of patients with right-hemisphere disease, using more complex linguistic material, we find a peculiar and instructive set of disorders.

Consider what happens when they listen to the story we have titled "Fireman Joe." First, the patient learns that Fireman Joe lived in Silver Springs, where children used to play near his firehouse. One day when the fire alarm went off, a little girl was actually playing on the fire engine. She was taken along to the scene of the fire, where she helped the fireman extinguish the fire. Afterward, the fireman thanked the little girl for her help.

After the story is read to the patients (and various control groups), we ask them to retell it and to answer questions about it. We find they are adept at relating the essential facts: they can remember the names of Fireman Joe and Silver Springs, and they often repeat entire sentences from the story verbatim rather than paraphrase the contents, as normal people would. Their retellings, however, are bizarre in a number of ways: they often repeat single sentences word for word but confuse the order of the sentences; their references to characters are often vague or erroneous; sometimes they leave out a whole section of the story that makes an important point.

The patients give other signs that their sense of the story has been disturbed. They often argue with points in it, saying, for example, that the little girl could not have been on the fire engine because "only authorized personnel are allowed." Or they inappropriately inject personal associations into their retellings: for instance, one patient volunteered that a relative of his had been hurt en route to a fire. There is also a lot of confabulation—that is, patients insert events that have no basis in the story. One told us that after the fire was over, the

313

fireman called the girl's mother to thank her for letting the child play on the fire engine.

In characterizing these deficiencies, we say that the patients have difficulty accepting the story on its own terms. To borrow from Coleridge, they are unable to adopt a "willing suspension of disbelief." They argue with points that should be accepted, even as they accept the bizarre elements that we sometimes put in just to see whether they have any sense of what is appropriate. The patients fail to respect the boundaries of the story, to accept its premises, but cross those boundaries at will to suit their own purposes.

Varying this technique, we discovered a number of other problems exhibited by right-hemisphere patients. For example, they have considerable difficulty coming up with the moral of a story. Either they simply repeat an element of the story or they seize upon a concrete feature of the story and convert that into the moral.

For example, in a cartoon story called "The Fence," two neighbors get into a fight and hurl garbage at one another over a fence until their houses fall apart. Later on, one neighbor tosses a flower over to the other neighbor's yard, and the story concludes with an exchange of flowers rather than brickbats. The story illustrates a variation of the golden rule, but when asked what the moral is, right-hemisphere patients either mention an event in the story ("Don't throw garbage") or embrace a superficially attractive but in fact inappropriate formula, like, "People who live in glass houses shouldn't throw stones."

Right-hemisphere patients not only crack jokes at inappropriate times but also have difficulty getting the sense of jokes told by others. Consider, for example, a vignette about Aunt Helen, which begins as follows: A parade was going down the street, and the two cousins were talking on the balcony. Said one to the other, "Here comes the parade, and Aunt Helen will miss it." "She's upstairs waving her hair," answered the other cousin.

Having heard that much of the joke, a patient is asked to choose the correct punch line from a set of four. The correct punch line goes: Said the first cousin, "Mercy, can't we afford a flag?" Right-hemisphere patients, however, frequently prefer an ending we have dubbed a non sequitur—in the case of this joke, "I wonder what's for dinner." Pressed to explain why they select such an ending, the patients indicate that a joke should end with a surprise. While they seem to have caught on to the fact that jokes often end with surprises, the patients fail to distinguish between endings that are surprising because they are "set up" (that is, they represent a twist on what has gone before) from endings that are surprising because they are totally irrelevant.

It is instructive at this point to recall the behavior of Justice Douglas in the months following his stroke. Like our patients, he could ostensibly carry on a conversation and, in fact, was capable of rapid and sometimes witty rejoinders. But one receives the clear impression that the Justice could not follow lengthy and complex argumentation, that he was prone to take off on tangents, to make irrelevant asides, to connect new events and situations to inappropriate precedents, and to attribute erroneous motivations to other speakers. Just as our right-hemisphere patients seem unable to make use of linguistic (or extra-linguistic) cues in "sizing up" a situation, Justice Douglas regularly seemed to "miss the point." Recently published evidence suggests that President Woodrow Wilson, following his right-hemisphere stroke in 1919, also exhibited some of the bizarre behaviors we have come to associate with massive right-hemisphere disease.

From these and other observations, we have come up with two ways of describing the difficulties that many such patients have with complex linguistic material. On the one hand, we can say that they lack a "plausibility metric": they seem unable to decide, given a specific event, whether or not it fits into an overall narrative structure. Hence they may either challenge items that are perfectly appropriate (the girl playing on the fire engine) or, on the other hand, go to extraordinary lengths to justify elements that really do not fit into a given context (an inappropriate punch line).

A related conclusion is that they lack the ability to set up a "scaffolding" for a story. They are unable to figure out the underlying architecture or composition of a story—the nature of and relationship between the various parts and characters. Instead, each part stands alone, a single brick unrelated to any other—or to the entire edifice. To put it another way, the "script" is missing or grossly deficient. The difficulties patients have in relating different portions of the story to one another and integrating them into a coherent whole may well depend upon spatial mechanisms that are the province of the right brain but are more abstract (or metaphoric) than those needed to conceive of location.

I should inject a few cautionary notes. First of all, these findings are not obtained with every right-hemisphere patient. They are particularly common, though, among those with large lesions in frontal por-

315

tions of the right hemisphere. Moreover, at least some of the symptoms described here have been encountered in other mentally disturbed patients, such as schizophrenics, and it is not yet clear how many language disabilities may be due solely to right-hemisphere damage and not to other forms of pathology. Nonetheless, the results obtained from right-hemisphere patients are different from those typical of other groups we have studied—for example, normal controls, aging controls, and left-hemisphere patients. We thus have some confidence that it is the left hemisphere that, when isolated, tends to miss the point in linguistic material.

It should be noted, finally, that while some split-brain patients do have linguistic skills in the right hemisphere, that hemisphere does not generally show great linguistic prowess on its own. While crucial for more general aspects of language, such as sensitivity to the moral of the story or to metaphors, this half of the brain seems in normal people to be quite primitive in handling the building blocks of language: the syllables, single words, syntax, and grammatical relations that are the mainstay of linguistic analysis remain the domain of the left hemisphere.

We can put our present research conclusions somewhat fancifully. If we imagine each hemisphere of the brain at a Marx Brothers movie, we might say that the left hemisphere alone—the robot described earlier—would be drawn to Groucho's wordplay; the right hemisphere, visually sensitive and alert to subtleties and nuances, might enjoy Harpo's antics. However, only with the two hemispheres working together, properly connected by the *corpus callosum,* can we enjoy the frantic interplay of *A Day at the Races* or *A Night at the Opera.*

What might these patterns in brain-damaged patients tell us about how the rest of us process language? Not very much, yet. We have all met people who are good at grasping facts but tend either to be too literal in interpreting them or to miss the point altogether. Likewise, we know others (often people with artistic talent of some sort) who are erratic in dealing with facts and do poorly on tests but who have an amazing ability to grasp the gist of a story, the subtle shadings of meaning. We can only speculate whether these differences can be traced to hemispheric specialization. One way to find out might be to test both types on standard measures of brain specialization, to see, for example, whether those who are good at sensing meanings are often left-handed or ambidextrous and look toward the left when pondering verbal material; both indices would suggest right-brain involvement in language for this group.

A final point may be made concerning rehabilitation. Armed with new insights into the problems that right-hemisphere patients face, is it possible to aid them to cope more successfully with their cognitive and linguistic impairments? So far as I know, no one has yet undertaken a program of rehabilitation that focuses specifically on some of the deficits outlined here. It is possible, however, to indicate some of the lines of assistance that might be attempted. First of all, given the penchant of these patients to be distracted and to draw inappropriate conclusions, it is crucial to be absolutely clear in talking with them, to leave no detail out, no stone unturned, and to make connections as explicit as possible. Relatedly, one should not assume that the patients have available to them the kinds of "daily scripts" on which most of us naturally rely: it is necessary to spell things out in the same way that one might for a visitor from another planet, a foreigner, or a speaking machine. A crucial step forward would be some acknowledgment or understanding on the patient's part that he has these difficulties: self-insight is often the first and most important step in rehabilitation.

Such self-insight will not be easy to come by in the case of severe right-hemisphere patients. Unfortunately, a tendency to deny one's deficits and to act as if one were perfectly normal is pervasive among right-hemisphere patients and seems to have characterized both Justice Douglas and President Wilson. The neurologist's old saw—"The nervous system never knows what's wrong with it"—is uncomfortably apt here.

Perhaps in the case of Justice Douglas there was no proper rehabilitative course to follow. But it seems clear to me that the rest of the world—the press, other Justices, and quite possibly those closest to him as well—would have been better able to deal with Douglas and to help him if they had been aware of how typical it is for patients with his kind of damage to behave (and speak) in just the manner that he did. Frank recognition—rather than polite coverup or denial—might in the long run have been more productive. In any case, the fact that Justice Douglas, and before him President Wilson, had major right-hemisphere strokes and yet remained in positions of authority for substantial periods of time, are issues with which individuals in a democratic society must contend. It may be more comforting to think that nothing has changed, that it is "all psychological." But the facts of brain organization and brain damage must be brought to bear if an informed decision is to be reached on a proper course of action in such delicate but consequential matters.

30

ARTISTRY AFTER BRAIN DAMAGE

THROUGHOUT my student days I was innocent of knowledge about (and, for that matter, devoid of interest in) the human brain. While not openly sympathetic to a "black-box approach," in which the nervous system is deliberately excluded from consideration, I felt no need to discover the "brain correlates" of the artistic behaviors I was trying to understand. In fact, when I was not conducting psychological experiments with children, I was content to talk with artists and ponder the way their developed skills produced fluent and highly original works of art.

But soon enough, I encountered an impasse, owing to one single fact: in competent artists, skills unfold with such fluency that it is extremely difficult for a nonprofessional to figure out the skills involved in artistry and how they are deployed. It was while confronting this dilemma that I chanced to hear the noted neurologist, Norman Geschwind, deliver a talk on the left and right hemispheres of the brain. At a time when laterality had not yet become the rage, Geschwind described several fascinating associations and dissociations that can be observed in brain-damaged patients. There is the paradoxical sparing of a capacity in the presence of widespread damage to the nervous system—for example, when an individual who seems unable to acquire any new information mysteriously retains the capacity to learn complex motor patterns. There is the equally startling devastation of a single ability in the repertoire of an otherwise competent individual, as when, for example, an individual who retains the ability to write, speak, and even to read numbers loses the ability to read letters and words.

Geschwind even touched upon what happens to competent artists when they suffer a stroke. To my astonishment I learned that an artist may suffer profound impairment of certain capacities—for example, becoming completely unable to express his thoughts in language—while still producing artworks of high quality. The opposite situation—isolated loss of artistry—also obtains, though less frequently.

In a moment of inspiration I felt things coming together. To work with brain-damaged patients and examine what happens to their ensemble of capacities might just provide answers to the puzzles I was confronting. If one could see how skills broke down, in what combination they occurred and recurred, which ones could be spared or destroyed in isolation, one might receive just those insights into the organization of skills which seemed beyond reach in the intact artist. In what for me marked a dramatic career shift, I elected to bracket my interest in developmental psychology and go to work at a hospital where I could study the fate of artistic skills under various conditions of brain damage.

In 1971 I became a full-time investigator at the Aphasia Research Unit of the Boston Veterans Administration Medical Center. At this site approximately thirty patients with brain disease are housed in a ward at any one time. Usually the majority are aphasic: that is, they have lost at least some linguistic capacities as a result of damage to the left (or dominant) hemisphere. But at any one time there is also an assortment of other patients, ranging from individuals with Korsakoff's disease—the patients who seem unable to learn anything except motor patterns—to individuals with pure alexia—the patients who have lost the ability to read while retaining all other linguistic functions. An interdisciplinary staff of clinicians and scientific researchers works with these patients, analyzing their disorders in detail and recommending a course of rehabilitation. The Boston Medical Center is one of the major sites for neurobehavioral studies in the world, and I have been most fortunate in having the opportunity to conduct my studies in this stimulating environment.

You can imagine my excitement when, during my second week at the Medical Center, I learned that a painter would be presented at the weekly "grand rounds." Here at last I would discover answers to the questions that had gripped me. However, my excitement was short-lived. I discovered that the painter had in fact been a house painter and had never undertaken anything more ambitious than a basement playroom. When I heard a few weeks later that we would observe a former singer, my excitement proved equally evanescent: in this case, our hapless patient was simply an individual who had sung in the high-school chorus but had displayed no particular musical flair since that time.

Fortunately for the arts, I have encountered very few artists during my decade at the medical center. This is in part because artists do not constitute a large part of the American population, in part because artists generally do not end up at a rehabilitation facility that caters primarily to individuals from lower socioeconomic groups. And so, making a virtue of necessity, I began to study more common forms of brain damage, such as aphasia, while hoping for the eventual opportunity to work with artists.

In two ways this hope has been realized. First of all, as my interest in the arts became known to other neuropsychological researchers, they have kindly brought to my attention artists who had come into their care. From these helpful collaborations—with the patients themselves no less than with the professional colleagues—I have learned much about the fate of artistry after brain damage. Second, after a period of time I came to realize that I did not have to wait to work exclusively with artists in order to answer many of the questions in which I was interested. Instead, I could simply devise artistic tasks that fell within the competence of normal "control" patients in the hospital and then administer these same tests to individuals who had sustained various forms of brain damage.

My reasoning was as follows. While most individuals are not artists, nearly all of us have attained some modest artistic skills. We can sing a song, make a drawing, tell a story. Artists build upon these basic skills. If we can examine how such relatively elementary abilities break down in normal patients after damage to the brain, we can receive valuable clues as to the organization of these same capacities in more highly skilled artists. Since hitting upon this insight, I have conducted a two-pronged line of research. I have examined the breakdown of art-related skills in normal individuals and, whenever possible, I have investigated the breakdown of more highly elaborated skills in artistic individuals. The findings I report here draw upon these twin sources of information.

Now after ten years of research it is opportune to take stock of the major conclusions that my colleagues and I have so far reached. We have had the opportunity to work with normal and talented individuals in three art forms: painting, music, and literature. In each case we have focused on the fate of artistic capacities following unilateral damage to the left or the right hemisphere. The story needs to be told separately for each art form. Yet, looking back at the artists as a group, we also find certain themes that together characterize artistry in a more general sense.

Painting

Before beginning my own work, I looked through the literature on painters who had sustained brain damage. And in reviewing the literature on those painters who had become aphasic as a result of damage to the left hemisphere, I encountered stunning claims. Several neurologists who had had the opportunity to work with aphasic painters claimed that not only did these painters retain their artistic capacity but that in fact their works of art *improved* in quality following the loss of language. Equally striking, some of these painters were said to be able to relearn to draw at a "premorbid level" using their nonparalyzed left hand.

While I was at first skeptical of these claims, chalking them up to wish fulfillment, my own experience has borne them out to a surprising degree. I have now seen the works of several individuals who became significantly and even permanently aphasic. In some cases their style does seem to have undergone a change—toward greater simplification and clarity—but I detected no significant decline in aesthetic quality or interest. Indeed, the remarks made by a major French painter who became aphasic seem particularly apt:

There are in me two men, the one who paints, who is normal while he is painting, and the other one who is lost in the mist, who does not stick to life—I am saying very poorly what I mean—There are inside me the one who grasps reality, life; and there is the other one who has lost his regard for abstract thinking . . . These are two men, the one is grasped by reality to paint, the other one, the fool, who cannot manage words anymore. (quoted in Alajouanine, p. 238)

It seems fair to say then, that while left-hemisphere disease can impair an individual's language and perhaps even his reasoning processes, there is no necessary compromise of visual graphic skills.

The story is instructively different in cases where an individual has

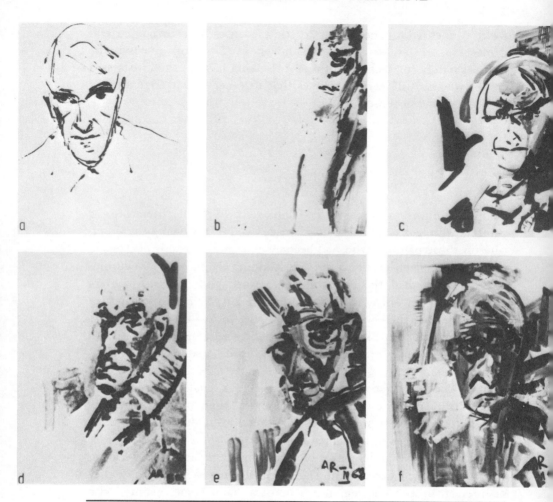

Figure 30.1. Self-portraits by Anton Räderscheidt before and after a stroke.

suffered unilateral right-hemisphere disease. Here we are indebted to pioneering work by the German neurologist Richard Jung, who collected works from four major German painters who had sustained right-hemisphere injury. Examination of the prestroke and poststroke paintings suggests to me a clear effect of the lesion. To begin with, these patients, who tend to neglect the left side of space in everyday life, also neglect the left side of the canvas, typically drawing incomplete figures. More significantly, the overall contour of objects is disrupted. The result is a fragmented and disconnected drawing, whose parts, while often recognizable, do not flow or fit together into an organized whole. Finally, and most dramatically, one detects a definite alteration in style. The paintings become more directly expressive, more raw and sensuous: it is as if an inhibitory mechanism has been released and the patients can now give freer vent to their most primitive, least disguised feelings. These trends can be seen in the accompanying set of six self-portraits by the German twentieth-century painter Anton Räderscheidt. The first was completed two years prior to his stroke; the remaining five were done at approximately two month intervals in the year following the stroke.

Such stylistic changes were actually noted by painting critics in the 1920s following the stroke of the well-known German expressionist Lovis Corinth. However, these changes were attributed to psychological factors, to Corinth's changing view of his life prospects rather than to the effects of damage to a certain locus in his brain. In my own view, however, it is more parsimonious to attribute the changes in Corinth's style to his right-hemisphere lesion. That is because one typically encounters a more primitive style following injuries of this sort, whereas one does not detect such a style change after other sicknesses or even, for that matter, following damage to the left hemisphere of the brain. We know from many other studies that the right hemisphere is "dominant' for emotional sensitivity and appropriateness. It may well be that lesions in this area undermine this sensitivity and, accordingly, give rise to a much rawer form of aesthetic expression.

Clinical studies of brain-damaged individuals can clarify other aspects of graphic activity. Consider, for example, the case of an amateur artist who suffered from visual agnosia. This is a rare condition where the patient exhibits a selective difficulty in recognizing objects presented visually—despite preserved language ability, preserved basic perceptual capacities, and the ability to recognize objects presented tactually. The patient exhibited a clear dissociation between the ability to recognize objects and the ability to draw them. When the patient recognized an object, he drew it in a flexible, free-hand, and highly legible style, which exploited his knowledge of the "schema"—the way in which an object of this sort is customarily drawn. In contrast, when (because of his agnosia) the patient did not recognize the object, he drew in an entirely different manner. Now he rendered the object far more accurately, but in a completely slavish way, recording every detail, including ones that were accidental and made recognition more difficult. The remarkable dissociation exhibited by this patient helps to answer a question that has long puzzled students of drawing: What is the role of "knowledge of an object" in affecting the way in which such an object is drawn? Does such knowledge help the artist, hinder him, or have no effect? Our patient documents that the capacity to draw in a completely realistic fashion does not depend upon knowledge of the identity of an object but in fact may even be disturbed or undermined by such knowledge.

We glean here in a brain-damaged individual intriguing support for the claims made by Betty Edwards in her recent book *Drawing on the Right Side of the Brain*. Edwards indicates that an individual may be able to draw more accurately if he holds an object upside down, and thus cannot recognize what he is drawing. Analogously, our agnosic patient demonstrates that these capacities can be teased apart, as if, owing to the ravages of brain disease, they resided in two different individuals.

Our principal insights about graphic activity come from studies of painters who have suffered an insult to the brain. However, we can also examine the drawings of once normal individuals who have sustained brain injury. Studies by Edith Kaplan of Boston's Veterans Administration Medical Center and Elizabeth Warrington of London's National Hospital indicate that drawings of individuals will change following unilateral damage to the brain, with the manner of change reflecting quite faithfully the site of the brain disease. Thus, when an individual suffers left-hemisphere disease, his drawings will tend to become simplified: details are left out but the overall contour will be recognizable (see the set of eight drawings on page 325). In many ways, in fact, the individual's drawings resemble those of a young child. In contrast, following right-hemisphere disease, an individual will retain the ability to render details but will have difficulty organizing them coherently into a single composition and will often produce disrupted or irregular contours (see the set of eight drawings on page 326). Thus we see in the normal individual manifestations of those symptoms that are more dramatically displayed by visual artists.

A final link between graphic artistry and right-hemisphere functioning can be discerned from a study of style sensitivity in unilateral left- and right-hemisphere patients. My colleagues and I found that left-hemisphere patients were quite successful at grouping paintings by their style; in fact, their performances often exceeded those of patients without brain damage. In sharp contrast, the right-hemisphere

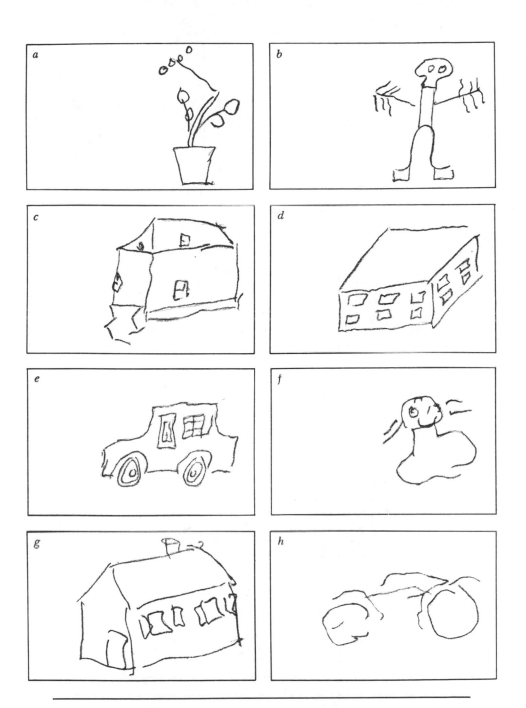

Figure 30.2. Free-hand drawings by right-handed patients with left-hemisphere lesions.

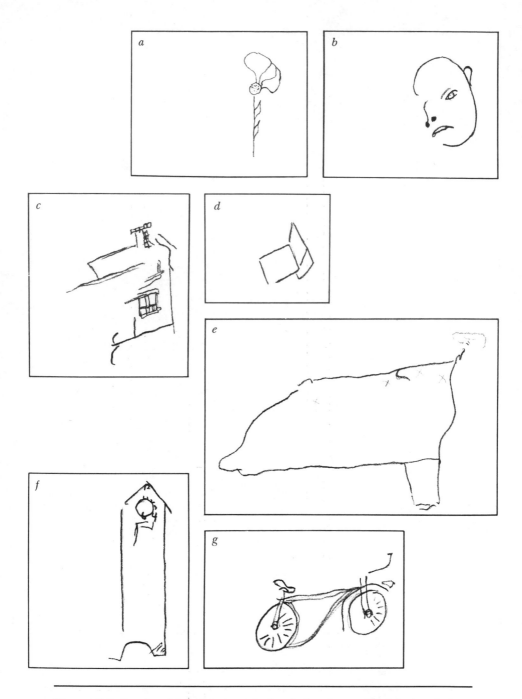

Figure 30.3. Free-hand drawings by right-handed patients with right-hemisphere lesions.

patients exhibited scant sensitivity to style. Instead they were overwhelmed by subject matter, attempting whenever possible to group paintings that had the same content even when they exhibited radically different styles. Even in an artistic task that is conceptual in nature, left-hemisphere disease proves less crippling than damage to those regions of the brain that are dominant for visual-spatial functioning.

Music

Complex as the saga of drawing is, an account of musical capacities following brain damage proves even more intricate. This is in part because of the great variety of musical capacities that can be studied: different roles—like performer, listener, composer; different instruments played with different parts of the body ranging from fingers on a piano, to lips on a clarinet, to the human voice; different types and degrees of training; and different profiles of innate ability. Each of these factors (operating alone or in concert) makes generalizations extremely difficult; and such characterizations are often disconfirmed following work with the next few patients.

Yet despite this dismaying variety, I feel justified in proposing some tentative generalizations about musical capacities following brain disease. In broad outline, these are reminiscent of the findings in the area of drawing. Perhaps the most important commonality lies in the fact that one can continue to be a highly competent musician despite significant injury to the left hemisphere of the brain. A case often quoted by neurologists is that of the renowned Russian composer V. Shebalin, who became severely aphasic following a stroke. Despite this malady, Shebalin continued his composing and teaching activities and was considered by critics to be as brilliant a composer as ever. No less an authority than the dean of Soviet composers, Dmitri Shostakovich, described Shebalin's fifth symphony as "a brilliant creative work, filled with highest emotions, optimistic and full of life." These sentiments were echoed by T. Khrennikov, another major contemporary Russian composer, who said, "We can only envy the brilliant creative activity of this outstanding man who, in spite of his illness, created the brilliant fifth symphony, replete with youthful feelings and wonderful melodies" (quoted in Luria, Tsvetkova, and Futer, p. 292).

This saga of continued musical productivity despite a significant aphasia is echoed in accounts of other patients. For example, a sixty-three-year-old Swiss pianist studied by neurologist Gil Assal suffered a severe Wernicke's aphasia, which left him unable to understand what others were saying and impaired his ability to express his own thoughts. Despite this difficulty, his musical capacities remained essentially intact. He could instantly recognize pieces of music and make all necessary corrections in a performance. Moreover, he could play pieces, including new ones, with no noticeable problem.

My colleagues and I had the opportunity to work with a major American composer of choral works who also suffered a significant Wernicke's aphasia. The Wernicke's aphasia cleared to a great extent, leaving only minor naming problems but a lingering severe reading disorder. Revealingly, however, the alexia was much more pronounced with linguistic materials than with musical notation. Our patient could hardly read a single word and yet could decipher musical notations quite well. Here is evidence that musical symbols and verbal symbols are processed by the nervous system in different ways. Much more significantly, he was able to compose in the same style and with the same skill as before his aphasia. No longer able to read texts, he had to memorize passages that he was setting, but this inconvenience did not seem to cramp his musical style in any way.

Taken together, these findings document that linguistic competence is no more a prerequisite for musical skill than it is for graphic skill. Nonetheless, there are cases on record where a severe aphasia has aborted an individual's creative activity. The most poignant is the case of Maurice Ravel, the distinguished French composer who at the height of his powers was stricken by Wernicke's aphasia. Like the pianist described earlier, Ravel retained his critical capacities; he could recognize melodies and point out when errors were made; his sense of pitch and musical judgment seemed as keen as before. However, in sharp contrast to his preserved discriminating powers, Ravel had difficulty in reading notes and performing from a score and, most notably, was unable to compose anymore. It is not clear from the case report exactly why Ravel could no longer compose. It is possible that he lost the motivation but more likely he either lacked new musical ideas or could no longer transmit them to others, through performance or scoring.

Little information is available on the effects of significant right-hemisphere disease on the musical capacities of well-known musicians. The redoubtable twentieth-century composer Igor Stravinsky may have suffered a right-hemisphere stroke at age seventy-five, but there seem to have been no noticeable sequelae in music or other cognitive domains. A much younger composer, whom my colleagues had the opportunity to study, presented a highly instructive picture of right-hemisphere disease. The composer retained his musical knowledge and continued teaching at a musical conservatory and writing books about music. However, in sharp contrast to the other musicians whose cases I have reviewed, this composer lost his interest in the creative process. He no longer felt motivated to compose; as he put it, he could no longer conjure up the appropriate atmosphere. Moreover, he conceded that he could no longer "conceive of the whole piece." This composer also noted that he did not listen to music for enjoyment as much as he had in the past and no longer experienced a rich set of associations while listening to music. His own post-morbid attempts at composition he correctly judged as uninspired and uninspiring.

It is risky to draw conclusions on the basis of a single case. Nonetheless, it is certainly worth noting that an individual with significant right-hemisphere disease, whose language remains at a high level and whose technical skills have been spared, seems to have undergone a profound alteration in his relationship to musical material and in his inclination to compose. Here we see a possibly instructive distinction between certain mechanics of musical ability and the motivation (or capacity) to produce a coherent work of art.

Our understanding of specific musical capacities has been enlarged by dichotic-listening studies with normal individuals and by a variety of investigations with once-normal individuals who have sustained brain injury. The general findings are quite straightforward. Most musical capacities seem to be represented chiefly in the right hemisphere; accordingly, performance is poorer in individuals who have sustained right-hemisphere disease. This "right-sided" dominance seems particularly true in the case of sensitivity to pitch and timbre, two of the most quintessentially musical forms of sensitivity. Sensitivity to rhythm seems to be housed in both hemispheres, though it is possible that the left hemisphere is somewhat more dominant for rhythm in most individuals.

But it is far too simple to conclude that music is principally a right-hemisphere function. Intriguing studies by Thomas Bever of Columbia University and also by other investigators suggest that as an individual becomes more skilled in music, capacities that were initially housed in the right hemisphere are found increasingly in the left hemisphere. Thus musically untrained individuals are far more likely than trained

329

individuals to exhibit right-hemisphere effects. It seems as if, with musical training, a significant proportion of skills migrate across the *corpus callosum* into the linguistically dominant hemisphere.

Even if this is true, the reasons for this shifting dominance remain obscure. It may be, for example, that more skilled individuals learn verbal labels for many musical functions, and these, of course, would be housed in the left hemisphere. It is also possible that any skill that becomes highly developed becomes more enmeshed in the dominant hemisphere, with the nondominant hemisphere being particularly useful for processing novel (not-yet-coded) kinds of information. All these findings underscore the need for caution in discussing the "typical" organization of music in the brain. In fact, hereditary factors may produce greater interindividual variation in the organization of music than, say, in the organization of linguistic or visual-spatial skills. This greater "variance," as a statistician would put it, might reflect the well-established adoptive value of musical abilities. Whereas visual-spatial and linguistic skills are clearly essential for the survival of the species, and thus might be organized in a more uniform way across diverse individuals, the reasons music has survived in all individuals, and has flourished in some, remain wrapped in obscurity. Nonetheless, it is not surprising that so many scientists strive to understand the nature and organization of musical capacities. Perhaps if we could account for these biologically mysterious abilities, other cognitive and affective puzzles would be more readily solved.

Literature

When I first began the study of artistry following damage to the brain, I harbored a hope: if an individual were especially gifted in an area, he might be able to escape the ravages of brain disease. It was at least a theoretical possibility that an individual who was a highly skilled user of words might prove less susceptible to a debilitating aphasia after left-hemisphere disease than an individual of unremarkable verbal skills.

Alas, this hope has proved to be completely unfounded. More so than other cognitive capacities, language is housed in a circumscribed area of tissue, and any individual, be he a Nobel laureate in literature or a taciturn down-Easter from Maine, will be significantly impaired by injuries in these areas. Indeed, the epitaph for my hypothesis was dramatically supplied by the French poet Charles Baudelaire, who after suffering a stroke had such impaired language that he could utter only the oath *cré nom*. His literary output was of course completely curtailed by his stroke.

This story could be retold for numerous highly articulate individuals who became aphasic following damage to the brain. In fact, I know of no instance where literary output endured despite significant aphasia. There are some cases of individuals who recovered from aphasia and could write serviceable prose. Indeed, in a few cases aphasics drawn from the clinical professions have recovered to the extent of being able (with or without help) to pen books about their difficulties. But two remarks must be made. First of all, the recovery almost always occurs in individuals who are quite young and whose symptoms have been alleviated almost immediately. Second, individuals who were once aphasic typically report subjective difficulties in producing language, be it written or oral. These impairments may not be apparent to the outside observer, yet the patient himself reports that he no longer has the immediate access to words or the facility in organizing them that he had in the years before his stroke.

Of course not all aphasias reduce verbal output. In the case of Wernicke's aphasia, which follows injury to the left temporal lobe, an individual may be more fluent than before. He can produce complex sentences, which, however, are largely devoid of meaning. One thus encounters a fascinating phenomenon: the styles of individuals with different aphasias bear at least a superficial resemblance to the styles of great writers. At the risk of caricature, one can point out that a Broca's aphasic, with a lesion in the left frontal lobe, bears certain surface resemblances to the extremely spare style of a writer like Hemingway: short, discrete sentences largely restricted to substantive words. In contrast, the patter of a Wernicke's aphasic has certain resemblances to the linguistically ornate style of an author like Faulkner, with long periodic sentences punctuated by relative clauses, gerunds, and many function words.

The linguist Roman Jakobson reports the case of the Russian novelist Gleb Ivanovich Uspensky, who in the last years of his life suffered from a peculiar speech disorder. Uspensky penned sentences like the following: "From underneath an ancient straw cap with a bleak spot on its shield there peeked two braids resembling the tusks of the wild boar; a chin grown fat and pendulous definitely spread over the greasy collars of a calico dicky and in thick layer lay on the coarse collar of the canvas coat, firmly buttoned on the neck." Jakobson notes that "the reader is crushed by the multiplicity of detail unloaded on him in a limited verbal space and is physically unable to grasp the whole, so that the portrait is often lost" (p. 80). Such instances remind us that it may be difficult in certain cases to distinguish a stylistic peculiarity from an actual limitation due to brain disease. And here, of course, we encounter the difference between a taciturn style like Hemingway's and the limited output of a Broca's aphasic. Whereas Hemingway chooses his words and frames his sentences deliberately, the Broca's aphasic has no choice regarding the style he adopts. Brain damage imposes what literary talent embraces.

Work with normal individuals who have suffered brain disease has fleshed out our understanding of literary creation in instructive ways. Individuals with unilateral right-brain disease may have superficial command of language but often display significant and severe impairments in the literary area. As I have noted in essay 29, right-hemisphere patients frequently prove unable to appreciate humor or metaphor or to get the points of stories. They are competent at remembering details, but in fact lose the sense of the overall piece and often are preoccupied with minor details at the cost of misconstruing a story or joke. And presented with a metaphor, they are more likely than an aphasic patient to take the trope literally and to miss the speaker's intent altogether.

It would be misleading to imply that these individuals have lost their metaphoric and humorous capacities altogether. Indeed, in spontaneous conversation they often show an inclination, even a penchant, for producing figures of speech or for making jokes. Yet, as we have noted, these jokes and figures of speech are inappropriate. They arise in situations in which they are not called for and they often make little sense to listeners. It is as if the literary resources continue to exist—even in abundance—but can no longer be marshaled for the right occasion. Similarly, it is not that the individual contents of a story are lost on a patient—in fact, memory for facts and syntax may be astoundingly good. Instead the patient seems unable to connect the parts of a story to one another; or he cannot relate these fragments to those organizing scripts or schemas that the rest of us automatically invoke when we encounter a new literary work.

The contrast between right-hemisphere and aphasic patients is particularly striking here. Aphasic patients do not tell jokes, make metaphors, or relate stories; their verbal output is simply too restricted. Nonetheless they show a surprising, even remarkably enduring sensitivity to the form and the purposes of such literary forms. Even when an aphasic can say very little about a joke or story, he can indicate by his laughter, his surprise, and by his brief paraphrases that he gets the point of the exercise. Even when he cannot paraphrase a metaphor, he can show by his comments or by pictorial matching that he appreciates the non-literal intent of the remark. In contrast to the right-hemisphere patient, the aphasic will rarely be deceived about the overall purpose of a joke or the moral of a story, even if he is unable to offer a precise précis.

Once again we encounter an instructive dissociation. The left hemisphere seems crucial for the mechanics of language, for the production and understanding of simple, single linguistic units. However, an aphasic with a preserved right hemisphere retains the capacity to understand what stories or jokes are about: in fact, given the redundancy and paralinguistic cues often embedded in such lengthier linguistic specimens, aphasic patients may surprise us by the extent to which they remain "with it." In right-hemisphere patients, alas, the story is different. The mechanics may be well preserved but the overall sense of what is going on and why it is going on are all too often lost. No story, let alone a poem or a novel, can be fashioned under such piecemeal circumstances.

If science advances through dismissing certain previously cherished hypotheses, we can claim some progress on the questions that animated my move to the Boston Veterans Administration a decade ago. First of all, any simple equation of an artistic function with a certain region of the brain has been proved untenable. Each art form (and for that matter, each brain region) is too complex for that. Nor does a high level of skill serve as a certain insurance policy against damage from brain disease. Certainly if a brain lesion occurs in specific loci, even the most talented artist will pay a fearsome price.

To dismiss another possibility, we have seen that each art form seems to be organized somewhat differently. Attempts in the press (and in scholarly journals) to bifurcate abilities in terms of "wholes" versus "parts" prove far too simple-minded to account for the variety of results reported here. Each art form seems to have its own evolution, its own neural representation, and its special ways of drawing upon (and inter-acting with) the full range of neural zones.

It is also possible to fashion a more positive characterization of artistry after brain damage. To begin with, we have seen that specific computational skills involved in particular art forms can be spared or destroyed in isolation. There is evidence for specific functions, represented in delineated neural regions, in the various art forms: the production of contour in drawing, the perception of pitch in music, the sensitivity to figures of speech in the literary realm. These and other capacities can be knocked out, or spared, depending on the nature and the locus of the brain disease. In some cases, the representation seems quite specific to an art form: musical capacities like pitch perception are mediated by areas that may be devoted exclusively to that function. But in other cases, artistry draws on much wider conceptual capacities: thus the same areas of brain that govern the production of contours are exploited more generally for a range of visual-spatial functions. The arts may harbor some areas of the brain for themselves, but they share many other zones with decidedly nonaesthetic pursuits.

Whether an artist will continue to produce works of art following damage to the brain and whether his style will remain the same cannot yet be reliably predicted. The data base is still too small. Nonetheless, one may speculate that if an individual suffers damage to the left hemisphere of the brain, and if he continues to produce at all, he is likely to fashion works similar to those produced prior to the stroke. In contrast, if damage occurs to the right hemisphere, the artist is more likely to exhibit a significantly different attitude or style of input. Computational capacities may be preserved, but there is likely to be altered motivation or a novel style, perhaps reflecting the disinhibiting effects of a lesion in the right hemisphere of the brain.

What remains a complete mystery for a student of neuropsychology are the most comprehensive aspects of artistic production. We can, to be sure, say something about the particular skills involved in artistry. We can even say something about the motivation and the style of an artistic work. But as for the overall conception, its sources, its execution, its evaluation—these remain as unilluminated by studies of brain damage as by studies of normal and talented individuals.

My own guess is that studies of localization of function may well be inappropriate here. To produce something well-organized, let alone something fresh and original, it may be necessary to have an essentially intact nervous system. Most of our nervous system is drawn upon simply to carry out routine functions. Only large amounts of "uncommitted" or "excess" cortex may allow an individual to go beyond workaday routine activity and to fashion newly conceived and highly original works of art. For these heights of artistry to be achieved, it does not suffice simply to have spared a certain limited area of brain: one needs to have all, or at least most, regions of the brain performing at top form. The destruction of significant areas of the brain makes it likely that these heights will no longer be attained, while revealing little about just how they have been achieved in the supremely gifted artist.

31

THE LIVES OF

ALEXANDER LURIA

CONSIDER two scientific careers. In the first, a gifted adolescent demonstrates an ability to do quality research in psychology, starts his own psychoanalytic discussion group, and launches a journal. By his early twenties he has mastered the psychological literature in several languages and corresponded with the great figures of his time, including Freud. During the next four decades he carries out brilliant investigations into the thought processes and emotions of children, criminals, Russian peasants, identical twins, and brain-damaged and retarded patients. By the last years of his life, he is beyond question the most distinguished psychologist in the Soviet Union.

The second career starts with a dynamic young researcher who is attempting to make a place for himself. Every time he chooses a field, he is forced by political considerations to abandon it and to move on to another that he knows little about. He is summarily fired from jobs, criticized and ridiculed in the press. He is heard praising scholars whom he considers fraudulent, while denouncing others whom he is known to admire. He comes to renounce even some of his own writings and to regard all of his good ideas as coming from others. By the end of his life, he considers his contribution totally ordinary and unremarkable.

Both these descriptions fit Alexander Romanovich Luria, who, after a stunning career, died in 1977 at the age of seventy-five. Most of us in the West knew only the first Luria, the incisive researcher who helped to reorient several fields of psychology. But with the publication in 1979 of his autobiographical essay, *The Making of Mind: A Personal Account of Soviet Psychology,* we have had a painful glimpse of a second Luria.

Read literally, Luria's autobiography reveals neither the first career—the highly original and productive scientist, nor the second—the tragic hero. Only by radical *deconstruction* of the text—a reading between Luria's own lines and a careful attention to the notes provided by Luria's friend and editor Michael Cole—does it become possible to piece together the main lines of Luria's life, to recognize his genuine contributions and his faults, and to arrive at an assessment of the man and what he accomplished. In re-examining Luria's career, we can also understand the agonizing choices faced by scientists working under totalitarian conditions and gain new insight into the subtle impact of such conditions on their individual psyches. And we can more fully appreciate the courage of a few, like the recently exiled physicist Andrei Sakharov, who refuse to bend or be silent.

The opening lines of Luria's book are prophetic: "I began my career in the first years of the great Russian Revolution. This single, momentous event decisively influenced my life and that of everyone I knew."

As if to defy this beginning, Luria's autobiography makes one of the most exciting—and horrible—periods of intellectual and political history sound like pages from the diary of a mediocre scholar. Despite the seductive subtitle, *A Personal Account of Soviet Psychology*, it has few personal references and is written in a style that reflects little passion or commitment. The book, which began as a script Luria was writing about his life for a documentary film by two Americans, has never been published in the Soviet Union, though a version is supposed to appear there soon.

Though Luria lived through Stalin's purges—and was almost a victim—Stalin's name is nowhere mentioned. Though he was at times viciously denounced by colleagues and even by friends, there is hardly a hint of this painful treatment. Though he eventually received countless honors in the Soviet Union and abroad, he protests that his abilities and contributions were unexceptional. Though people who knew him say he was sophisticated in political argument, he is equally self-deprecating in this area: "Properly speaking, I never really mastered Marxism to the degree I would have liked. I still consider this . . . a major shortcoming in my education."

Luria was the son of a middle-class Jewish doctor who became a university professor, but whose career had been held back by conditions under the czar. As a young man Luria had welcomed the chance to participate in a revolution and to help shape the energies it unleashed. Indeed, some of the excitement of those epochal days can be sensed in the early chapters of Luria's book, when he talks of working tirelessly with his colleagues to forge a new Soviet psychology that, building on the wisdom of Marx, would prove of service to humankind.

Luria's early correspondence with Freud, as well as his meeting with the distinguished Russian physiologist Vladimir Bekhterev, show the young scholar, barely in his twenties, touching all the right bases. In addition to writing books, editing journals, and stimulating social movements, he was at the advanced age of twenty-one invited to assume a major position at the Moscow Institute of Psychology. We should all be so ordinary!

All this happened before an event that Luria considers a turning point in his intellectual formation: his encounter in 1924 with the redoubtable young Soviet scholar Lev Vygotsky. By all accounts, Vygotsky was a genius: a master of many subjects, a fount of novel conceptions, a visionary able to lecture for hours at a time without notes. When he died of tuberculosis at the age of thirty-eight, Vygotsky left more than eighty unpublished manuscripts. Of this figure, Luria once remarked: "All that is good in Russian psychology today comes from Vygotsky."

With Alexei Leontiev and a few other colleagues, Luria and Vygotsky began to enact a program that did revolutionize Soviet psychology. However, the golden years of the self-styled "troika" did not last. By the early 1930s the works of both Luria and Vygotsky were being strongly criticized in the Russian psychological journals. In 1936 the Central Committee of the Communist Party decided effectively to abandon psychological research. Vygotsky had already been dead for two years, and Luria, out of a job, had little choice at the age of thirty-four but to find a new career.

He attended medical school and finished his studies in neuropsychology just before the Second World War. Entrusted with the care of battle victims during the war, Luria mastered the symptoms that accompany various brain lesions and pioneered in forms of rehabilitation for wounded soldiers. But once again, following a further shake-up in Russian psychology after the war, he was fired from his position at the Neurosurgical Institute, and at the age of fifty had to launch yet another career, this time as a student of mental retardation.

The Lives of Alexander Luria

In the wake of the thaw in Russia after Stalin's death in 1953, Luria was once again allowed to assume more comfortable research—as a sometime student of child psychology and as an expert on aphasia and other brain disorders. But by this time he had grown extremely cautious. He became the mute man of the autobiography, the man of unquestionable scientific powers who apparently saw himself simply as an instrument of larger forces. As he declares in the book's final words: "People come and go, but the creative sources of great historical events and important ideas and deeds remain. That is perhaps the only excuse I had for writing this book."

Compelled to change his career several times, shifted from institution to institution like a foster child, Luria might well have lacked coherence and unity in his life. In fact, however, certain basic themes and procedures ran through all of his work.

While still an unformed teenager, Luria had already realized that any comprehensive psychology must speak both to what human beings can know (their cognitive powers) and to the forces that make them act in a certain way (their motivation). Upon first reading Freud, he was excited by the confirmation of the vital role played by the unconscious in motivating behavior. Yet, eager to place psychology on a solid scientific footing and loyal to the Pavlovian emphasis on elementary reflexes, Luria sought to wed Freud's insights to more empirical methods.

Luria invented a technique for measuring a person's emotional state and underlying emotional tone. Deceptively simple, the method consisted of having an individual free-associate to a list of words presented by the experimenter. Some of the words used were deliberately neutral in tone; others might be expected to tap an emotional reaction or conflict within the individual—for example, the word *rob* when presented to a suspected thief; the word *grade* heard by someone about to take an examination. The verbal technique was combined with a motor test in which the individual had to squeeze a rubber bulb while free-associating to the target word. Under normal circumstances, a person will say the word that comes first to mind and will be able, at the same time, to squeeze the bulb in a quick and smooth manner. But if someone is experiencing stress while contemplating the meaning of the word, Luria reasoned, then he is likely to give a bizarre verbal response or to exhibit some uncertainty or irregularity in the squeezing of the bulb, or perhaps display both of these symptoms.

Luria found irregular rhythms of squeezing in those individuals who had conflicts: he was able to distinguish by this simple method between suspected and actual murderers, between randomly chosen individuals and students awaiting an exam. Though in later life he dismissed this method as "just an early lie detector," it was, in fact, of major importance. Never before had the intricate interplay between a person's knowledge (command of linguistic meaning) and unconscious anxieties (which surround sensitive topics) been so convincingly documented in a psychological study.

Bulb pressing also turned out to be a useful method of studying the mental lives of young children, of brain-damaged adults, and of other populations. Luria devised tasks in which individuals were asked to press the bulb when, say, a green light went on or when an experimenter uttered a given target phrase; or they were instructed not to press it when, say, a red light went on, a green light went off, or the experimenter said another phrase. (Note Luria's reliance on a simple, conditioned response, such as a bulb press, and on the linkage between language and actions—both mainstays of Soviet psychology.)

Initially it was impossible to keep young children from pressing the bulb. As long as the bulb was in a two-year-old's hand, the child would press it. Later on, pressing the bulb came partially under the control of language. If an experimenter uttered something, the child would press the bulb; however, bulb pressing would occur even when the child was told, "Don't press the bulb"—thus, rather than controlling behavior through meaning, the language simply had an "impelling" function.

By the age of three or four, the actual meanings of the words exerted some effect, but only when they in some way mimicked the task the child was supposed to carry out. So when the child was told, "Press, press," the two separately stressed syllables exerted the desired effect: the child would press twice. However, when the same meaning was conveyed with a less rhythmic phrase, "Please press the bulb twice," the child could not be counted on to carry out the task correctly. Only at the age of five or six did children carry out the commands correctly. For only then could they attend exclusively to the meaning, ignoring the cadence and relying on pure verbal mediation to "press when the green light is on, but not in the presence of the red light."

In detailing this sequence, Luria was carrying out a program launched originally with Vygotsky. The two psychologists sought to describe nothing less than the evolution of complex human behavior, which originates in simple reactions to stimuli and slowly but inexorably comes under the control of the symbol system of language. Ultimately, language, once a mere handmaiden of action, comes to control it. To Soviet psychologists, stimulated by Marx's view of culture, the regulation of action through the use of language was distinctly human, making possible higher-level achievements of intention, will, and consciousness of self.

Even as such behaviors developed, however, they could break down. In a profoundly important series of studies with brain-damaged patients, Luria documented the various ways in which an individual once proficient in the verbal control of voluntary behavior might fail. Sometimes, as in demented patients, failure would be due to perceptual problems; sometimes, as in those with Parkinson's disease, to motor deficits; sometimes, as in aphasics, to an inability to understand language.

The most illuminating cases, however, were those of patients who suffered from none of these deficits and yet still failed to carry out the desired sequence of actions. Such people had adequate perception (they could see the stimuli), understood the commands (they were able to paraphrase an instruction), and had normal motor abilities (they were capable of carrying out the required motions). What they could not do was to use language to direct their own behavior. They could respond to isolated commands but could not assume initiative in their own lives. With his colleague Eugenia Homskaya, Luria demonstrated that such people suffer from damage to the frontal lobes, which are crucial to control of voluntary behavior.

By combining the data from children and from brain-damaged adults, Luria could formulate a persuasive account of major elements of human cognition. He saw the brain (and the mind) as a series of structures that are reorganized several times in the course of development, with increasingly higher centers ultimately taking over mental functions. Young children—and many brain-damaged adults—were at the mercy of more primitive perceptual systems (you act when you see a light) and of primitive uses of language (you act when you hear some words, any words). The more highly developed individual could control behavior by attending to meaning, and then by planning sequences of behavior in the right order, revising these plans, reflecting upon them, and monitoring results.

In what may well be one of his enduring contributions, Luria would tease behaviors into their component parts and then attempt to use the spare "working" parts of the mental apparatus to provide a "functional replacement" for parts of the cortex that had been destroyed. In the case of retarded patients, for example, Luria would use simple systems of behavior that were relatively intact in order to accomplish tasks that, in normal individuals, could more readily be accomplished by other functioning systems. Similarly, if individuals with frontal-lobe damage could no longer regulate behavior on their own, Luria would provide them with a series of outside stimuli—carefully arrayed objects, printed cards, rhythmic slogans—that, by providing a kind of external regulation, would in effect substitute for internal regulation. With the aid of such shrewd insights, Soviet rehabilitation efforts were often strikingly successful.

Interest in "levels of mind" and varieties of mentation led Luria to other well-known studies. He spent many years collaborating with a man named S. V. Sherashevsky, who possessed an incredible memory. Luria described Sherashevsky, who was essentially incapable of forgetting anything, in a charming memoir, *The Mind of the Mnemonist*. Luria also undertook intensive studies of identical and fraternal twins, seeking to unravel the vexed effects of nature and nurture. Not content with conventional studies of twins, Luria examined the curious phenomenon of twin language—the extraordinary ways in which twins sometimes develop their own means of communicating with each other. In addition, he introduced the important distinction between "natural" forms of knowledge in identical twins (such as sheer memory capacity) and "cultural" knowledge (for example, the skill of employing mnemonic aids).

But to our contemporary sensibility, Luria's most fascinating writings documented his expedition in 1931 to work with preliterate peasants in the remote areas of Uzbekistan. Luria's interest was twofold: to document the operations of the "primitive mind" as manifest in individuals who led a simple life and had no education; and at the same time to compare their performance with that of educated individuals in order to determine both the degree and the way that primitive cognition is supplanted by more sophisticated forms of reasoning.

Luria's method for eliciting revealing testimony from his informants is reminiscent of the ingenious probes used by Piaget with children. Again and again, he demonstrated that the Uzbekistanis organized, experienced, and answered questions in ways that differed fundamentally from those of the educated Westerner or Easterner. Asked simply to repeat the syllogism, "Precious metals do not rust. Gold is a precious metal. Does it rust or not?," one peasant answered, "Precious metals rust. Do precious metals rust or not?" Another syllogism was: "In the far north where there is snow, all bears are white. Novaya Zemlya is in the far north and there is always snow there. What color are the bears there?" To this problem, one peasant responded, "There are different sorts of bears. . . . I've never seen a black bear; I've never seen any others. . . . Your words can be answered only by someone who was there." Introducing a classification task in which the peasants were asked to select from four pictures—of three adults and a child— the one that didn't belong, the experimenter commented, "Clearly the child doesn't belong in this group." But a peasant responded, "Oh, but the boy must stay with the others. All three of them are working, you see, and if they have to keep running out to fetch things, they'll never get the job done; but the boy can do the running for them." Asked to pick from a set of three objects—a saw, a log, and an ear of grain—the one that goes with an ax and a sickle, another subject replied, "If you want them to be the same, you'd have to pick the ear of wheat. A sickle reaps grain, so this ear will be plucked by this sickle."

What gave Luria's reports their power were not the isolated quota- tions—similar curiosities could probably be gathered by interviewing enough people anywhere—but rather their number and consistency. The peasants' responses revealed a general insensitivity to abstract forms of classification, a resistance to reasoning through language. Only those individuals who had entered school displayed some sensitivity to the kinds of issues posed by the syllogisms. Only they could deal with the hypothetical, with linguistic contradictions, or with superordinate, "umbrella" categories, like "furniture" or "clothing."

Luria was excited by the discoveries of his expedition. In one wonder- ful moment, after testing the peasants for the presence of optical illu- sions (which German psychologists considered universal), Luria wired back to Vygotsky: "The peasants have no illusions!"

His research should have won him the same kind of acclaim in the Soviet Union that was being accorded to Piaget in the Western world. But what happened? Luria was severely denounced upon his return to Moscow. A critic spoke of "pseudoscientific, reactionary, anti-Marxist, and anti-working-class theory [that], in practice, leads to the anti-Soviet conclusion that the political policy of the Soviet Union is carried out by people and classes who think primitively, unable as they are to engage in abstract thought."

So discouraged was Luria by this reception that he failed to publish the results of his expedition; rather, as with many other lines of research that he had conducted in his youth, he simply kept them on file in his own home. Only after repeated urgings by Michael Cole in the

1960s, and only after a trial-balloon version of this research had been favorably received, did Luria dare to produce a slim monograph and issue his findings—almost forty years after the initial expedition.

Nature and nurture, language and thought, cognition and emotion, development and breakdown, higher order and more primitive functions, theory and practice—these are some of the themes that ran through Luria's various lives and give them a measure of coherence. Other psychologists have treated many of these themes, and others have also investigated some of the same populations, but few of them did so with as much elegance and theoretical power as Alexander Luria. But now, with the hindsight of current psychological knowledge, what can we say about his most enduring contributions?

Luria's legacy can only be evaluated, I think, in the light of the history of Soviet psychology and its relation to Western psychology. When Luria first began to study psychology, work in Russia was primarily of two sorts. On the one hand, there was the materialist tradition of Pavlov and Bekhterev. The mind, in this view, was fundamentally physical, thought was built out of reflexes, and there was nothing special about consciousness, will, or intention (if such mentalistic entities existed at all). Another equally venerable point of view, distinctly in the European tradition (though also tied to certain strands of nineteenth-century Russian thought), emphasized consciousness and other special features of man's nature and seriously questioned whether there could be an objective science of psychology.

Luria, Vygotsky, and their closest associates took as their task the fusion of these two traditions. They wished to find an objective material basis for the highest human achievements and aspirations. Their study of primitive forms of mentality exerted particular impact because it suggested a means of ascending from reflex to thought, from elementary percepts and action to abstract language, from mere reaction to pensive planning.

And, supplying a needed philosophical premise from Marx and Engels, the Soviet psychologists proposed that the single factor that made man special—enabling him to transcend his animal heritage—was the surrounding cultural context. Left to themselves, human beings were just intelligent apes. But drawing on their past cultural inventions, men and women could expand their intellect, their knowledge, and their consciousness to even greater heights.

Even as cognitive and developmental psychologists have become more dominant in the West, the Luria-Vygotsky axis, while still controversial, has exerted ever-increasing influence in the Soviet Union. To the extent that the peculiar Soviet blend of cognitive psychology gains in international sway—the interest in motor-language programs, the study of neuropsychological disorders, the search for different levels of mentation, the belief in functional systems that can be reorganized in the light of various kinds of stress—Luria's place in twentieth-century psychology will be secure.

When it comes to the specifics of his contributions, however, the results may be somewhat more mixed. By Anglo-American standards, Luria's reporting of his experiments was rather loose, and his findings have not always proved replicable. The broad outlines of his point of view are frequently confirmed—the details less so. To my mind, this has less to do with the facts of his investigations than with the style of psychological writing that he adopted. For Luria, as for many scholars in the European tradition, a comprehensive theoretical framework was essential to integrate comfortably the results of one's studies, to generate ideas for new experiments, and to refute all competing approaches. Thus Luria is reported to have provoked visiting students repeatedly asking, "So what about your interesting result? What theory does it fit into? What point of view does it prove?"

This may be the weakness of the two areas of Luria's research that I know best: the relationship between language and behavior in children, and the types of aphasia in adults. The reported studies and observations in the two fields fit beautifully into his guiding framework. Unfortunately, however, nature is not always so neat. Luria ignored certain kinds of language disturbance in adults and certain patterns in responding on the part of children when they clashed with his theoretical expectations. The pressures to appear as a doctrinaire Pavlovian may have made Luria see phenomena with greater clarity than they actually possessed. Given a free community of scholars, one can count on rival researchers to ferret out the distortions; and, indeed, other scholars in aphasia and child development have already pointed out Luria's excesses. But if such "wishful seeing" is the price to be paid for engaging an extraordinary mind, it certainly was worthwhile in Alexander Luria's case.

In the view of a Russian colleague who knew Luria quite well for twenty years, the renowned scholar reacted to political events in his country by becoming an inveterate "avoider." Of course, in avoiding trouble, in being careful about what he said in print or even privately, he was hardly special in Soviet Russia. It is we in the West—generally free to write what we believe in—who occupy the privileged and, it must be admitted, somewhat atypical situation. Which of us, faced with the same threats, would have acted any differently from, or perhaps even as honorably as, Luria?

I can understand why Luria in his autobiography does not mention Stalin, the brutal criticism of his work, or those decisive meetings of bureaucrats at which his fate was more than once determined. Even if there were no censorship, he would have found it painful to write about those events.

I find it less easy to understand, however, why so many of the good ideas in Luria's book are attributed to Russians and so little credit is given to his Western colleagues. It is obvious to any reader of Luria, for example, that his thoughts about aphasia were strongly influenced by the American linguist Roman Jakobson. Yet Jakobson gets only one mention in the entire volume, even as lesser Soviet figures are cited ad nauseam.

Nor am I comfortable with the stories asserting that Luria, in his later years, did not speak of his Jewishness, and that he acted in a less than exemplary fashion toward colleagues who came to be out of favor with authorities. There are stories of how he refused to support younger scholars who did not toe his line or to speak up for friends who were under attack; how he even, on occasion, joined in their denunciation; how he, somewhat high-handedly, attempted to promote his own work while blocking the efforts of those who disagreed with him. These are rumors, to be sure, and some of them are very difficult to substantiate or disprove. Moreover, they must be balanced with stories of Luria's kindness, particularly to scholars from abroad, but also to members of his own research team. Yet, in any assessment of the man, the rumors cannot be totally ignored.

Michael Cole relates a poignant anecdote about Luria at the lowest point of his career, at the time when he had been dismissed from the Neurosurgical Institute and was essentially without any support whatsoever. Luria came home one evening, went into his study, put his head on his desk, and wept. According to Luria's wife, Lana Pimenovna, it was the one occasion when his optimism and confidence in his ability to overcome all obstacles failed him.

In my own view, much more was stilled in Luria. As a result of his experiences, he had finally lost a sense of perspective on what he had done and on how much he had done. In his book he was perhaps not consciously dissembling; he honestly could no longer comprehend what had happened. So often in his life did he have to change jobs, jargon, explanations, credits, and blame, that he had lost a sense of where he had been and where he was going.

Indeed, there are but two passages in the book where Luria seems truly alive. The first is in his description of the early days of Soviet psychology, when, with his good friends Vygotsky and Leontiev, a young and preternaturally energetic Luria set out to remake the scientific world. The second is in the touching final chapter, in which Luria indicates his own sympathy—which he obviously kept well under wraps—for what he calls "romantic science," a pursuit that avoids reducing living facts to mathematical schemas and preserves "the wealth of living reality." Luria alludes to his own attempts at romantic science in his case study of the mnemonist and in an equally touching memoir about a brain-injured soldier, *The Man with the Shattered World.* The supreme irony is that Luria cherished this approach to individuals, demonstrated it daily in his clinical investigations, and yet steadfastly avoided it in his own autobiography.

Alexander Luria began his career as a scientist interested in fusing and explicating the human polarities of emotion and thought. While not fully succeeding, he went further toward that goal than nearly any other scholar. In his *Making of Mind* he gives a rational account of his activities but has lost sight almost completely of the forces that spawned them and that governed his behavior. His story is incomplete, for as Vygotsky wrote in *Thought and Language,* "To understand another's speech, it is not sufficient to understand his words—we must understand his thought. But even that is not enough—we must also know its motivation" (p. 151).

I hope Luria would have had sympathy with an effort to probe beneath his words for the feelings that gave life to them—and to him.

347

PART V

THE HEIGHTS OF CREATIVITY

INTRODUCTION

TO MY REGRET, I have had little opportunity to engage in sustained studies of the creative process as it unfolds in acknowledged masters. This remains the task for other occasions, if not for another lifetime. But I am heartened by the fact that some researchers have at last been able to bring the tools and insights of cognitive psychology to bear upon the work of individuals whose accomplishments are indisputably of the highest order. I have in mind here the pioneering work of Herbert Simon and his colleagues with master-level chess players; the incisive examinations of poets' work by my long-time colleague at Project Zero, David Perkins; and, most especially, the path-breaking examination of the creative process in science by Howard Gruber.

As an epilogue to the more intensive studies of children and brain-damaged patients presented in the earlier sections, and as a kind of promissory note to future work, I want to conclude this volume with two essays on creative work at its heights. The first is a description of research on creativity in the adult years, which focuses on the methods devised by Howard Gruber. These methods have thus far been used principally in connection with scientific thinkers, but they lend themselves readily to artists and other creative individuals as well. Then, in a speculative conclusion to this collection, I find in a casual reflection expressed by Mozart some cues about the nature of creative work. Mozart's remark suggests to me that there are at least some commonalities between the mundane processes in which we all engage and the creative powers of the world's greatest geniuses.

351

32

CREATIVITY IN THE

ADULT YEARS

INDIVIDUALS continue to develop throughout their lives. The contributions of a Charles Darwin, a Pablo Picasso, or a Katharine Hepburn certainly deepen in the decades after adolescence. But until recently psychologists who study human development have focused almost entirely on the period of life before the age of twenty. Moreover, the measures on which they have relied in their studies have almost all been brief tasks—learning word lists, mastery of a maze—which can be surmounted in a manner of minutes (and which are even more rapidly forgotten). Even the most illustrious developmental psychologist of our time, Jean Piaget, had nothing to say about mental life in the adult years, and little to say about achievements that unfold over the course of years. Indeed, when Piaget's student Howard Gruber mentioned his wish to study creativity, Piaget responded skeptically, though not without sympathy, "It touches everything."

Now, however, inspired by Piaget's scientific example, Gruber and his students have gone on to examine major creative achievements in the adult years. Gruber, a psychologist at Rutgers University, spent a decade examining the emerging creativity of Charles Darwin and then authored the award-winning *Darwin on Man*. Where other psychologists concerned with creativity had devised simple paper-and-pencil tests which they administered to scores of subjects, Gruber instead pored over a set of notebooks kept by Darwin during the years 1837–39—the period usually judged to be the time when the theorist of evolution made his most seminal discoveries.

The spirit of Piaget can be discerned in Gruber's description of Darwin's method of work. Darwin was seen as a persistent, active, fully engaged person. Counter to the conventional view of creativity as a mystical, irrational process, Darwin experienced no sudden epiphany of inspiration, no wholly novel thoughts or theories. Instead, Darwin marshaled endless lists of thoughts, images, questions, dreams, sketches, comments, arguments, and notes to himself, all of which he continually organized and reorganized. It was all part of a mammoth, painstaking effort to understand the way living processes have yielded the plethora of plant and animal species in the natural world. Key themes were introduced, discussed, and sometimes abandoned only to be revisited at a later time. Pivotal insights were anticipated in earlier scribbles, and occasionally discovered twice. One can even estimate the pace of this creative activity: whereas for normal individuals a mental illumination occurs perhaps once a week, for Darwin, who worked tirelessly on his projects, it seems to have occurred on an almost daily basis.

As Gruber sees it, the student of creativity must reconstruct the mental life of the creative individual at various points in the development of his work. Snapshots of this evolving mental life cannot be read off directly, even in the case of a note-maker as compulsive as Darwin. "In his notebooks, Gruber reports, "ideas stumble over each other in a seemingly chaotic fashion. The underlying order is something to be constructed, not observed." Accordingly, the theorist of creativity has to identify certain enduring motifs—in the case of Darwin, themes such as origins, variations, survival, natural selection, heredity—and produce a series of "cognitive maps" that capture the thinker's view of his project at various points in its own evolution.

After his expeditions into the mind of Charles Darwin, Gruber moved on to another equally daunting figure in science, his own mentor Jean Piaget. He is now engaged in a comprehensive study of the development of Piaget's ideas, one that will examine not only Piaget's own formidable intellectual trajectory but also his collaborations during a period of more than sixty years with a huge array of scholars. In addition, Gruber has inspired colleagues and coworkers to undertake intensive case studies of other creative individuals, in the arts as well as the sciences; and as a result of these efforts, certain emerging generalizations about the creative life can now be offered.

Gruber conceives the "whole thinking" person as harboring a number of interacting subsystems. One subsystem involves the organization of knowledge. A creative person seeks to relate various facts and theories scattered across his area of concern in order to come up with a coherent and comprehensive synthesis. Moreover, a creative individual typically spawns a network of enterprises—a complex of searches that engages his curiosity over long periods of time. These activities usually sustain one another and give rise to an incredibly active creative life. As the individual's focus changes, he may attend specifically to certain forms of information and self-consciously neglect others. He is capable of bracketing problems that lead to blind alleys, or even of "destroying problems" that threaten to take him too far away from his chosen network of hypotheses. But in the long run the creative individual will predictably return to the major nodes in his network of enterprises in order to construct the most comprehensive system possible.

In addition to this congeries of activities, the creative individual also pursues (or is pursued by) a number of dominant metaphors. These figures are images of wide scope, rich, and susceptible to considerable exploration, exposing the investigator to aspects of phenomena that might otherwise remain invisible to him. Often the key to the individual's most important innovations inhere in these images. In Darwin's case, the most fecund metaphor was the branching tree of evolution, on which he could trace the rise and fate of various species. However, during various periods he also viewed nature as a tangled bank, physical organs as inventions or contrivances, and natural selection as 100,000 wedges trying to force adapted structures into gaps in nature.

Gruber's students have uncovered other such metaphors of wide scope. According to Jeffrey Osowski of Rutgers University, William James had a penchant for viewing mental processes as a stream or river, rather than in terms of the associationist images of a train or a chain. In the view of Martha Moore Russell of the Educational Testing Service, any consideration of John Locke should focus on his falconer, whose release of a bird symbolized the quest for human knowledge. Finally, in conveying his own emerging view of the creative process, Gruber finds himself attracted to the Mosaic image of the bush that is always burning but never consumed.

Another system operating in the "whole" person is concerned with a guiding purpose. The individual's quest cannot be viewed merely as a reflection of unconscious motivations or accidental career choices.

Rather, the creator is animated by a series of self-conscious problems and projects which he is determined to monitor regularly and to carry through to successful completion. The individual determines which skills he needs in order to achieve his purposes and works tirelessly to develop and perfect them. In the process he transforms himself until what might be difficult for other persons becomes second nature to him. He may also feel the need to discover new sets of peers who can educate him about what currently concerns him, and he needs the strength to abandon these collaborators (at least in a professional sense) when he moves on to a new area of concern.

The individual's sense of purpose—his goal-directedness—guides the choice of a whole set of enterprises and dictates which to focus on at a given time, which to abandon, when to develop a new set of skills, and when to fall back upon tried and true ones. As Gruber puts it, the individual resembles a well-coordinated juggler, who is able to keep a number of objects in mind (or hand) at a particular moment and who actually sustains pleasure from his ability to carry out such a juggling feat—though the ultimate goal of creating new objects or making fresh discoveries always remains regnant.

A total system stems from the creator's affective life. The individual experiences a strong, almost primordial tie to the subjects of his curiosity. Einstein, Darwin, Piaget—all felt a special intimacy with the natural world. In each case, a loving dialogue with nature, dating back to childhood, was transformed into a scientific journey. The creative individual comes to love his work—indeed, cannot thrive without it. And the kind of pleasure he derives from making scientific discoveries, from solving a puzzle of nature, or from completing an artistic work can be compared in a non-facetious way with the kind of pleasure most individuals gain from sexual involvement with someone they love.

Gruber reminds us of the difficulty and loneliness of any creative undertaking. Despite the pleasure that individuals obtain from their work, they are typically embarked on a solitary voyage, where the chances of failure are high. To pursue this risky tack, they must be courageous and willing to deviate from the pack, to go off on their own, to face shame or even outright rejection. It requires a strong constitution to go it alone in creative matters, and most innovative people at times experience a strong need for personal, communal, or religious support.

How does Gruber's highly original approach relate to that of others who have studied creativity? One obvious comparison is with the psychoanalyst Erik Erikson, who has traced the development of ideological innovators—individuals like Mahatma Gandhi and Martin Luther—who successfully introduced new world views. In many ways Erikson's heroes resemble Gruber's—persons of tremendous energy whose worlds featured numerous highly interconnected activities and concerns. But where Gruber's focus is largely cognitive, Erikson centers on motivation and affect. The psychoanalyst sees the individual's societal concerns as growing out of his own personal and familial conflicts. The ideological innovator contrives a meaningful personal solution which, in light of widespread cultural concerns during his lifetime, happens to make profound sense to an entire population. Whether Erikson's approach can be reconciled with Gruber's is not known, but both men stand out in their spurning of the glib generalization and in their total immersion in the facts and themes of each "case" that they examine.

Another issue, of particular moment to Piagetians, is whether the actual quality of creative thought processes changes beyond adolescence. In Piaget's view, the highest level of thinking, which he called the stage of formal operations, is attained in adolescence, and while new discoveries are certainly possible, the fundamental way in which thought occurs will not change, even in a Darwin or an Einstein. However, some commentators influenced by Piaget have proposed an additional cognitive capacity, that of problem-finding; this proclivity, clearly pivotal for those who launch scientific revolutions, may only come to the fore in later periods of life and seems qualitatively different from the logical capacities limned by Piaget. The ability to come up with new problems and to decide which are most susceptible to solution defies analysis in strict Piagetian terms.

Yet another puzzle concerns the relation of creative breakthroughs to the overall organization of an individual's mental and social life. Is creativity most likely to occur during certain phases of life (such as the mid-life crises described by Daniel Levinson and Erik Erikson)? Does it presuppose the highest stage of moral or personality organization, the kind of autonomous, principled individual described by developmentalists Lawrence Kohlberg of Harvard and Jane Loevinger of Washington University? May it occur unexpectedly in an otherwise unremarkable person, or must it be part of the life-fabric of an unusual individual?

The incidence of extreme creative behavior is so unusual that perhaps it can occur only under very special circumstances. Gruber's colleague, David Feldman of Tufts University, in fact speaks of the necessity for "co-incidence"—that conjunction of genetic, familial, motivational, and cultural factors which must all be present if the efforts of an Einstein, a Darwin, or a Beethoven are to come to fruition. Nor is it likely that one creative individual could be substituted for another. Leonardo da Vinci could not have become Darwin, Beethoven could not have become Einstein. Finally, the emergence of creative persons (as we know them) may presuppose a certain view of the individual on the part of the culture and of the individuals themselves. Possibly the creative individual is an invention of the post-Renaissance society in the West. Such an exceptional person may be unknown in those cultures that place a much higher premium on adaptation to a culturally endorsed model of behavior. And perhaps in our own culture, the time of the creative hero may be passing.

33

THE COMPOSITIONS OF

MOZART'S MIND

WOLFGANG AMADEUS MOZART once described in a letter his manner of composing. It was most natural to compose, he said, when he was in a cheerful mood—traveling in a carriage or strolling after a hearty meal. "When and how my ideas come, I know not; nor can I force them," he explained. But the ideas he found to his liking were easily retained, and soon he was able to fashion an appealing piece of music out of their parts—"to make a good dish of it," as he put it. Mozart proceeded to characterize his activities in a most intriguing way:

All this fires my soul, and provided I am not disturbed, my subject enlarges itself, becomes methodized and defined, and the whole, though it be long, stands almost complete and finished in my mind, so that I can survey it, like a fine picture or a beautiful statue, at a glance. Nor do I hear in my imagination the parts *successively*, but I hear them, as it were all at once (*gleich alles zusammen*). What a delight this is I cannot tell! (quoted in Ghiselin, p. 45)

The claim to hear an entire piece of music—which may take twenty or thirty minutes to perform—in one's head at one moment in time when it has not even been composed seems incredible. Only because Mozart was one of the great geniuses—and perhaps the greatest prodigy—of all times has this letter been taken seriously at all (and some musicologists have in fact disputed its authenticity).

But even assuming that Mozart wrote the letter and that he was not exaggerating or boasting, the question arises of precisely *what* he meant? How can one hear something, as it were, in one's mind's ear? And how can one go on to contrive a composition entirely cerebrally and then, defying time, attend to it in its entirety in one's head at a single moment? We will never know the answers to these questions: Mozart has long been dead, and it is in any case unlikely that he could have amplified the comments made in the letter. For those interested in the creative process, however, it is worth our pondering what Mozart might have meant by this strange phrasing. And in the course of this "mental experiment," it should be possible to glimpse some of the concepts and some of the issues that are being pondered today by investigators of "mental representation"—by that growing tribe of researchers known as cognitive scientists.

To begin, it is worth recalling what else we know about Mozart's processes of composition, and considering how his procedures compare with other notable feats of creative activity. Beyond doubt Mozart composed with great ease and rapidity. There is no other way to account for the production of more than six hundred pieces of music, including forty-one symphonies and some forty-odd operas and masses, during barely three decades of creative life, except by invoking an extraordinary fluency. Mozart's colleagues and contemporaries confirm that he wrote with astonishing efficiency. As a biographer Alfred Einstein reported, "All witnesses of Mozart at work agree that he put a composition down on paper as one writes a letter, without allowing any disturbance or interruption to annoy him, the writing down, the 'fixing' was nothing more than that—the fixing of a completed work, a mechanical act" (p. 142). Yet, while confirming Mozart's own introspective account, observers and biographers have been quick to point out that Mozart was anything but careless or unduly hasty. Rather, when given an assignment, he thought about it for long periods of time, would try out various combinations on the piano, hum them to himself, and contemplate how to accommodate the musical idea (or theme) to the rules of counterpoint and to the peculiarities of particular texts, performers, and instruments.

There are on record other composers who produced works as rapidly, but there are also numerous contrasting cases. Like Mozart, Beethoven was a fluent and skillful improviser, but he composed only with much more overt difficulty. In addition to keeping a notebook replete with discarded themes and false starts, Beethoven would score a piece numerous times—revising, rejecting, crossing out in his impetuous and messy hand. While Mozart's rapidly produced scores seldom contained erased passages—and indeed were practically of "camera-ready" quality—Beethoven's sketchbooks chronicled painful, even tormented sieges of creation. Certainly Beethoven's agonies during the throes of creation—rather than Mozart's seemingly seamless composing activity—served as the model of the suffering romantic artist in his garret.

Accounts of creation in other media echo the same contrasts. For every fluent Mozart, Trollope, or Picasso, who poured forth works with unceasing fecundity, and for every Edgar Allan Poe, who claimed to plot out his works with mathematical precision, one encounters reports of a Dostoevsky, who reworked his novels numerous times, a Thomas Mann, who struggled over three pages a day, or a Richard Wagner, who had to work himself up into a nearly psychotic frenzy before finally finding himself able to put pen to score.

One recourse in such a state of affairs is to discard such introspective accounts altogether. Alternatively, one can assume that these differences signal variations in personality, style, or introspective candor, rather than fundamental differences in approach to creation. As yet another possibility, individuals may intend different meanings by the same phrases. For example, the twentieth-century American composer Walter Piston once reported to a friend that a piece on which he had been working was almost completed. "Can I hear it then?" his friend asked. "Oh, no," Piston retorted, "I haven't yet selected the notes." Far from being ironic, Piston apparently meant that he had planned out the abstract structure of the piece—the number of movements, the principal shifts in orchestral color, the various forms to be employed, and so on—but had still to decide upon the specific vehicles with which to embody his musical conception.

But is it possible to supersede speculation in such matters? Can we actually attain insight into the process of composition by one, two, or even the whole federation of composers? Can we construct models of the composer's mnemonic capacities, his perceptual acuity, his planning strategies, his manner of projecting how a theme will develop or an orchestrated section will sound? And can we apply the accumulated understanding to a specific case of composition—figuring out, for example, whether Mozart could actually conjure up the details of a piece in his head or could only have been referring (Piston-fashion) to the overall conception? Was he endowed with a more capacious memory and more vivid acoustic imagery than other composers, or was he simply able to realize a general conception more rapidly in the course of putting pen to paper? These are some of the challenges that cognitive scientists have posed for themselves. And while members of this group are far from able to model the thought processes of a Mozart, or even of lesser mortals engaged in more mundane activities, the ways in which they have been approaching such issues prove instructive.

Composing a piece of music extends beyond the competence of most individuals (including most cognitive scientists). One promising avenue for conceptualizing this process is to ponder what is involved in less formidable activities. Consider, for example, the way that you plan a dinner party, particularly if you have in the past often planned such parties. You must think about what food to eat, in what order, how much of each dish to prepare, when to cook and serve each, whom to invite, where to seat them before, during, and after the meal, which individuals are likely to grate on one another and which should get along, which decorations to display, what to wear, and much more. Such planning can reach a fine degree of specificity. I have known hosts and hostesses who have worried about who is left-handed and who smokes, about which topics of conversation to raise at the beginning of the meal and which to avoid, how big a portion to allot each individual as an appetizer so as to make sure he will "have room" for the entree. *

Or consider your procedure if you are asked to write a letter of recommendation on behalf of a colleague, particularly if, like me, you often feel besieged by this assignment yet want to make certain that the letter exerts a beneficent effect. I have a plan that I generally follow in writing such letters. I begin by indicating the circumstances under which I have met the individual, how well I know him, what the nature of our relationship (professional and personal) has been. A second paragraph usually describes the growth of that individual over the period of time that I have known him and indicates the kinds of work and issues that occupy a central place in that person's professional life. A third paragraph will review the person's principal scholarly

---

* Sometimes life imitates art. After writing this essay, I came across a forty-page monograph by cognitive psychologist Richard Byrne: "Planning Meals: Problem Solving on a Real Data-Base."

accomplishments so far and his future promise. (An optional paragraph will focus on teaching abilities.) A fourth paragraph will touch on the individual's personal dimensions—what kind of a colleague he makes, how he gets along with others, whether he has a good sense of humor, is reliable, responsible, and so on. (An optional paragraph will detail problems or weaknesses.) The final paragraph is summative: it recapitulates what I find most outstanding about the individual, explains (or explains away) any difficulties I have mentioned, and attempts to integrate my assessment of the individual as a scholar and future contributor to the field with his qualities as a person, friend, and colleague. I may also suggest some comparisons with others of comparable age, background, and ambition and offer to provide further information.

Of course, like the hypothetic meal served above, this "model" or "prototypical" letter is deliberately skeletal. It can be modified to a greater or lesser extent, depending upon a variety of considerations, including how much time I have to devote to the effort and how positively I feel about the person. The challenge I pose myself is to modify this basic scaffolding (designed to serve most purposes) so that it clings to the particular individual I am describing.

In confronting data like this—the host planning a party, the colleague writing a letter of recommendation—a cognitive scientist would likely adopt the following perspective. He would say that the host and the teacher have general schemas—abstract mental representations of what a party or a letter should be like. These schemas are sufficiently general and abstract to apply to a variety of parties, a series of letters. Some "slots" of the schemas are relatively inflexible—drinks always have to be served, a letter always opens with a salutation. Other "slots" of the schemas are quite flexible—the foods to be served or the issues with which the job candidate has been engaged may be entirely different from one "embodiment" of the schema to another. But in general the diverse embodiments of the schemas share at least a family resemblance with one another. Moreover, the realization of each future instance is helped immeasurably by the prior existence of the schema— the mold with its recesses of various shapes and sizes into which particular ingredients are poured.

While it might seem sacrilegious to compare these mundane activities with the composing of *Don Giovanni* or the *Jupiter Symphony*, I find that the concept of a schema, with its modifications and elaborations, at least provides a useful point of entry. Mozart could not have written his major works—let alone composed them with so little apparent strain—had he not written thousands of fragments of music before. Mozart lived, moreover, during a time when the rules for musical composition were much more clearly spelled out than they are today: there existed definite formulas for writing a symphony, and these formulas were quite sharply constrained. It was possible for almost anyone of a musical bent (including Frederick the Great!) to write a passable piece of music. (At the same time, contemporary ears find it difficult to detect differences among the various compositions of the schools that surrounded Mozart and Haydn. The "second rank" creators in an era typically produce works that are most faithful to and make the least interesting departures from the "schema of the time.")

We can assume, then, that once Mozart had decided to write a symphony, many of the most important decisions had in fact been made in advance—just as was the case with our more modest contemporary examples. What the general schema did not supply were all the glorious themes or the detailed elaborations that differ significantly across several hundred works. Even as the assignment to planners of parties inheres in making a distinctive addition to the repertoire of galas, Mozart's challenge was to come up with some promising themes for the opening of each movement; to "play" these themes in his mind against the backdrop of the compositional schema to which he was restricted (and indebted); and then to fashion those exciting departures and deviations that made each symphony different from the others, while still remaining, as he put it, *Mozartisch*.

I should make a number of points about this model. To begin with, it is, in the jargon, a "top-down" (rather than a "bottom-up") approach. We do not assume that party planning (or letter writing or symphonic composing) begins afresh with the first element (the greeting at the door) and then proceeds moment to moment until the last event (saying good night). Nor do we assume that the individual begins with the most specific details (what flowers to buy) and then moves to more general considerations (who to invite, what kind of cuisine to serve). Rather, we assume that the overall plan for the item to be schematized already existed before its actual instantiation; and that it is the creator's task to draw upon and exploit a prior schema so as to produce a distinctive, if not distinguished, member of its class.

Under this plan a cognitive scientist need not prejudge how specifically the schema has been articulated in the mind of the individual before he "goes public"—for example, writing down words on a page or making a first phone call. Presumably some individuals (or all individuals at some time) make only the most general kinds of decisions before beginning to implement the schema, while others have effected the most detailed decisions in advance before any public behavior can be observed. Thus, if I am in a hurry and do not care much about the letter, I may simply type out a draft with hardly any forethought and correct only the most glaring infelicities before sending it off. On the other hand, if much is riding on the letter, I may plan it out painstakingly in advance, prepare a number of drafts, and circulate it among colleagues before sending it off. This disparity in care does not ensure a difference in overall quality—I have written some fine letters off the top of my head and some mediocre letters despite ample anguish. However, the amount of planning probably does correlate with the extent to which the letter deviates from a schema. It is very difficult to produce a novel instance of the schema without considerable planning and adjusting, even as it is unlikely that a carefully fashioned letter will turn out to be virtually identical to those produced at other times.

Let us, then, renew contact with the possible meanings of Mozart's remark. If the composer simply meant that he had some general ideas about the piece of music in his mind and that he could monitor its deviation from other instances in a few particulars, but that actual details remained to be worked out, his remarks would be relatively unproblematic. After all, if we can plan a letter or a party with only minimal specificity, why should one of the outstanding composers of all times, who certainly spent more time composing than we do in these mundane activities, experience undue difficulties in anticipating the broad outlines of a composition even before he had written it out?

But clearly, if we are to believe the reports of his contemporaries, Mozart meant that he did a great deal more than plan the broad outlines. He would have us believe that he could plan out the whole piece in detail, element by element, before putting a mark on the page (how else could he write it out so quickly and smoothly?), and he would have us believe the even more remarkable claim that he could actually perceive it—hear it!!—in the orchestral chamber of his mind.

What are we to make of these claims? I do not have much difficulty with Mozart's apparent ability to envision—or "en-audit"—an entire piece in his own mind before writing it down. His remark testifies to a superlative planning capacity and a nearly infallible memory, to the extent that he did not need the aid of a notebook in order to keep the various fragments in his own mind. Aided by his own composing background and by the existence of powerful schemas, including the schemas based on his own previous works, he was able to make suitable annotations and specifications in his mind. As a result, the piece in all of its individuality could be conceptualized beforehand and then simply transcribed. Even if Mozart did not plan out every single detail beforehand—and I rather doubt that he did—it did not matter, for he was superbly (and justifiably) confident that the details would follow rather easily. If worst came to worst, and he had to abandon a section (or if best came to best, and he conjured up a splendid new idea), Mozart, like any prepared genius, would exploit this opportunity.

And as for the second claim, to hear the whole piece *gleich alles zusammen*? If Picasso had claimed that he could see a whole canvas in his head before producing it, this would not astonish us, for even though one cannot actually survey a whole scene without an eye movement, one can certainly envision a quite detailed scene at a single mental moment. The difference between Picasso and us inheres in the fact that we are by and large restricted (except in dreams) to scenes we have already seen. Our hypothetical Picasso could anticipate scenes that he was only subsequently going to paint.

Where Mozart differs is in his claim to hear a whole piece simultaneously. Here, across the chasms of time and space, I would presume to read Mozart's mind and say that he did not mean this statement literally: Mozart was not, I submit, able to hear an entire twenty-minute piece within a second or two. Rather, Mozart seems to have employed a metaphor here, but one of some accuracy and power. What Mozart meant, I think, was that the entire organization, the distinctive architectonic of the piece of music was fully articulated in his mind. The crucial decisions about where sections of a piece would begin and end, where instruments would enter, when themes would recur, could all be grasped at one moment in time (just as the entire scenario of the dinner party might seem immanent to one of us after we had pondered it for a considerable period of time).

But what about the actual sound quality of the music? Surely it is different to envision a canvas à la Picasso, or a party à la host, than to imagine a whole piece of music that ordinarily unfolds in hundreds of measures over a period of time. Mozart may have intended one of two points. He may have meant that he was perceiving the piece of music in an essentially *amodal* way—that is, rather than hearing it, seeing it, or feeling it, he just apprehended its organizational structure in terms of more abstract, nonsensory properties (such as beginnings, climaxes, countersubjects, return of the theme). Or he may have meant that he could hear, as it were, almost at the same time the major themes of the music and the ways in which they were treated and elaborated upon at the critical moments in the piece. It is as if all the "subjects" of a fugue, which are usually introduced one at a time over several measures, could be played at the same time in one's mind, so that their potential manipulation for purposes of harmony and counterpoint might be perceived with near simultaneity. Put overly simply, Mozart may have heard the whole melody as if it were an enormously rich chord.

Can we get any further clarifications from descriptions of Mozart's own writing practices? Thanks to his frequent changes in ink and varying colors of ink, we can confirm that Mozart was almost totally a "top-down" kind of composer. He never wrote out specific sections of a movement, complete in all voices, but rather proceeded in a stubbornly holistic way. He always wrote out the primary theme—for example, the one introduced by the first violins—in its entirety and only subsequently revisited this section to fill in the subordinate parts. As Alfred Einstein tells us:

In a work of chamber music or a symphony, he fixes first the principal voices, the melodic threads, from beginning to end, leaping as it were from line to line, and inserting the subordinate voices only when he "goes over" or "overhauls" the movement in a second stage of the procedure. (p. 143)

Yet even Mozart allowed for surprises. Einstein indicates that sometimes during the seemingly half-mechanical labor of filling in (or filling out) the details, Mozart would invent a new fragment, become excited, and then seek to integrate this fragment into other aspects of the piece. The voice of genius is never still.

Even armed with detailed suggestions of how Mozart composed, we are still besieged by questions. For example, one might still contend that, rather than simply proceeding from a schema already well worked out in his mind, Mozart might have had all the details worked out, but simply for convenience decided to write out the major parts of the piece first and fill in details later. (Indeed, on occasion Mozart would ask one of his assistants to fill in the most mechanical details of a piece.) Here some of the experimental innovations of cognitive psychology might eventually offer illumination. If Mozart were to reappear today, we might ask him in the interests of science to carry out some feats: to write out the contemplated piece with full detail from the first measure to the second, third, and so on; to write out the last part of the piece first; to carry through the entire score of a subsidiary instrument first; or even to write the complete piece backwards. If he could execute all these tasks perfectly, we would have to conclude that Mozart had in his head the fully printed score of the piece and was really only an amanuensis—a slavish transcriber. If, however, as appears likely, Mozart would succeed when required to furnish the principal themes, while having difficulties with highly detailed assignments (like writing out the middle portion of the development section for the piccolo), then we would receive confirmation that Mozart was embodying a well-developed schema that nonetheless still allowed certain flexibility. In other words, while he probably anticipated more of the notes than Piston had when the latter's piece was "almost done," Mozart's composing procedures were at least in part constructive and not totally mechanical.

My own efforts at a cognitive exegesis suggests that Mozart had made all of the key decisions about his piece beforehand and could, upon request, provide all the principal themes and variations. All the same, the details of the specific execution of individual parts awaited the time when he was actually scoring the composition.

It can justly be pointed out that this exercise—which is, in broad outlines, one method of attack favored by contemporary cognitive science—leaves out the most important and most mysterious aspects of composition. Why did Mozart compose? Why in the style that he favored? Where did his themes come from? In particular, how can we account for the intrinsic beauty of the arias of *Don Giovanni* or the opening bars of the piano solo in his C-minor concerto, as well as for the ingenious—or genius—transformations he wrought with these themes? How can we account for the startling differences among pieces, the specific "ideas" that nonetheless bear the unmistakable stylistic signature of Mozart? Some of these questions are within the purview of cognitive science, others might well be ruled "out of court," but the sad truth is that we scarcely know how to think about them at the present time.

A description of the composer's mental processes, of course, in no way detracts from the beauty and subtlety of the work itself. For instance, psychologists must take note of, but as yet have few means of explaining, Mozart's remarkable musical talents, his incredible energy, his motivation to write the greatest music of his time, his uncanny dramatic sense, his fabled powers of concentration, his sometimes quixotic but always vital manner. Little as psychology has to say about Mozart's miraculous mind, it has even less insight into his fascinating character.

Yet I do not feel discouraged. The notion of a schema within its realization and elaboration represents a significant advance over the rigidly atomistic approaches of an earlier time. The willingness to countenance what might be involved in the composition of a letter—or even a sonata—is a beneficent development. The discovery and specification of similarities between mundane activities and the creative outpourings of a master is also healthy—some analogous principles may well be at work, even though the rate and scale renders them in some ways incomparable. The suggestive ties between creation and memory, between invention and repetition, cradle important insights. Sophisticated methods of interviewing creative artists in order to gain purchase on their problem-solving procedures may also eventually bear fruit, as should attempts to simulate such problem-solving (and problem-finding) activities on a computer.

A research program that seeks to illuminate such heights of creativity should not (and in my experience does not) affect our experience and enjoyment of the works themselves: these remain glorious, whether or not we understand something of the schematizing activity that generated them. A teacher of mine once responded to a student who was concerned that biochemistry would undermine religion, "We are not here to denigrate God—we are here to glorify molecules."

REFERENCES

Alajouanine, T. "Aphasia and artistic realization." *Brain* 71 (1948): 229–41.

Arnheim, R. *Visual thinking.* Berkeley: University of California Press, 1969.

———. *Art and visual perception: The new version.* Berkeley: University of California Press, 1974.

Bate, W. J. *Samuel Johnson.* New York: Harcourt Brace Jovanovich, 1977.

Bernstein, L. *The unanswered question.* Cambridge, Mass.: Harvard University Press, 1976.

Bettelheim, B. *The uses of enchantment.* New York: Alfred A. Knopf, 1976.

Byrne, R. "Planning meals: Problem solving on a real data-base." *Cognition* 5 (1977): 284–332.

Cassirer, E. *An essay on man.* New Haven: Yale University Press, 1944.

———. *The philosophy of symbolic forms.* 3 vols. New Haven: Yale University Press, 1953–59 (original German publication 1923–29).

Chukovsky, K. *From two to five.* Berkeley: University of California Press, 1968.

Comstock, G. et al. *Television and human behavior.* New York: Columbia University Press, 1978.

Edwards, B. *Drawing on the right side of the brain.* New York: St. Martin's Press, 1979.

Einstein, Alfred. *Mozart: His character, his work.* New York: Oxford University Press, 1945.

Feldman, D. *Beyond universals in cognitive development.* Norwood, N.J.: Ablex Publishers, 1980.

Freud, S. *On the psychopathology of everyday life.* New York: Macmillan, 1914 (original German publication 1904).

Gablik, S. *Progress in art.* New York: Rizzoli International, 1976.

Gardner, H. *The arts and human development.* New York: John Wiley & Sons, 1973.

———. *Artful scribbles.* New York: Basic Books, 1980.

Ghiselin, B. *The creative process.* New York: Mentor, 1959.

Gombrich, E. H. *Art and illusion.* Princeton, N.J.: Princeton University Press, 1961.

———. *The sense of order.* Ithaca: Cornell University Press, 1979.

Goodman, N. *Languages of art.* Indianapolis: Hackett Publishing Co., 1976.

———. *Ways of worldmaking.* Indianapolis: Hackett Publishing Co., 1978.

Gruber, H. *Darwin on man.* 2d ed. Chicago: University of Chicago Press, 1981.

Jakobson, R. In Jakobson, R. and Halle, M. *Fundamentals of language.* The Hague: Mouton, 1956.

References

Kant, I. *Critique of judgment.* Translated by J. H. Bernaid. London: Macmillan, 1892 (original German publication 1790).

———. *Critique of practical reason.* Translated by Lewis W. Beck. Indianapolis: Bobbs-Merrill Co., 1956 (original German publication 1788).

Kessen, W., Levine, J., and Wendrich, K. A. "The imitation of pitch in infants." *Infant Behavior and Development* 2 (1978): 93–99.

Kosinski, J. *Being there.* New York: Bantam Books, 1980.

Langer, S. *Philosophy in a new key.* Cambridge, Mass.: Harvard University Press, 1942.

———. *Mind: An essay on human feeling.* 2 vols. Baltimore: Johns Hopkins University Press, 1967, 1972.

Lévi-Strauss, C. "Linguistics and anthropology." In C. Lévi-Strauss. *Structural anthropology.* New York: Basic Books, 1958 (essay originally delivered in 1952 and published in 1953).

———. *Tristes tropiques.* New York: Atheneum Publishers, 1963 (original French publication 1955).

———. *Mythologiques.* 4 vols. Paris: Plon, 1964–1971 (translated into English and published by Harper & Row, New York).

———. *The savage mind.* Chicago: University of Chicago Press, 1966 (original French publication 1962).

———. *The raw and the cooked.* New York: Harper & Row, 1969.

———. *La voie des masques.* Paris: Plon, 1979.

Lowenfeld, V. *Creative and mental growth.* New York: Macmillan, 1947.

Luria, A. R. *The mind of the mnemonist.* New York: Basic Books, 1968.

———. *The man with the shattered world.* New York: Basic Books, 1972.

———. *Cognitive development.* Cambridge, Mass.: Harvard University Press, 1976.

———. *The making of mind: A personal account of Soviet psychology.* Cambridge, Mass.: Harvard University Press, 1979.

———, Tsvetkova, L. S., and Futer, D. S. "Aphasia in a composer." *Journal of Neurological Sciences* 2 (1965): 288–92.

Mander, G. *Four arguments for the elimination of television.* New York: William Morrow & Co., 1978.

Meyer, L. *Emotion and meaning in music.* Chicago: University of Chicago Press, 1956.

Milgram, S. Conversation. *Psychology Today* June 1974: 71–80.

Nottebohm, F. "Brain pathways for vocal learning in birds: A review of the first ten years." *Progress in Psychobiology, Physiology and Psychology* 9 (1980): 85–124.

Piaget, J. *Logique et connaissance scientifique.* Paris: Encyclopédie de la Pléiade, 1967.

———. *Biology and knowledge.* Chicago: University of Chicago Press, 1971 (original French publication 1967).

Piatelli-Palmarini, M., ed. *Language and learning.* Cambridge, Mass.: Harvard University Press, 1980.

Perkins, D. *The mind's best work.* Cambridge, Mass.: Harvard University Press, 1981.

Pitcher, E. and Prelinger, E. *Children tell stories.* New York: International Universities Press, 1963.

Pritchett, V. S. *The cab at the door.* London: Chatto and Windus, 1968.

Rosenberg, J. *On quality in art.* Princeton, N.J.: Princeton University Press, 1967.

Rousseau, J. J. *The Émile of Jean Jacques Rousseau.* Edited by W. Boyd. New York: Columbia Teachers College, 1962 (original French publication 1762).

References

Schilpp, P. A., ed. *The philosophy of Ernst Cassirer.* Evanston, Ill.: The Library of Living Philosophers, 1949.

Selfe, L. *Nadia.* New York: Academic Press, 1977.

Simon, H. *Models of thought.* New Haven: Yale University Press, 1979.

Ungerer, T. *The three robbers.* New York: Atheneum Publishers, 1962.

Vygotsky, L. S. *Thought and language.* Cambridge, Mass.: M.I.T. Press, 1966.

Winn, M. *The plug-in-drug.* New York: Viking Press, 1977.

Wölfflin, H. *Principles of art history.* New York: Dover Publications, n.d. (original German publication 1915).

Woodward, B. and Armstrong, S. *The brethren.* New York: Simon & Schuster, 1979.

NAME INDEX

Name Index

Skinner, B. F., *xi*, 7, 13, 228, 233
Sklar, Bernard, 304–5
Smith, Ann, 110–27
Sparks, Robert, 276
Sperry, Roger, 282, 311
Stalin, Joseph, 337, 339, 346
Stein, Gertrude, 63
Steiner, George, 74
Stravinsky, Igor, 36–37, 58, 528
Sturgis, Katherine, 56

Terman, Lewis, 193, 198
Thorpe, W. H., 146
Töppfer, Rodolphe, 92
Trollope, Anthony, 260
Turner, Joseph, 72

Ungerer, Tomi, 238
Urban, Wilbur, 50
Uspensky, Gleb Ivanovich, 331

van Gogh, Vincent, 193
Velletri-Glass, Andrea, 307
Vibbert, Martha, 255
Vygotsky, Lev, *xii*, 338, 340, 343–44, 347

Wagner, Richard, 36, 360
Wapner, Wendy, 313
Warrington, Elizabeth, 324
Werner, Heinz, 149
Wernicke, Carl, 291
Whitehead, Alfred North, 50
Whorf, Benjamin Lee, 274

Wilson, Brent and Marjorie, 254
Wilson, Woodrow, 314, 317
Winn, Marie, 234
Winner, Ellen, 103–9, 158–67
Wittgenstein, Ludwig, 50
Wolf, Dennie, 110–27, 149, 171–73
Wölfflin, Heinrich, 78
Wordsworth, William, 193
Wright, John, 236–37

Yeats, William Butler, 196

Zaidel, Eran, 312

375

SUBJECT INDEX